Captopril and Hypertension

Topics in Cardiovascular Disease

Series Editors:

Edmund H. Sonnenblick
Albert Einstein College of Medicine, New York

and

William W. Parmley
University of California Medical School, San Francisco

NUCLEAR CARDIOLOGY: Principles and Methods
Edited by Aldo N. Serafini, Albert J. Gilson, and William M. Smoak

THE PRACTICE OF CORONARY ARTERY BYPASS SURGERY
Donald W. Miller, Jr.

THE PULMONARY AND BRONCHIAL CIRCULATIONS IN CONGENITAL HEART DISEASE
Colin M. Bloor and Averill A. Liebow

CAPTOPRIL AND HYPERTENSION
Edited by David B. Case, Edmund H. Sonnenblick, and John H. Laragh

Captopril and Hypertension

Edited by
David B. Case
New York Hospital/Cornell Medical Center
New York, New York

Edmund H. Sonnenblick
Albert Einstein College of Medicine
The Bronx, New York

and

John H. Laragh
New York Hospital/Cornell Medical Center
New York, New York

Plenum Medical Book Company
New York and London

Library of Congress Cataloging in Publication Data

Main entry under title:

Captopril and hypertension.

(Topics in cardiovascular disease)
Revised, updated, and reorganized papers, originally presented at a symposium held at Henry Chauncy Conference Center, Princeton, N. J., sponsored by the Squibb Institute for Medical Research.
Includes index.
1. Hypertension–Chemotherapy–Congresses. 2. Captopril–Testing–Congresses. 3. Hypotensive agents–Congresses. I. Case, David B. II. Sonnenblick, Edmund H. III. Laragh, John H. IV. Squibb Institute for Medical Research, New Brunswick, N.J. V. Series.
RC685.H8C36 616.1'32 80-23373

Softcover reprint of the hardcover 1st edition 1980
227 West 17th Street, New York, N.Y. 10011

Plenum Medical Book Company is an imprint of Plenum Publishing Corporation

ISBN-13: 978-1-4615-9181-8 e-ISBN-13: 978-4615-9179-5
DIO: 10.1007/ 978-4615-9179-5

Contributors

Michael J. Antonaccio, Ph.D., Director, Pharmacology, The Squibb Institute for Medical Research, Princeton, New Jersey 08540

Steven A. Atlas, M.D., Assistant Professor of Medicine and Assistant Attending Physician, Cardiovascular Center and Division of Cardiology, New York Hospital–Cornell Medical Center, New York, New York 10021

Emmanuel L. Bravo, M.D., Research Division, Cleveland Clinic Foundation, Cleveland, Ohio 44106

Hans R. Brunner, M.D., Associate Professor of Medicine, Université de Lausanne, and Director of Nephrology and Hypertension, Department of Medicine, Hôpital Cantonal Universitaire, CH-1011 Lausanne, Switzerland

David B. Case, M.D., Associate Professor of Medicine, Cardiovascular Center and Division of Cardiology, New York Hospital–Cornell Medical Center, New York, New York 10021

Hong Son Cheung, M.S., Assistant Research Fellow, The Squibb Institute for Medical Research, Princeton, New Jersey 08540

Jay N. Cohn, M.D., Professor of Medicine and Head, Cardiovascular Division, University of Minnesota Medical School, Minneapolis, Minnesota 55455

David W. Cushman, Ph.D., Senior Research Fellow in Pharmacology, The Squibb Institute for Medical Research, Princeton, New Jersy 08540

Harriet P. Dustan, M.D., Director, CVRTC, University of Alabama Medical Center, Birmingham, Alabama 35294

Haralambos Gavras, MD., Associate Professor of Medicine, Boston University School of Medicine, and Head, Hypertension Section, Boston City Hospital, Boston, Massachusetts 02118

Irene Gavras, M.D., Assistant Professor of Medicine, Boston University School of Medicine, and Hypertension Section, Boston City Hospital, Boston, Massachusetts 02118

Norman K. Hollenberg, M.D., Ph.D., Professor and Director of Physiologic Research, Department of Radiology, Harvard Medical School, and Senior Associate in Medicine, Renal Division, Peter Bent Brigham Hospital, Boston, Massachusetts 02115

Zola P. Horovitz, Ph.D., Vice President and Associate Director, The Squibb Institute for Medical Research, Princeton, New Jersey 08540

G. R. Keim, D.V.M., Director of Drug Safety Evaluation, The Squibb Institute for Medical Research, New Brunswick, New Jersey 08903

Hans J. Keim, M.D., Instructor in Medicine, Johannes Gutenberg-Universität, I. Medizinische Klinik und Poliklinik, 6500 Mainz, Germany

Glenn R. Kershaw, M.D., Clinical Fellow in Hypertension, Boston University School of Medicine, and Hypertension Section, Boston City Hospital, Boston, Massachusetts 02118

James R. Knill, M.D., Vice President for Medical Affairs, The Squibb Institute for Medical Research, Princeton, New Jersey 08540

John H. Laragh, M.D., Hilda Altshul Master Professor of Medicine; Director, Cardiovascular Center; and Chief, Division of Cardiology, New York Hospital–Cornell Medical Center, New York, New York 10021

Doris N. McKinstry, Ph.D., Director, Clinical Pharmacology, The Squibb Institute for Medical Research, Princeton, New Jersey 08540

E. Eric Muirhead, M.D., Professor of Pathology and Clinical Professor of Medicine, University of Tennessee Center for the Health Sciences, Memphis, Tennessee 38163

Miguel A. Ondetti, Ph.D., Associate Director, The Squibb Institute for Medical Research, Princeton, New Jersey 08540

W. S. Peart, M.D., F.R.C.P., F.R.S., Medical Unit, St. Mary's Hospital, London W2 1NY, England

Bernard Rubin, Ph.D., Senior Research Group Leader, The Squibb Institute for Medical Research, Princeton, New Jersey 08540

Emily F. Sabo, B.S., Research Assistant in Biochemistry, The Squibb Institute for Medical Research, Princeton, New Jersey 08540

Jean E. Sealey, Ph.D., Associate Professor of Physiology in Medicine, Cardiovascular Center and Division of Cardiology, New York Hospital–Cornell Medical Center, New York, New York 10021

Richard L. Soffer, M.D., Professor of Medicine and Biochemistry, Cornell University Medical College, New York, New York 10021

Edmund H. Sonnenblick, M.D., Professor of Medicine and Chief, Division of Cardiology, Albert Einstein College of Medicine, Bronx, New York 10461

Patricia A. Sullivan, R.N., Cardiovascular Center and Division of Cardiology, New York Hospital–Cornell Medical Center, New York, New York 10021

Robert C. Tarazi, M.D., Research Division, Cleveland Clinic Foundation, Cleveland, Ohio 44106

Stephen Textor, M.D., Research Staff, Research Division, Cleveland Clinic Foundation, Cleveland, Ohio 44106

Charles P. Tifft, M.D., Assistant Professor of Medicine, Boston University School of Medicine, and Hypertension Section, Boston City Hospital, Boston, Massachusetts 02118

G. A. Turini, M.D., Department of Medicine, Université de Lausanne, and Department of Medicine, Hôpital Cantonal Universitaire, CH-1011 Lausanne, Switzerland

Robert A. Vukovich, Ph.D., Director, Division of Developmental Therapeutics, Revlon Health Care, Tuckahoe, New York 10707

B. Waeber, M.D., Department of Medicine, Université de Lausanne, and Department of Medicine, Hôpital Cantonal Universitaire, CH-1011 Lausanne, Switzerland

John M. Wallace, M.D., Professor of Medicine, University of Texas Medical College, Galveston, Texas 77550

J. P. Wauters, M.D., Department of Medicine, Université de Lausanne, and Department of Medicine, Hôpital Cantonal Universitaire, CH-1011 Lausanne, Switzerland

Preface

This monograph was developed from a collection of papers that were originally presented at a symposium entitled "Pathogenesis of Hypertension" held at the Henry Chauncy Conference Center, Princeton. New Jersey. These manuscripts were subsequently revised, updated, and reorganized in a manner suitable for this publication. The symposium was planned to stimulate interest among investigators and clinicians alike in the potential for a new class of drugs called converting enzyme inhibitors in clinical medicine. The meeting was sponsored by the Squibb Institute for Medical Research, whose pioneering biochemical and pharmaceutical research had led to the development of the first orally active converting enzyme inhibitor.

It is hoped that this monograph will cohesively pull together the thesis that the identification, quantification, and containment of the renin factor in hypertension can be a powerful diagnostic and therapeutic strategy in clinical medicine. In addition, the sequence of studies presented in this manuscript will serve to demonstrate how basic biochemical and physiological research produces fundamental and critical information on which subsequent major advances in clinical pharmacology and medicine can be based.

This monograph is divided into three sections. The first is a general discussion of the effects of several specific hormones on the mechanisms of hypertension. The second section specifically develops the background for the development of angiotensin-converting enzyme inhibitors and contains some preclinical experience. The third section describes the experience that has been gained using converting enzyme inhibitors both diagnostically and therapeutically in man and their potential for the future.

David B. Case, M.D.

New York, New York

Contents

Part I
Humoral and Physiological Mechanisms in Hypertension

Chapter 1

Blood Pressure Homeostasis 3

Robert A. Vukovitch and James R. Knill

Chapter 2

Mechanisms of Hypertension Induced by Electrolyte-Active Steroids . . 15

Emmanuel L. Bravo, Harriet P. Dustan. and Robert C. Tarazi

Chapter 3

The Relationship of the Renal Medulla to the Hypertensive State 25

E. Eric Muirhead

Chapter 4

The Influence of Various Neurological Defects on the Release of Renin in Normal Man 39

W. S. Peart

Chapter 5

Angiotensin as a Determinant of Renal Perfusion and Function 57

Norman K. Hollenberg

Chapter 6

Systemic Vascular Resistance: Regulation and Effect on Left Ventricular Function 77

Jay N. Cohn

Part II
Angiotensin-Converting Enzyme: Its Role and Development of Inhibitors

Chapter 7

Physiological, Biochemical, and Immunologic Aspects of Angiotensin-Converting Enzyme 89

Richard L. Soffer and Edmund H. Sonnenblick

Chapter 8

Design of New Antihypertensive Drugs: Potent and Specific Inhibitors of Angiotensin-Converting Enzyme 103

David W. Cushman, Hong Son Cheung, Emily F. Sabo, and Miguel A. Ondetti

Chapter 9

Captopril (Capoten®; SQ 14,225) (D-3-Mercapto-2-methylpropanoyl-L-proline): A Novel Orally Active Inhibitor of Angiotensin-Converting Enzyme and Antihypertensive Agent 115

Bernard Rubin, Michael J. Antonaccio, and Zola P. Horovitz

Chapter 10

Toxicologic and Drug Metabolic Studies of SQ 14,225 in Animals 137

G. R. Keim

Chapter 11

Captopril: An Oral Angiotensin-Converting Enzyme Inhibitor Active in Man 149

Hans R. Brunner, Haralambos Gavras, B. Waeber, G. A. Turini, and J. P. Wauters

Part III
Clinical Use of Converting Enzyme Inhibitors

Chapter 12

The Renin System in High Blood Pressure, from Disbelief to Reality: Converting Enzyme Blockade for Analysis and Treatment 173

John H. Laragh

Chapter 13

Experiences with Blockade of the Renin System in Human Hypertension Using Converting Enzyme Inhibitor SQ 20,881 and Saralasin 185

David B. Case, Hans J. Keim, John M. Wallace, and John H. Laragh

Chapter 14

The Use of SQ 20,881 Converting Enzyme Inhibitor (Teprotide) for Diagnostic Purposes in Hypertension 201

Haralambos Gavras, Irene Gavras, Stephen Textor, Charles P. Tifft, Glenn R. Kershaw, and Hans R. Brunner

Chapter 15

Clinical Experience with Blockade of the Renin–Angiotensin–Aldosterone System by an Oral Converting Enzyme Inhibitor (SQ 14,225, Captopril) in Hypertensive Patients 211

David B. Case, Steven A. Atlas, John H. Laragh, Jean E. Sealey, Patricia A. Sullivan, and Doris N. McKinstry

Index 231

Part I · Humoral and Physiological Mechanisms in Hypertension

Chapter 1

Blood Pressure Homeostasis

Robert A. Vukovich and James R. Knill

The circulatory system is a closed-loop system in which cardiac output is dependent upon adequate venous return. Distribution of this output to the various organ systems in amounts appropriate to their needs is accomplished by constriction or relaxation of vascular smooth muscle. Within this closed system, a pressure gradient is discerned, with pressure greatest in the aorta and lowest in the vena cavae.

The flow of blood through the anatomic complexity of the circulatory system can be described rather simply using hydraulic principles. Several basic interrelationships apply among flow, pressure, and resistance. Flow is a measure of volume per unit of time; blood pressure is a measure of the force exerted by blood per unit area of vessel wall; and resistence to blood flow is the impediment to flow and is due, among other things, to function loss. These three factors are related by the following equation:

$$\text{Blood flow} = \frac{\text{Pressure}}{\text{Resistance}}$$

It is apparent that the volume of blood moving through an artery or vein is directly proportional to the pressure drop across a given segment (the pressure gradient) and inversely proportional to the resistance within that segment. That is to say, if flow through a vessel is to remain constant, changes in vascular resistance must be accompanied by inversely proportional changes in pressure.

The reduction in pressure which accompanies blood flow through a vessel results from friction between blood and vessel wall and is proportional to the length of the vessel. Blood flow is laminar, i.e., blood plasma and formed elements move fastest through the center of a vessel and

ROBERT A. VUKOVICH, Ph.D. · Division of Developmental Therapeutics, Revlon Health Care, Tuckahoe, New York 10707. JAMES R. KNILL, M.D. · Division of Medical Affairs, The Squibb Institute for Medical Research, Princeton, New Jersey 08540.

$$\text{Flow} = \frac{\pi \Delta P r^4}{8 l v}$$

ΔP = Pressure gradient l = Tube length
r = Tube radius v = Fluid viscosity

FIGURE 1. Poiseuille's law of hydraulics.

slowest, because of friction, when closest to the vessel wall. This can be linkened to fluid sheets sliding one over the other. A more technical description of the factors responsible for friction losses in blood flow is related by Poiseuille's law (Figure 1).

In the application of Poiseuille's law of hydraulics to the circulatory system, certain concessions must be made. First, blood flow through the circulatory system is pulsatile, not constant. Second, blood vessel walls are elastic and distensible, not rigid. Third, blood flow may not always be laminar. It is because of these factors that Poiseuille's law can only be applied qualitatively to the systemic circulation.

Vessel diameter, it can be seen, plays an important role in determining blood flow through that vessel. It can be observed that the flow of blood is greatest through the largest vessels (e.g., aorta) and least through the smallest vessels. That is to say, pressure gradients become much steeper as arteries branch off from the aorta and become smaller, especially at the level of the arterioles and capillaries. In addition, flow from capillaries to the great veins is accompanied by a decrease in resistance.

The total resistance to blood flow through blood vessels connected in series is given in the equation:

$$R_{\text{TOT}} = R_1 + R_2 + \ldots + R_n$$

It can be appreciated that total resistance is equal to the arithmetic sum of the individual resistances of each vessel.

For vessels connected in parallel, the total resistance is described as:

$$R_{\text{TOT}} = 1/(R_1 + R_2 + \ldots + R_n)$$

Total resistance to flow through vessels connected in parallel is equal to the arithmetic sum of the reciprocals of the individual resistances. In other words, the total resistance to flow is less than that of any one of the vessels alone in any circuit in which vessels are connected in parallel.

In Figure 2,[1] the systemic circulation is depicted as consisting of a number of circuits connected in parallel. Each circuit delivers blood flow to one specific organ group. Blood flow from the arterial to the venous side within a given circuit is through vessels which are connected in series. The total resistance through each series circuit is equal to the sum of the individual resistances to flow. This should be compared with the calculation of total resistance for the general circulation, a parallel system, which is equal to the reciprocal of the sum of the reciprocals of the individual resistances.

Consideration of arterial pressure regulation should include an understanding of the structure and function of the individual vascular bed

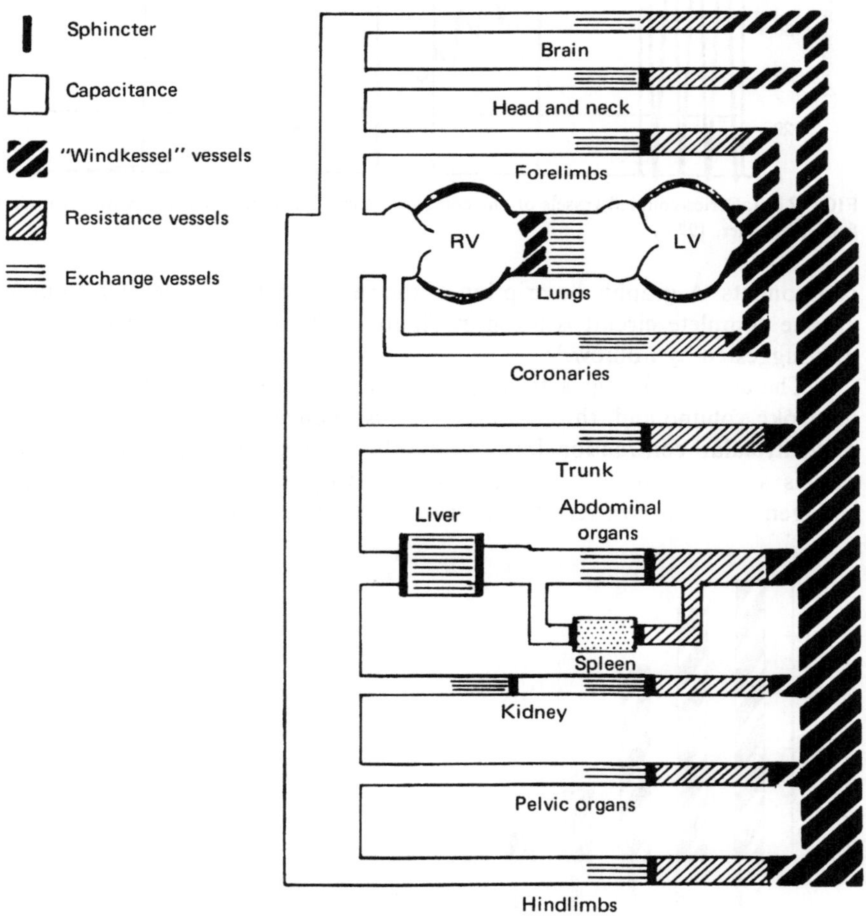

FIGURE 2. Schematic diagram of the systemic circulation illustrating circuits connected in parallel and in series.(Reprinted with permission from Silber and Katz, 1975.)

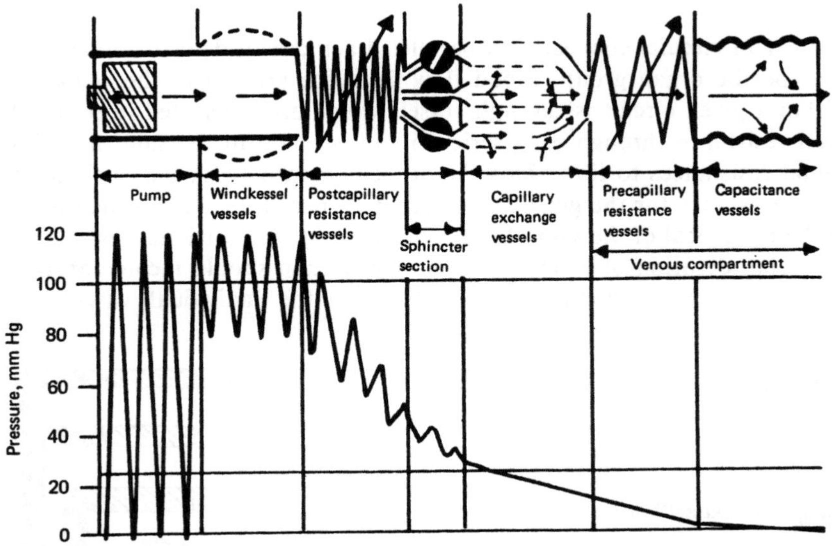

FIGURE 3. Series-coupled vessels of one complete vascular circuit.(Reprinted with permission from Detweiler, 1973.)

components. A graphic description of the series-coupled vessels which make up one complete circuit is given in Figure 3.[2] This functional classification was suggested by Folkow.[3]

The aorta and large arteries are capable of absorbing the kinetic energy of stroke volume and, through function loss, convert the intermittent pulses of ventricular contraction into a smoother, more continuous flow. These vessels serve as shock absorbers because they contain much elastic and collagen material. Wetterer[4] has estimated that over 50% of the dampening

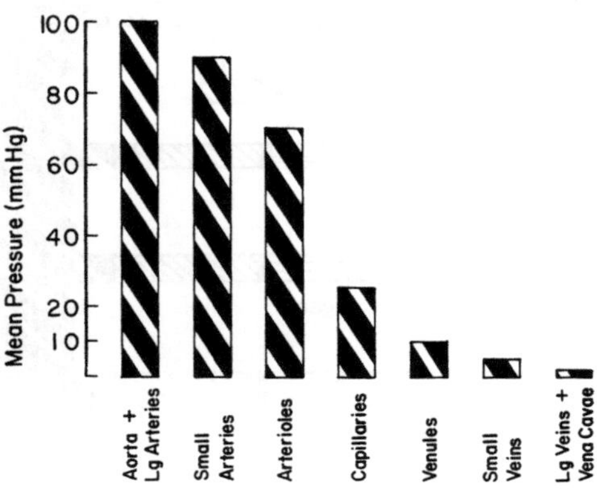

FIGURE 4. Mean pressure within the systemic circulation. (Redrawn from Silber and Katz, 1975.)

function of Windkessel vessels may be attributed to the aorta itself. Windkessel vessels are followed by resistance vessels. Precapillary resistance vessels are the small arteries and arterioles. Arteriolar smooth muscle imparts sphincter properties to the terminal portions of arterioles which can reduce, increase, or totally block blood flow to various capillary beds. Post-capillary resistance is determined by the venules and small veins. Capacitance vessels are comprised of the venous compartment. Through the action of a unique valvular system, a unidirectional flow of blood is directed toward the heart under low pressure.

Figure 4 graphically depicts the mean arterial pressure within various parts of the systemic circulation.[1] It can be seen that the greatest resistance to flow occurs in the arterioles, capillaries, and venules as demonstrated by the greatest drop in pressure. The tonus of the precapillary resistance vessels can be increased or decreased by locally produced substances, by the action of vasomotor nerves, or by pharmacologic agents.

Blood flow to various organ systems is directly proportional to both the velocity of blood through a given vessel segment and the cross-sectional area of the segment. Expressed another way, blood velocity is directly proportional to the volume flow and inversely proportional to the square of the vessel diameter. This means, for example, that blood velocity is greatest in the aorta and least in the capillaries.

In terms of volume flow, Figure 5[2] illustrates the resting and maximal flows of various circuits within the systemic circulation. Secretory and excretory organs receive blood supplies greater than those required for their nutritional benefit. The excess capacity is necessary in order that these organs fulfill their exocrine or excretory function.

Satisfactory venous return to the heart is essential in order to maintain adequate cardiac output and tissue perfusion. Such venous return and tissue

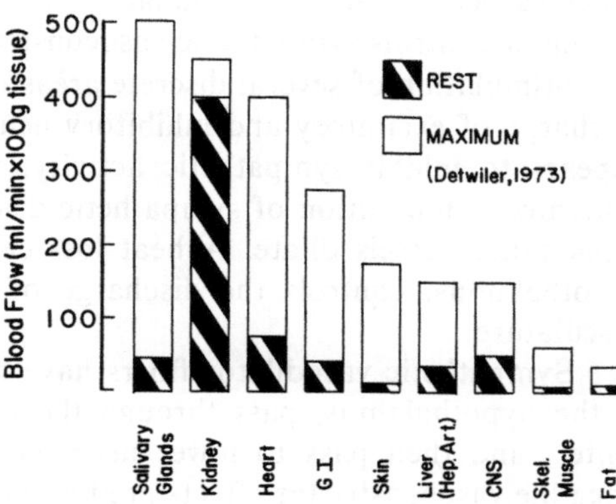

FIGURE 5. Resting and maximal blood flow in various organs. (Redrawn from Detweiler, 1973.)

perfusion are the net result of a delicate balance between vasoconstriction and vasodilation. Several mechanisms operate to effect this balance. Autoregulation is one such mechanism. It has been suggested[5,6] that tissue oxygen concentration is an important factor regulating local blood flow. Both relaxation and constriction of precapillary sphencters occur in response to local tissue oxygen levels. Mediators of this response could include local production of metabolites, prostaglandins, and kinins. Many other vasoactive substances have been implicated; however, their precise contribution to local autoregulation remains to be determined.

In spite of the complex nature of the autoregulatory system, it does not play the major role in normal blood pressure homeostasis. In normotensive man, the central nervous system plays the dominant role. Vasoconstrictor fibers belonging to the thoracolumbar or sympathetic nervous system originate within the lateral horns of the spinal gray matter and extend from T-1 to L-2 or L-3. Arterioles are innervated by vasoconstrictor fibers which originate within this portion of the autonomic nervous system. In addition to regulating arteriole diameter, these fibers also exert strong control over heart size and capacitance vessels. In this way, venous return and cardiac output can be regulated to meet body demands. In addition, the cutaneous vasculature is also innervated by these fibers, and, through their regualtion, heat loss from the body can be controlled. These sympathetic fibers can exert their influence segmentally, regionally, or in a generalized fashion, affecting all of the vessels they innervate, depending on the stimulus. The sympathetic outflow is principally under the control of higher centers located in the medulla, hypothalamus, and cortex. This association is shown in Figure 6.

A vasomotor center located in the floor of the fourth ventricle in the medulla has two discrete areas designated as a pressor area (lateral) and a depressor area (medial). Experimental stimulation of these areas produces either vasocontriction of vasodilation, respectively. The medullary vasomotor center controls sympathetic vasoconstrictor fibers only.

Stimulation of several discrete areas of the hypothalamus results in the discharge of excitatory and inhibitory neurons. The anterior hypothalamus appears to inhibit sympathetic activity; when it is excited electrically, a generalized diminution of sympathetic discharge occurs, and resistance and capacitance vessels dilate. A heat loss center, also located in the anterior hypothalamus, controls the discharge of sympathetic fibers to cutaneous vasculature.

Sympathetic vasodilator fibers have their origin in the cortex, synapse in the hypothalamus, pass through the medulla outside of the vasomotor center, and then pass to lower neurons. Their function remains obscure, since the vasoconstrictor effects predominate over vasodilation.

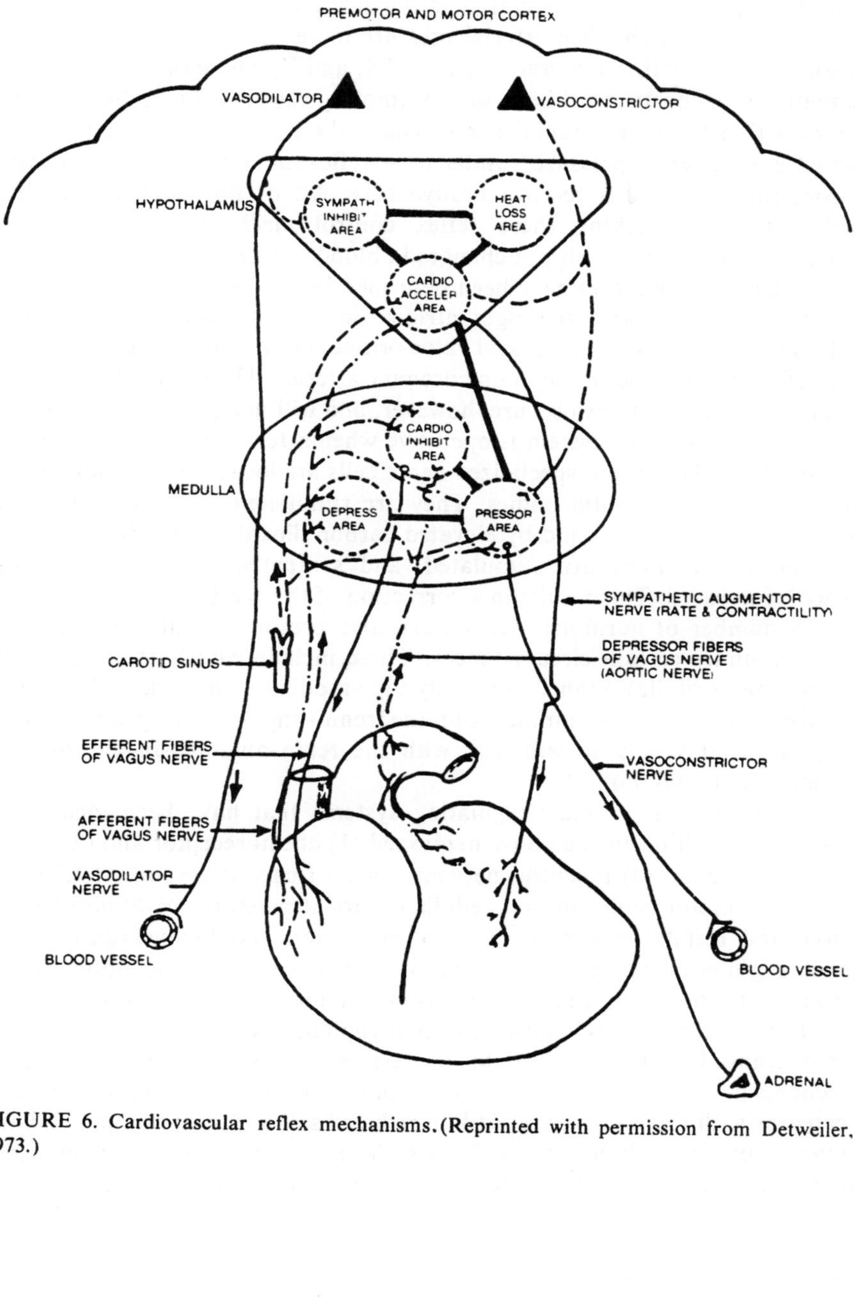

FIGURE 6. Cardiovascular reflex mechanisms. (Reprinted with permission from Detweiler, 1973.)

Experiments have shown that the fundamental control of arterial pressure is reflexly controlled by the action of the arterial pressure itself on stretch-sensitive receptors designated as baroreceptors or pressoreceptors.[7] These receptors, located principally in the aortic arch and carotid sinus, are stimulated by stretch when arterial pressure increases. Impulses flow to the vasomotor center through cranial nerves IX, and X, where they inhibit sympathetic vasonconstrictor fibers, thus promoting vasodilation. Other efferent fibers within the tenth cranial nerve reduce the heart rate. Therefore, any increase in arterial pressure results in a reflex inhibition of sympathetic vasoconstriction and a relative bradycardia. All of this happens rapidly, within seconds, making these reflex control mechanisms of principal importance in reversing abrupt changes in blood pressure.

Other baroreceptors have been described in the walls of the vena cavae and their junction with the right atrium, in the pulmonary veins, in the pulmonary artery, at the tricuspid valve orifice, in the wall of the left atrium and left ventricle, and in the main coronary arteries. They physiological role of these reflexes remains obscure, however, and will not be discussed here.

A chemoreceptor system is operative when arterial pressure falls below about 80 mm Hg. These specialized nerve cells are located in the root of the aortic and in the carotid bodies. They are stimulated by poor delivery of oxygen to the receptors and by elevated carbon dioxide levels. Sympathetic vasoconstrictor fibers are stimulated, and sympathetic discharge to the heart is increased. This results in a correction of the pressure.

A number of hormonal factors can also profoundly influence arterial pressure under certain circumstances. These include catecholamines (from the adrenal medulla), kinins (especially the vasodilator, bradykinin), prostaglandins, serotonin, histamine, and the renin–angiotensin system. Other chapters in this volume will deal with the renin–angiotensin–aldosterone system and bradykinin.

Other arterial pressure-regulating systems that have been identified[8] include, in addition to the abovementioned (1) chemoreceptor and (2) baroreceptor reflexes, (3) a central nervous system ischemic response (ischemia of the vasomotor center in the medulla occurs at pressures of 40 mm Hg or lower and results in a marked vasoconstriction and tachycardia), (4) a renin–angiotensin vasoconstrictor mechanism, (5) a stress–relaxation mechanism (arteriole walls relax when distended for a period of time), (6) a capillary–fluid shift mechanism (elevated capillary bed pressures result in a rapid transudation of fluid into the tissue spaces), (7) an aldosterone mechanism, and (8) a renal–body fluid mechnism wherein pressure decreases within the kidney result in a reduced salt and water output and an increase of body fluid. Figure 7 lists these mechanisms and shows the approximate pressure ranges within which they are said to be operative.

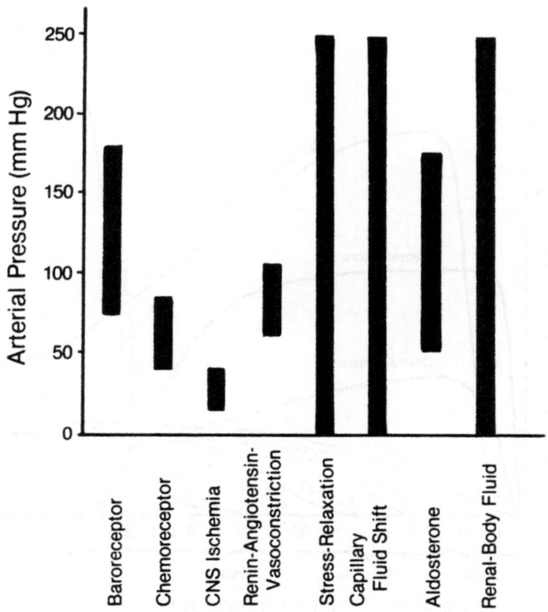

FIGURE 7. Arterial pressure regulatory mechanisms and the approximate pressure ranges within which they are operative.(Reprinted with permission from Guyton et al., 1972.)

As can be seen, only three mechanisms operate throughout all pressures. The other five mechanisms regulate arterial pressure within discrete pressure ranges.

The concepts of feedback gain and infinite gain have been suggested by Guyton et al.[8] to explain arterial pressure regulation. These workers employ computerized systems analysis in an attempt to determine the interrelationships among the above control mechanisms. The parameter, feedback gain, is defined as the quotient of the amount of arterial pressure correction by the amount still to be corrected. Infinite gain is defined as feedback gain which corrects a pressure change completely.

In Figure 8 are shown the temporal relationships between the onset of an abrupt arterial pressure change and the maximum correction effected by each of the above mechanisms. Only one mechanism, the renal–body fluid mechanism, has infinite gain. The basic premise is that elevated arterial pressure is accompanied by an increase in the renal output of salt and water until pressure is normalized. It should be pointed out that the renal–body fluid mechanism requires several hours of operation before significant effects on blood pressure are realized. Acute correction of pressure is

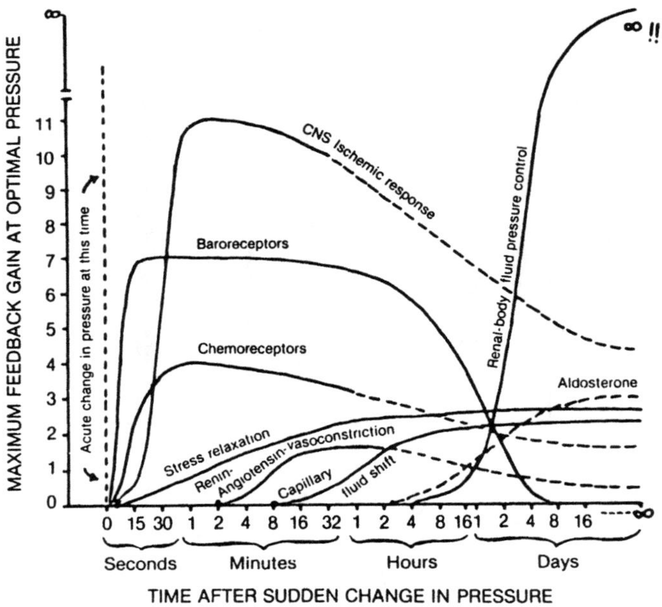

FIGURE 8. Temporal relationship between onset of abrupt arterial pressure drop and maximum correction effected by regulatory mechanisms. (Reprinted with permission from Guyton et al., 1972.)

effected by the baroreceptor and chemoreceptor reflexes, whereas long term blood pressure homeostasis is a function of renal–body fluid balance.

It is important to note that renal function must be adequate and remain unchanged and salt and water intake should be fixed at a constant daily rate in order to render the renal–body fluid mechanism capable of infinite gain.

In conclusion, blood pressure homeostasis is achieved through the concerted influence of central, chemical, hormonal, and renal mechanisms. Derangements in any one or more of these systems can result in an impairment of the corrective process and the development of hypotension of hypertension.

References

1. Silber EN, Katz LN: *Heart Disease*. New York, Macmillan, 1975.
2. Detweiler DC: *Physiological Basis of Medical Practice*. Baltimore, Williams & Wilkins Co, 1973.
3. Folkow B: Range of control of the cardiovascular system by the central nervous system. *Physiol Rev* 40(Suppl 4):93, 1960.

4. Wetterer E: Die Wirking der Herztatigkeit auf die Dynamik des Arteriensystems. *Verhandl Dtsch Ges Kreislaufforsch* 22:266, 1956.
5. Stainsby W.N.: Local control of regional blood flow. *Ann Rev Physiol* 35:151, 1973.
6. Carrier O, Walker JR, Guyton AC: Role of oxygen in autoregulation of blood flow in isolated vessels. *Am J Physiol* 206:951, 1964.
7. Heymans C, Neil E.: *Reflexogenic Areas of the Cardiovascular System*. London, J & A Churchill, Ltd , 1958.
8. Guyton, AC, Coleman TG, Cowley AW, et al: Arterial pressure regulation. *Am J Med* 52:584, 1972.

Chapter 2

Mechanisms of Hypertension Induced by Electrolyte-Active Steroids

Emmanuel L. Bravo, Harriet P. Dustan, and Robert C. Tarazi

The role of electrolyte-active steroids in the development and maintenance of hypertension remains unclear. Observations accrued from the deoxycorticosterone acetate–saline (DOCA–saline) hypertensive rat[1-3] may have little clinical relevance because, in this model, hypertension is induced by reducing renal mass and by the administration of large amounts of salt together with DOCA. On the other hand, clinical studies in the syndrome of primary aldosteronism are difficult to assess, since data have been obtained in patients with established hypertension[4] or following discontinuance of spironolactone.[5]

To obtain information concerning hemodynamic and humoral adjustments that occur in hypertension resulting from electrolyte-active steroids, we studied a dog model that can be produced by long-term oral administration of metyrapone without reducing renal mass or increasing salt intake.[6] In this model, ACTH overdrive leads to increases in deoxycorticosterone (DOC) secretion and is associated with suppressed plasma renin activity (PRA) and significant hypokalemia.[7] Sequential determinations of hemodynamic indices, of plasma catecholamines, and of responses to adrenergic blocking drugs and to altered salt intake allowed a balanced assessment of the factors involved in the development and maintenance of this type of hypertension.

Studies were performed on intact, trained, conscious male mongrel dogs with chronic indwelling iliac artery catheters whose diet contained 100–120 mEq of sodium and 60 mEq of potassium per day.[6] In all studies, metyrapone was administered orally in doses of 100 mg/kg per day. Methods for the measurements of cardiac output (CO) and other derived

---

EMMANUEL L. BRAVO, M.D., and ROBERT C. TARAZI, M.D. Research Division, Cleveland Clinic Foundation, Cleveland, Ohio 44106. HARRIET P. DUSTAN, M.D. · CVRTC, University of Alabama Medical Center, Birmingham, Alabama 35294.

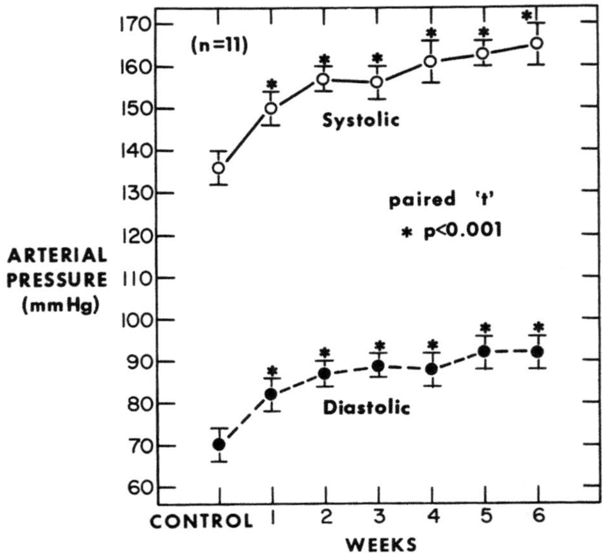

FIGURE 1. Response of arterial blood pressure to metyrapone administration (100 mg/kg per day) in dogs receiving a normal sodium intake.

hemodynamic indices, of extracellular fluid volume (ECF), and of plasma catecholamines have been described previously.[6] Student's *t*-test for paired observations was used for statistical analysis of the data. Results are presented as mean values ± SE.

The response of arterial blood pressure to metyrapone administration is depicted in Figure 1. All dogs showed significant increases in blood pressure within 7–10 days which were maintained as long as the drug was given, in some instances up to 56 weeks. The hemodynamic patterns observed with the rise in blood pressure are illustrated in Figure 2. In order to handle the large amount of data obtained by biweekly determinations for 8 weeks in 11 dogs, the values were calculated as follows: Period I refers to the first 2 weeks of treatment when blood pressure tended to be labile, and Period II to the last 4 weeks of treatment when the blood pressure was stable. Each point represents the mean of at least three observations. Three different hemodynamic patterns were recognized: (1) in five dogs the hypertension was associated from the onset with significant elevations of CO and remained so during the period of observation. ECF was significantly increased. (2) Sequential changes in three dogs showed initial increases in CO followed by a rise in TPR and decreases in CO. (3) In the third group, total peripheral resistance (TPR) was elevated from the onset and remained

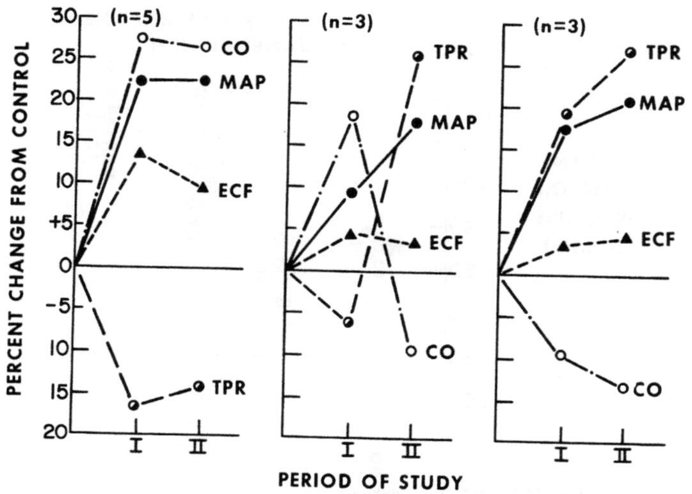

FIGURE 2. Hemodynamic characteristics of metyrapone-induced hypertension in the dog during the labile and established phases of hypertension.[6]

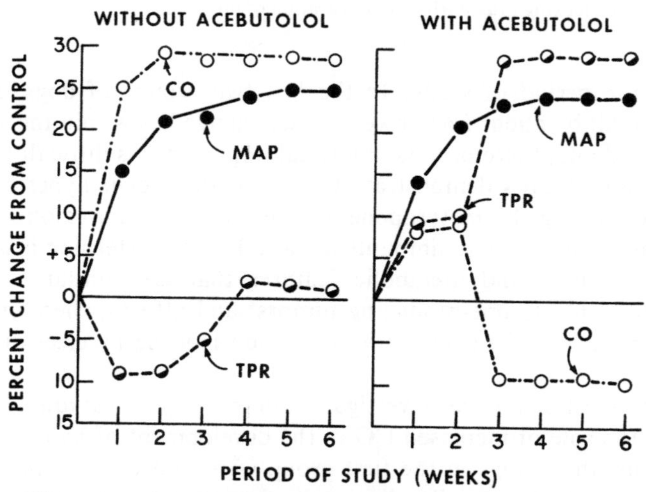

FIGURE 3. Effect of pretreatment with acebutolol on the hemodynamic response to metyrapone administration.[6]

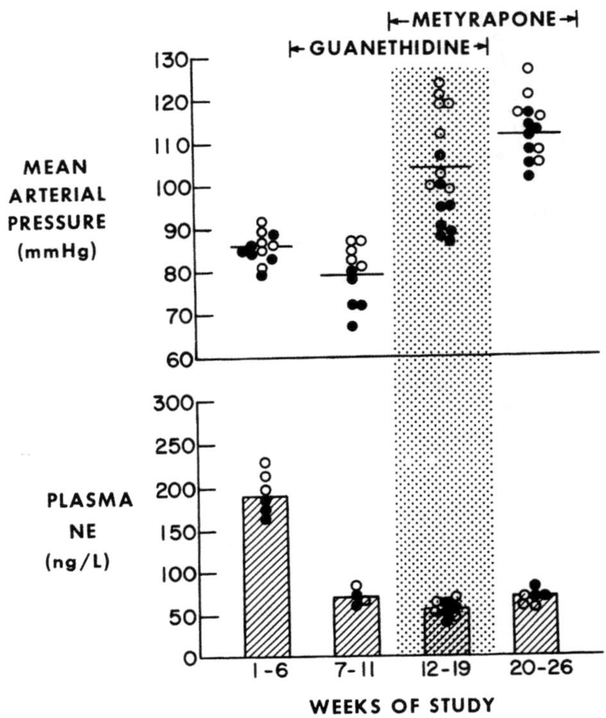

FIGURE 4. Response of blood pressure and plasma NE to pretreatment with a peripherally acting adrenergic blocking drug during administration of metyrapone.[6]

so during the period of study. In the last two groups of dogs, ECF was increased in all by about 5%; however, this change lies within the sensitivity of the method and, therefore, its biological importance is difficult to assess.

The above results demonstrate that DOC-dependent hypertension can be produced in dogs by metyrapone without need of nephrectomy or of the administration of excessive amounts of salt. This hypertension is associated with hemodynamic and metabolic features that are similar to those in patients with aldosterone-producing tumors[4] and affords, therefore, a convenient approach to the study of hypertension induced by electrolyte-active steroids.

Three questions were investigated in subsequent studies. The first concerned the role of increased CO in the development of hypertension. To evaluate this, three dogs in the first group were pretreated with acebutolol (30 mg/kg per day), a cardioselective β-adrenergic blocking drug, prior to reinstitution of metyrapone. Figure 3 shows that arterial blood pressure rose to similar value in spite of the fact that the rise in CO was effectively prevented by acebutolol. The development of hypertension under the latter conditions was, therefore, related to marked increases in TPR.

The second question which we attempted to answer concerns the relationship between enhanced activity of the peripheral nervous system and the hypertension induced by electrolyte-active steroids.[1-3] In these studies, the importance of adrenergic influences was investigated by the use of adrenergic blocking drugs which act at different sites in the nervous system. The administration of guanethidine (5 mg/kg per day), a peripherally acting adrenergic drug, did not affect blood pressure, although plasma norepinephrine (NE) was decidedly reduced (Figure 4). The subsequent addition of metyrapone did not alter plasma NE concentration and led to the same rise in blood pressure as in untreated animals. Following cessation of guanethidine, the blood pressure did not rise further, nor did plasma NE increase. In separate studies the administration of clonidine (30 μg/kg per

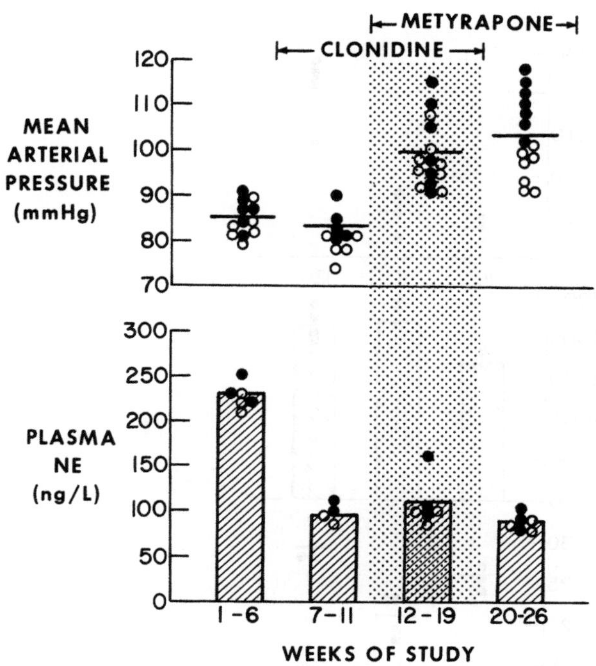

FIGURE 5. Response of blood pressure and plasma NE to metyrapone administration during pretreatment with a centrally acting adrenergic drug.[6]

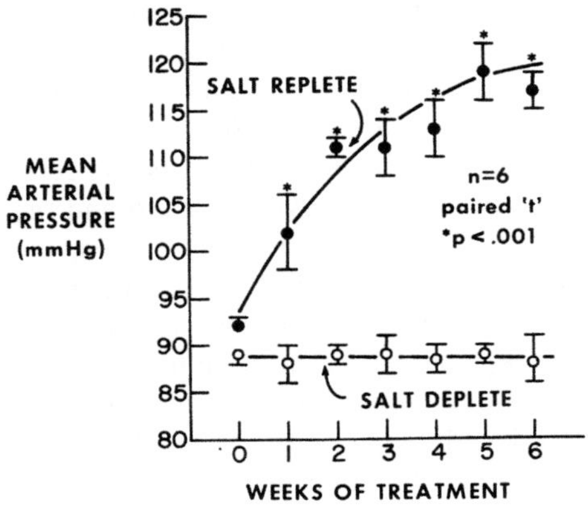

FIGURE 6. Effect of salt on the blood pressure response to metyrapone administration.[6]

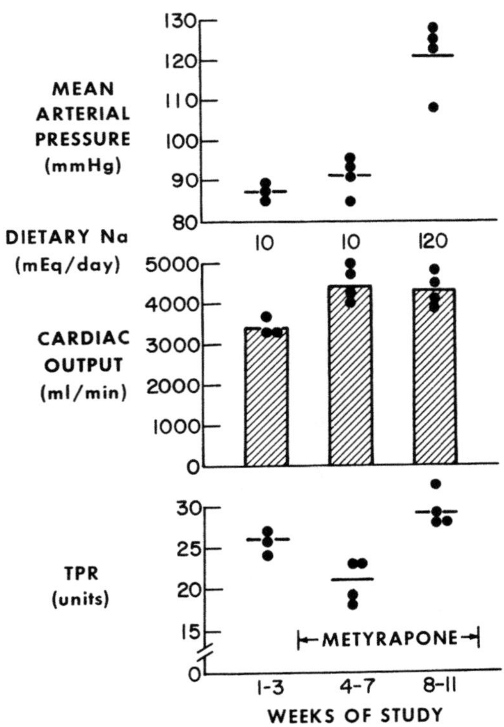

FIGURE 7. Hemodynamic response to dietary sodium manipulation during treatment with metyrapone.

day), a centrally acting adrenergic drug, for the same duration led to similar responses. These findings are depicted in Figure 5. These observations suggest that a major role for the sympathetic nervous system appears unlikely. However, they do not preclude the possibility that even minute concentrations of circulating plasma NE may contribute to enhanced reactivity of peripheral resistance vessels which had undergone structural changes as a result of chronic hypertension.[7]

A third question to consider is the role of salt in the pathogenesis of hypertension. Salt provided a necessary adjunct to DOC in producing the maximum blood pressure effect. As illustrated in Figure 6, sodium deprivation was singularly effective in preventing the development of hypertension induced by metyrapone administration. Reinstitution of the usual salt intake resulted in prompt increase in mean arterial pressure (MAP). The rise in blood pressure was associated with increased TPR while CO remained unchanged (Figure 7). These results suggest a vital role for sodium in producing these peripheral vascular changes.

Insofar as the mechanisms by which hypertension developed in these dogs are concerned, our observations do not support a major role for either increases in CO or enhanced activity of the sympathetic nervous system. However, they indicate some interaction between sodium and electrolyte-active steroids in the production of hypertension.

To account for the development and maintenance of hypertension in these dogs, a possible sequence of events could focus on the arterial wall in which altered membrane permeability would give rise to increased vascular reactivity (Figure 8). Considerable evidence has accumulated indicating that induction of hypertension in rats with DOCA and saline leads to altered membrane properties of vascular smooth muscle and that such changes occur prior to establishment of hypertension.[9-13] Increased membrane

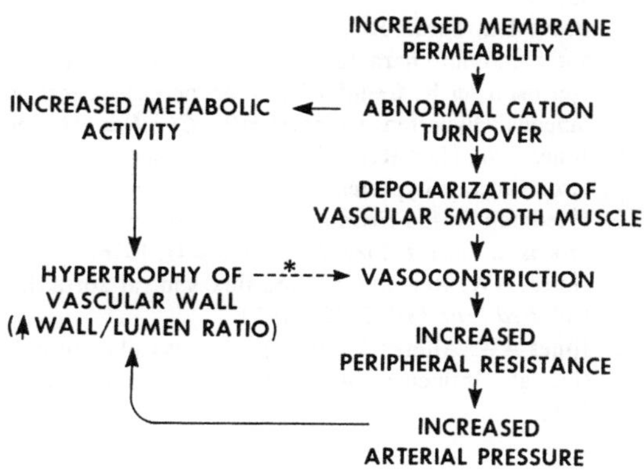

FIGURE 8. A hypothesis regarding the role of peripheral vascular changes in the initiation and maintenance of hypertension induced by electrolyte-active steroids.*, Increased reactivity.

permeability could result in abnormalities of cation turnover which, by partially depolarizing the muscle cell membrane, could lead to vasoconstriction and elevated peripheral resistance. Such changes would be expected to increase metabolic activity and may provide an early signal for vascular smooth muscle hypertrophy. This, when combined with rising arterial blood pressure, could lead to thickening of the media and raise the wall/lumen ratio.[14] This structural adaptation, implying enhanced reactivity, could be crucial for both potentiating and maintaining the hypertensive process.

These studies suggest that in this form of steroid-induced hypertension neither cardiac factors nor the sympathetic nervous system appears to play a prominent role in the development and maintenance of hypertension. The demonstration of salt as a necessary adjunct to deoxycorticosterone in producing hypertension indicates some interaction between salt and electrolyte-active steroids that remains to be elucidated.

References

1. Volicer L, Scheer E, Hilse H, et al: Turnover of norepinephrine in the heart during experimental hypertension in rats. *Life Sci* 7:525–532, 1968.
2. DeChamplain J, Farley L, Cousineau D, et al: Circulating catecholamine levels in human and experimental hypertension. *Circ Res* 38:109–114, 1976.
3. Reid JL, Zivin JA, Kopin IJ: Central and peripheral adrenergic mechanisms in the development of deoxycorticosterone-saline hypertension in rats. *Circ Res* 37:569–579, 1975.
4. Tarazi RC, Ibrahim MM, Bravo EL, et al: Hemodynamic characteristics of primary aldosteronism. *N Engl J Med* 289:1330–1335, 1973.
5. Wenting GJ, Man in't Veld AJ, Verhoeven RP, et al.: Volume–pressure relationships during development of mineralocorticoid hypertension in man. *Circ Res* 40:I-163–I-170, 1977.
6. Bravo EL, Tarazi RC, Dustan HP: Multifactorial analysis of chronic hypertension induced by electrolyte-active steroids in trained, unanesthetized dogs. *Circ Res* 40:I-40–I-45, 1977.
7. Bravo EL, Tarazi RC, Dustan HP: Metyrapone-induced hypertension in dogs: I. Humoral and metabolic characteristics. (Submitted for publication).
8. Hermsmeyer K: Cellular basis for increased sensitivity of vascular smooth muscle in spontaneously hypertensive rats (SHR). *Circ Res 38*(Suppl II):53–57, 1976.
9. Jones AW, Hart RG: Altered ion transport in aortic smooth muscle during deoxycorticosterone acetate hypertension in the rat. *Circ Res* 37:333–341, 1975.
10. Friedman SM, Friedman CL: Cell permeability, sodium transport and the hypertensive process in the rat. *Circ Res* 39:433–441, 1976.
11. Jones AW: Reactivity of ion fluxes in rat aorta during hypertension and circulatory control. *Fed Proc* 33:133–137, 1974.
12. Jones AW: Altered ion transport in vascular smooth muscle from spontaneously hypertensive rats: Influences of aldosterone, norepinephrine and angiotensin. *Circ Res* 33:563–572, 1973.

13. Berecek KH, Bohr DF: Vascular reactivity in the DOCA-hypertensive pig. *Circ Res* 42:764–771, 1978.
14. Folkow B, Hallback M, Lundgren Y, et al: Importance of adaptive changes in vascular design for establishment of primary hypertension, studied in man and in spontaneously hypertensive rats. *Circ Res* 32–33(suppl II):2–16, 1973.

Chapter 3

The Relationship of the Renal Medulla to the Hypertensive State

E. Eric Muirhead

Introduction

The kidney appears to relate to the hypertensive state via two opposing actions, what Braun-Menendez termed the prohypertensive and antihypertensive renal actions.[1] According to current views, the prohypertensive renal action results primarily from (1) activation of the renal pressor system(s) (mainly the renin–angiotensin system), and (2) failure of the kidney to prevent Na–volume loads (because of disease or absence or the excessive action of mineralocorticoids, primarily aldosterone). It is our view that the antihypertensive renal action also results from a dual renal effect, namely (1) the relief of Na–volume loads by the excretory process and (2) activation of a renal antipressor system existing primarily in the renal medulla. Moreover, it is proposed that this antipressor system resides, to a great extent, in the renomedullary interstitial cells (RIC).

It is the purpose of this chapter to consider evidence in favor of the RIC antipressor system.

Nonexcretory Antihypertensive Action of Whole Kidney

This term was used by Grollman to encompass a function of the kidney unrelated to the ability of this organ to regulate electrolyte–water balance, to protect the pH of the blood, and to excrete wastes and other unwanted substances. By different types of renal manipulations, the existence of this function has been supported by work in several laboratories.[2-5] More recently, we have derived additional data in support of such action by the whole kidney. The clip of the one-kidney, one-clip Goldblatt hypertensive (1KGH) rat was removed (unclipping procedure) under one of four different conditions; controls had a sham operation.[6] (1) Unclipping alone was

E. ERIC MUIRHEAD, M.D. · Departments of Pathology and Medicine, University of Tennessee Center for the Health Sciences, Memphis, Tennessee 38163.

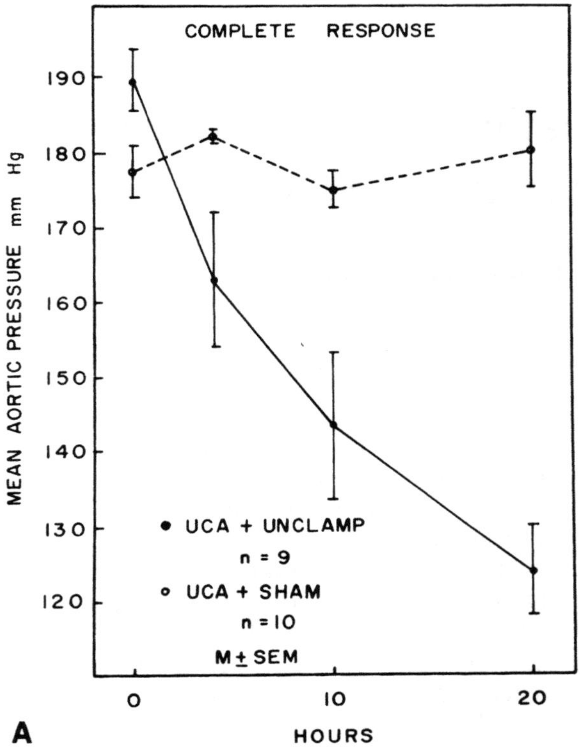

FIGURE 1. (A) Effect of unclipping a one-kidney, one-clip Goldblatt hypertensive rat (1KGH) after anastomosis of the ureter to the vena cava (UCA) (solid line) as opposed to a sham operation (broken line). The mean arterial pressure receded to normal levels within 20 hr.

associated with a normal arterial pressure within an average of 3 hr, while at the same time, a prominent diuresis–natriuresis occurred. (2) Ureterovenous anastomosis followed by unclipping was attended by a normal arterial pressure within an average of 20 hr (Figure 1). (3) Unclipping plus an intravenous saline infusion equal to or exceeding the Na–volume loss via the diuresis–natriuresis also normalized the arterial pressure within an average of 20 hr (Figure 1). Thus, the results of (2) did not occur because of substances entering the circulation via the ureterovenous anastomosis. (4) Ureterovenous anastomosis plus a Na–volume load (saline intravenously in an amount equal to 1.25–5% of the body weight) followed by unclipping was associated with normalization of the arterial pressure within approximately 48 hr. Sham-operated controls had no change in arterial pressure over the

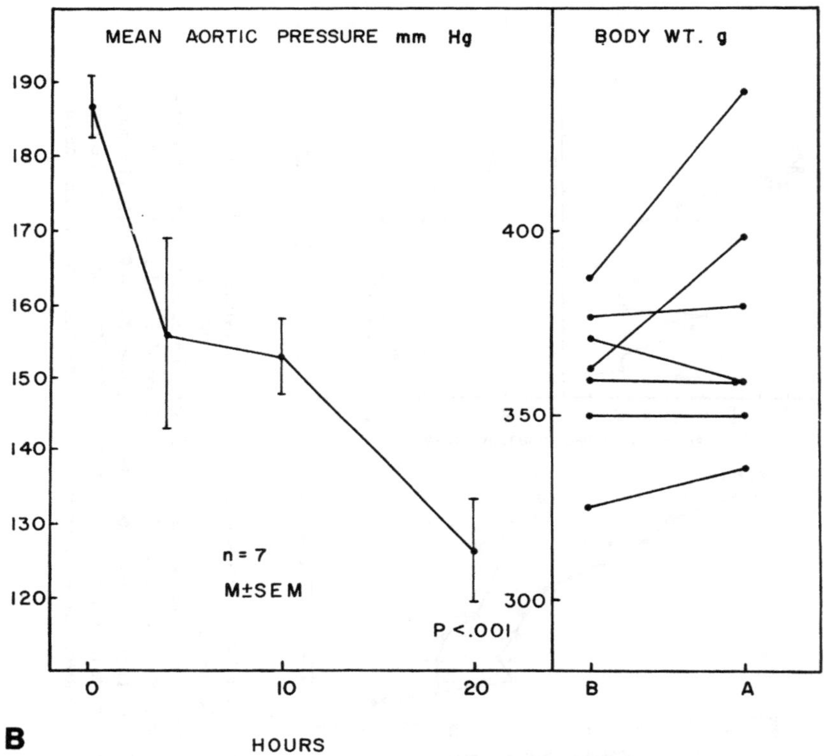

(B) Effect of an intravenous saline infusion begun prior to unclipping in 1KGH rats. The saline infusion was maintained at a rate that either equaled or exceeded the Na loss via the urine. The MAP reached normal values in the same manner as following UCA. Body weight either remained the same or increased except for one example in which body weight decreased after the pressure had normalized.

same time intervals. These observations are considered to support a nonexcretory antihypertensive renal function, at least as related to the excretion of Na and reduction of fluid volume. Further, diuresis–natriuresis appeared to accelerate this function but was not essential for it.

Nonexcretory Antihypertensive Action of Renal Medulla

Transplants of fragmented renal medulla (Tr Med) have been shown to exert an antihypertensive action in studies conducted in at least six separate laboratories (Figure 2).[7-15] The antihypertensive effect has been found in a variety of experimental hypertensive states. It is noteworthy that these

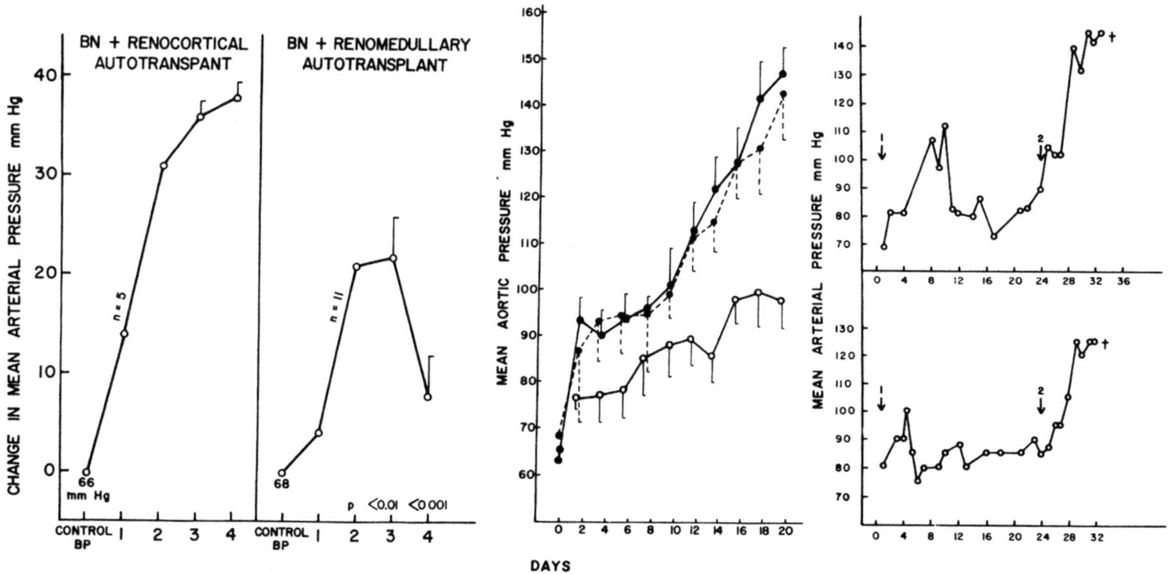

FIGURE 2. The first two panels on the left demonstrate protection by renomedullary tissue against hypertension from bilateral nephrectomy of the rabbit plus extreme Na loading (9 mEq/kg per day). Transplants of fragmented renal cortex failed to prevent the hypertension (first panel), while transplants of fragmented renomedullary tissue (second panel) slowed the rise in pressure during the first two days and then reverted the pressure toward control levels by the fourth day. (From Muirhead et al.[11]) The middle panel displays protection against malignant hypertension (MH) of the rabbit. ●——●, MH alone; ●- - - -●, MH plus renocortical transplants; ○——○, MH plus renomedullary transplants. (From Muirhead et al.[10]) The Panel on the extreme right shows that when Tr Med, which protect against MH, were removed (arrow 2), the arterial pressure elevated sharply, and the animals died in MH. (From Muirhead et al.[10])

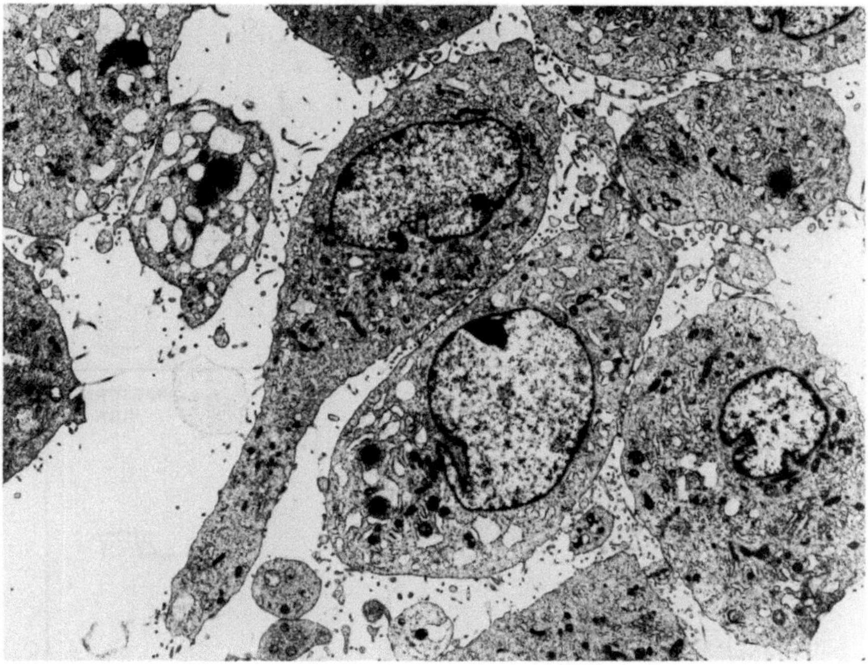

FIGURE 3. The appearance of RIC as grown in monolayer tissue culture (EM photograph, ×2400). The main features of RIC in situ within the kidney are retained, including osmiophilic granules, cisternae, and elongated cytoplasmic processes. (From Muirhead et al.[20])

transplants, incapable of forming urine, exert an antihypertensive action against extremely Na-loaded renoprival hypertension and malignant hypertension. Similar transplants of renal cortex do not exert this effect. Tr Med, in time, consist mostly of RIC and capillaries. The RIC appear to be the elements of the renal medulla exerting this action.

Monolayer Tissue Culture of RIC (TCric)

Monolayer tissue cultures of RIC were derived from Tr Med[16,17] (Figure 3). The derivation of such culture has been confirmed in at least three other laboratories[18,19] (F. Russo-Marie, personal communication).

Nonexcretory Antihypertensive Action of Transplants of Cultured RIC (Tr TCric)

The cultured RIC (TCric) were injected subcutaneously as transplants (20×10^6 to 50×10^6 cells) into hypertensive animals,[21,22] including 1KGH,

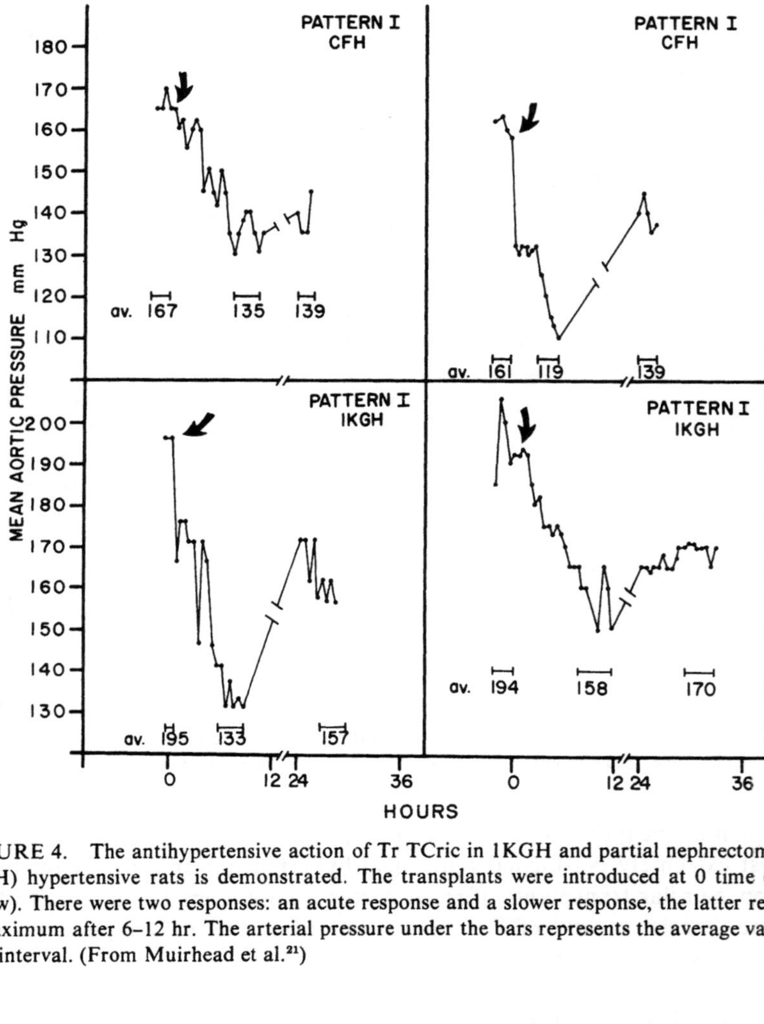

FIGURE 4. The antihypertensive action of Tr TCric in 1KGH and partial nephrectomy–salt (CFH) hypertensive rats is demonstrated. The transplants were introduced at 0 time (at the arrow). There were two responses: an acute response and a slower response, the latter reaching a maximum after 6–12 hr. The arterial pressure under the bars represents the average value for that interval. (From Muirhead et al.[21])

2KGH, partial nephrectomy–salt, and angiotensin–salt types. The Tr TCric exerted a powerful antihypertensive action, on occasions within 6–12 hr (Figures 4 and 5). In time, these transplants consisted mostly of RIC and capillaries and had the appearance of an endocrine organ. The antihypertensive action of cultured RIC occurs in the absence of natriuresis–diuresis. This experiment has been confirmed in at least one other laboratory (D. W. DuCharme, personal communication).

The implications of these observations are self-evident. The RIC most likely exert their antihypertensive action by secreting a substance(s) that cir-

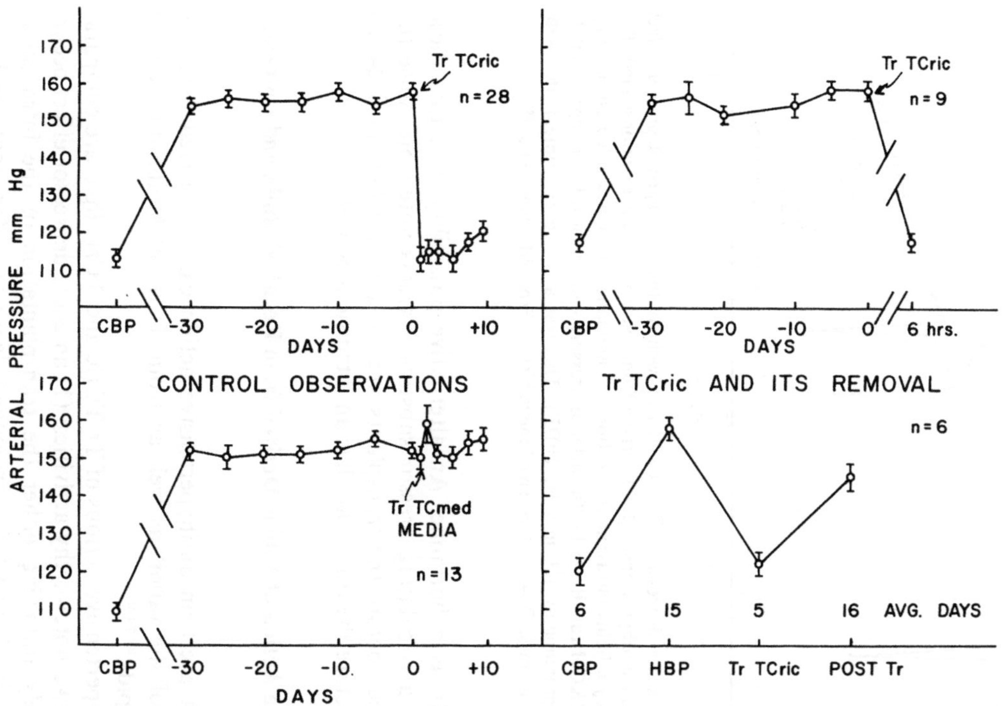

FIGURE 5. A summary of the effect of Tr TCric in angiotensin–salt hypertension. Upper left panel shows lowering of the arterial pressure by the transplant within 24 hr and maintenance of this effect for an additional 10 days. Upper right panel shows the antihypertensive effect within six hr. Left lower panel depicts controls receiving a tissue culture transplant not containing RIC; there was no change in arterial pressure. The right lower panel shows return of the arterial pressure toward the original hypertensive state after removal of the Tr TCric. (From Muirhead et al.[23])

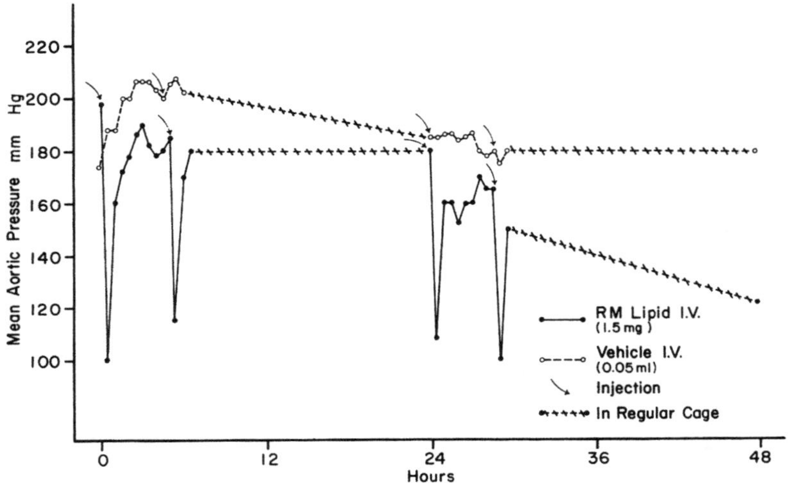

FIGURE 6. The acute depressor effect (ADE) as well as the prolonged depressor effect (PDE) induced by the antihypertensive lipid derived from renal medulla are demonstrated. The ADE was induced by a bolus intravenous injection and amounted to an acute depression of up to 100 mm Hg in 1KGH rat. By 48 hr, the arterial pressure had changed from approximately 180 mm Hg to approximately 120 mm Hg (PDE). This was a paired experiment: ●——●, received the lipid at arrows, O----O, received the vehicle). (From Muirhead et al.[26])

culates and acts as a hormone. An alternative possibility, i.e., that these cells neutralize a circulating pressor substance, seems untenable, since the action may occur before the transplants are vascularized (within 6–24 hr) and therefore before the transplant has an intrinsic blood flow.

Antihypertensive Action of Lipids Derived from Renal Medulla and Cultured RIC

Lipids that exert an antihypertensive action can be derived from the renal medulla of the rabbit as well as from TCric of lapine and murine origin (TCric lipid).[22,24,25]

The antihypertensive actions of Tr TCric and TCric lipid are comparable. There are two noteworthy activities: (1) an acute depressor effect occurring immediately following either the transplantation or the intravenous injection of the lipid, and (2) a prolonged depressor effect that reaches a maximum within 6–12 hr and may last up to 24 or more hr (Figures 6 and 7). The observation that the cultured cells and the lipid extracted from the same cells exert similar antihypertensive actions suggests, but does not prove, that the lipid may be the mediator of the cell function. At any rate, it is considered proper to proceed with this hypothesis as the primary one.

The antihypertensive lipids derived from the renal medulla and from TCric do not appear to belong to the known prostaglandins that are extracted from the kidney, and especially the renal medulla. Thus, there is the distinct possibility that a new class of antihypertensive lipids may be forthcoming.

A Possible Relationship between the Antihypertensive RIC System and the Prohypertensive Renin–Angiotensin System

We have standardized malignant one-kidney, one-clip hypertension of the rabbit by the application of a rigid narrow clip to the left renal artery and removal of the right kidney.[10] Under these conditions, the mean arterial pressure describes a reproducible time course. A lethal termination

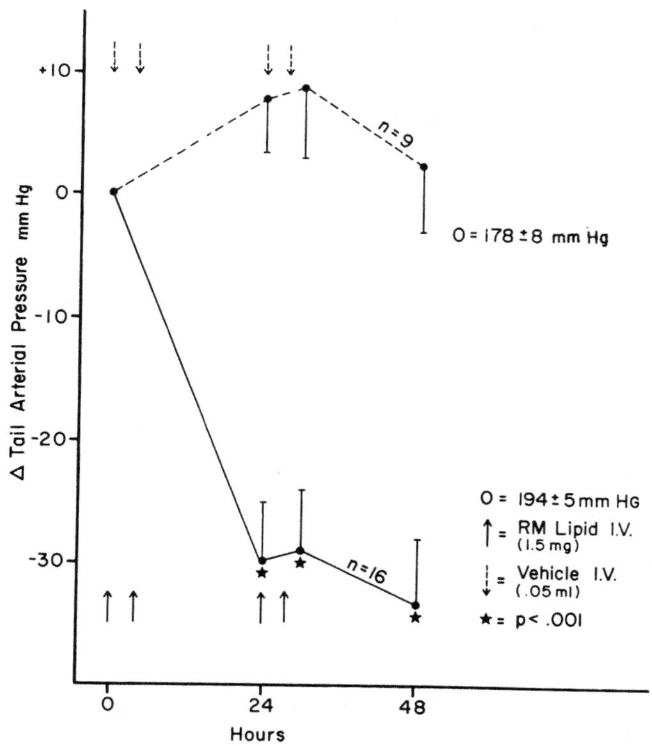

FIGURE 7. The antihypertensive action of the renomedullary lipid as determined in 1KGH rats by the tail pressure method is shown. The arrows indicate four doses of either the lipid (●——●) or the vehicle (●----●). The acute depressor effect has been deleted. The arterial pressure was significantly depressed at 24, 30, and 48 hr following the first injection. (From Muirhead et al.[26])

invariably occurs within 3 weeks. The mean arterial pressure changes from 60–70 mm Hg to 80–105 mm Hg within 24–36 hr and then lingers at the latter levels for 10–14 days. During the third week, the arterial pressure rises sharply to lethal levels (130–150 mm Hg). The animals die after between 16 and 22 days and display three additional features of malignant hypertension (MH): hypertensive encephalopathy, renal insufficiency (uremia), and diffuse fibrinoid necrosis of small arteries and arterioles of the viscera.

Two separate manipulations were superimposed on the narrow clip–nephrectomy procedure: (1) autotransplantation of the renal medulla from the removed right kidney,[10] and (2) multiple daily im injections of the converting enzyme inhibitor teprotide, SQ 20,881 (1 mg/kg every 6–8 hr).[27] As shown in Figure 8, both manipulations prevented the malignant phase of the hypertensive state and in a similar manner. The early rise of the arterial pressure was not prevented, but the lethal rise of the third week was prevented. None of the animals receiving either the Tr Med or the SQ 20,881 died (all controls died). Moreover, following either removal of the Tr

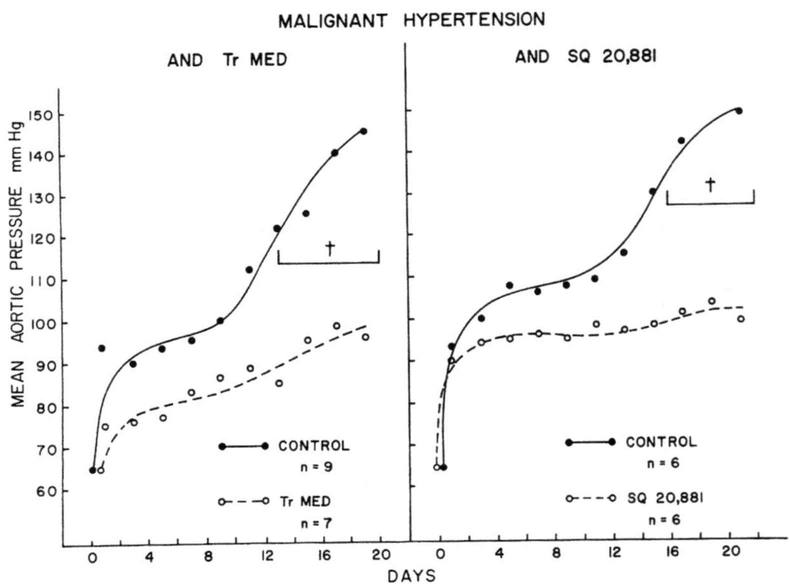

FIGURE 8. A comparison of the action of Tr Med and the converting enzyme inhibitor SQ 20,881 in MH. ●——●, Sequence of arterial pressure change in the control rabbits subjected to the MH procedure. O----O, Protection against MH by Tr Med in the left panel and by SQ 20,881 in the right panel. The similarity in results is apparent. All control animals died by 16–22 days. All animals receiving either Tr Med or SQ 20,881 survived this interval. (Modified from Muirhead et al.[10] and Muirhead et al.[27])

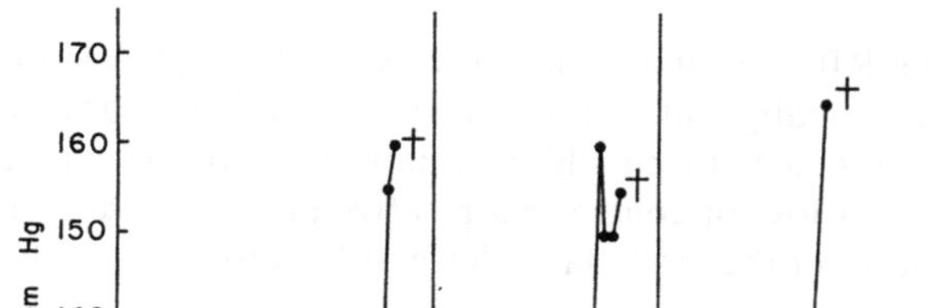

FIGURE 9. When SQ 20,881 was discontinued after it had protected against MH for 3 weeks (arrow), the arterial pressure elevated sharply, and the animals died of MH. The sequence is similar to that following removal of Tr Med that had protected against the same hypertensive state (see Figure 1). (From Muirhead et al.[27])

Med or cessation of treatment with SQ 20,881, the arterial pressure rose sharply, and the animals died with MH (Figures 2 and 9). It is to be recalled that SQ 20,881, by inhibiting kininase II (converting enzyme), inhibits the renin–angiotensin system and potentiates the kinin system.

The similarities between the curves following Tr Med and SQ 20,881 of Figure 7, indicating a protection against MH, could be fortuitous. Other possibilities, however, could pertain including the existence of a relationship between the antihypertensive RIC system and the prohypertensive renin–angiotensin system. Two hypotheses appear worthy of further consideration: (1) that the proposed antihypertensive renomedullary hormone of the RIC in some fashion antagonizes the pressor effects of angiotensin, and (2) that the renin–angiotensin (RA) system suppresses the action of the RIC antihypertensive system. Thus, in MH the RA system could suppress the function of RIC within the clipped kidney, a feature that is, at least temporarily, overcome by the extrarenal transplant of renal medulla.

Conversely, the RIC hormone could interfere with the RA system during its build-up in the malignant phase. These hypotheses are not mutually antagonistic. Thus, if both possibilities pertain, then a vicious prohypertensive build-up from loss of control via positive and negative factors could be an integral feature of the malignant phase of hypertension.

Summary

A nonexcretory antihypertensive function of the kidney has been supported by a variety of manipulations of the kidney. The antihypertensive action of transplants of fragmented renal medulla (Tr Med) and of transplants of cultured renomedullary interstitial cells (Tr TCric) suggests that this function is exerted, at least in a major way, by the renal medulla and its interstitial cells (RIC). The antihypertensive action of Tr TCric appears to have two components: a rapid one (not always detected) and a slow one (reaching a maximum between 6–12 hr and 3–6 days). Lipid extracts of TCric and renal medulla also exert an antihypertensive action.[22] At least two antihypertensive lipids can be derived from renal medulla,[28] one is polar (antihypertensive polar renomedullary lipid or APRL), and the other is neutral (antihypertensive neutral renomedullary lipid or ANRL). APRL exerts both a rapid and a slow action in lowering the arterial pressure of hypertensive recipients. ANRL exerts mainly the slow component. APRL is semisynthetic while ANRL is a natural product. The actions of these lipids are similar to those of Tr Med and Tr TCric. These lipids are not classic prostaglandins.

The antihypertensive action of Tr Med (mainly RIC) and Tr TCric (entirely RIC) most likely results from the secretion of a hormone by the cells of the transplants. The extracted antihypertensive lipid is the most eligible candidate for this hormonal action.

The antihypertensive action of the RIC and its putative hormone could, in part, oppose the prohypertensive action of the RA system and Na–volume loads. There remains also the possibility that the RA system suppresses the action of the RIC system. With the tools now available (TCric, TCric lipid, and the refined renomedullary antihypertensive lipid), these hypotheses can be subjected to critical evaluation.

References

1. Braun-Menendez E: The prohypertensive and antihypertensive actions of the kidney. *Ann Intern Med* 49:717–731, 1958.
2. Grollman A, Muirhead EE, Vanatta J: Role of the kidney in the pathogenesis of hypertension as determined by a study of the effects of bilateral nephrectomy and other

experimental procedures on the blood pressure of the dog. *Am J Physiol.* 157:21–30, 1949.

3. Floyer MA: Further studies on the mechanism of experimental hypertension in the rat. *Clin Sci* 14:163–181, 1955.
4. Kolff WJ, Page IH, Corcoran AC: Pathogenesis of renoprival cardiovascular disease in dogs. *Am J Physiol* 178:237–245, 1954.
5. Muirhead EE, Jones F, Stirman JA: Hypertensive cardiovascular disease of dog, relation of sodium and dietary protein to ureterocaval anastomosis and ureteral ligation. *Arch Pathol* 70:108–116, 1960.
6. Muirhead EE, Brooks B, Brosius WL: The antihypertensive non-excretory renal control of sodium volume loading. *Clin Res* 32:630A, 1974.
7. Muirhead EE, Stirman JA, Jones F: Renal autoexplantation and protection against renoprival hypertensive cardiovascular disease and hemolysis. *J Clin Invest* 39:266–281, 1960.
8. Muirhead EE, Brown GB, Germain GS, Leach BE: The renal medulla as an antihypertensive organ. *J Lab Clin Med* 76:641–651, 1970.
9. Tobian L Jr, Azar S: Antihypertensive and other functions of the renal papilla. *Trans Assoc Am Physicians* 84:281–288, 1972.
10. Muirhead EE, Brooks B, Pitcock JA, Stephenson P: Renomedullary antihypertensive function in accelerated (malignant) hypertension. Observations on renomedullary interstitial cells. *J Clin Invest* 51:181–190, 1972.
11. Muirhead EE, Brooks B, Pitcock JA, Stephenson P, Brosius WL: The role of the renal medulla in the sodium-sensitive component of renoprival hypertension. *Lab Invest* 27:192–198, 1972.
12. Manthorpe T: The effect on renal hypertension of subcutaneous isotransplantation of renal medulla from normal or hypertensive rats. *Acta Pathol Microbiol Scand* [*A*] 81:725–733, 1973.
13. Susic D, Sparks JC, Machado EA: Salt-induced hypertension in rats with hereditary hydronephrosis: The effect of renomedullary transplantation. *J Lab Clin Med* 87: 232–239, 1976.
14. Solez K, D'Agostini RJ, Buono RA, Vernon H, Wang AL, Finer PM, Heptinstall RH: The renal medulla and mechanisms of hypertension in the spontaneously hypertensive rat (SHR). *Am J Pathol* 85:555–567, 1976.
15. Manger WM, Van Praag D, Weiss RJ, Hart CJ, Hulse M, Rock TW, Farber SJ: Effect of transplanting renomedullary tissue into spontaneously hypertensive rats (SHR). *Fed Proc* 35(3):556, 1976.
16. Muirhead EE, Germain GS, Leach BE, Pitcock JA, Stephenson P, Brooks B, Brosius WL, Daniels EG, Hinman JW: Production of renomedullary prostaglandins by renomedullary interstitial cells grown in tissue culture. *Circ Res* 31 (*suppl* II):161–172, 1972.
17. Murihead EE, Germain GS, Leach BE, Brooks B, Stephenson P: Renomedullary interstitial cells (RIC), prostaglandins (PG) and the antihypertensive function of the kidney. *Prostaglandins* 3:581–594, 1973.
18. Zusman RM, Keiser HR: Prostaglandin biosynthesis by rabbit renomedullary interstitial cells in tissue culture. *J Clin Invest* 60:215–223, 1977.
19. Dunn MJ, Staley RS, Harrison M: Characterization of prostaglandin production in tissue culture of rat renal medullary cells. *Prostaglandins* 12:37–49, 1976.
20. Muirhead, EE, Germain, GS, Pitcock, JA, Brooks, B, Leach, BE: The renal medulla and the hypertensive state, in Fregly J, Fregly MS (eds): *Oral Contraceptives and High Blood Pressure.* Gainesville, Florida, Dolphin Press, pp. 301–314.
21. Muirhead EE, Germain GS, Armstrong FB, Brooks B, Leach BE, Byers LW, Pitcock

JA, Brown P: Endocrine-type antihypertensive function of the renomedullary interstitial cells. *Kidney Int* 8 (*Suppl* 5):122–133, 1975.
22. Muirhead EE, Rightsel WA, Leach BE, Byers LW, Pitcock JA, Brooks B: Reversal of hypertension by transplants and lipid extracts of cultured renomedullary interstitial cells. *Lab Invest* 36:162–172, 1977.
23. Muirhead, EE, Leach, BE, Pitcock, JA, Germain, GS, Byers, LW, Armstrong, FB, Brown, P: The antihypertensive action of renal medullary interstitial cells grown in tissue culture. *Acta Physiol Lat Am* 24:163–169, 1974.
24. Muirhead EE, Leach BE, Byers LW, Brooks B, Daniels EG, Hinman JW: Antihypertensive neutral renomedullary lipids (ANRL), in Fisher JW (ed): *Kidney Hormones*. London, Academic Press, 1970, p. 485.
25. Muirhead EE: The case for a renomedullary blood pressure lowering hormone, in Berlyne GM (ed): *Contributions to nephrology*. Basel, Karger, 1978, vol. 12, pp. 69–81.
26. Muirhead, EE, Rightsell, WA, Leach, BE, Byers, LW, Pitcock, JA, Brooks, B: The renal medullary antihypertensive function and its candidate antihypertensive hormone. *Ann Acad Med Singapore* 5:36–44, 1976.
27. Muirhead EE, Brooks B, Arora KK: Prevention of malignant hypertension by the synthetic peptide SQ 20,881. *Lab Invest* 30:129–135, 1974.
28. Prewitt RL, Leach BE, Byers LW: Brooks B, Lands WE, Muirhead EE: Antihypertensive polar renomedullary lipid, a semisynthetic vasodilator. *Hypertension* 3:299–308, 1979.

Chapter 4

The Influence of Various Neurological Defects on the Release of Renin in Normal Man

W. S. Peart

Introduction

The factors that have been implicated in renin release are shown in Table 1; they may be divided into acute and chronic factors as illustrated by the difference between the rise of plasma renin activity on standing compared with the slower increase under the influence of sodium deprivation. In examining the situation in normal man, it is important to try to incorporate the findings from various other types of experimental studies, ranging from the isolated perfused kidney to the kidney perfused in situ with and without an intact tubular system. Much more is known about the acute situation in man and animals and, while this is sometimes difficult to interpret, the chronic situation with some exceptions is not very well understood. Again, in trying to understand the normal situation in man, it is necessary to draw on pathological changes and to see how they may reveal some of the important mechanisms in the normal physiological state.

It is customary, indeed time honored, to look at the diagram of the glomerulus with its afferent and efferent arterioles and the macula densa (Figure 1) and to pose the usual question as to whether renin release depends mainly upon a baroreceptor at the level of the afferent arteriole,[1] and whether this can be distinguished from the influence of changes in urinary composition at the macula densa.[2-4] The difficulty in normal man or in an animal with intact kidneys is, of course, that whatever change is produced in the renal artery pressure is very quickly reflected in changes of urinary composition, and while by various maneuvers it is possible to dissociate renal artery pressure from urinary composition, the results have

W. S. PEART, M.D., F.R.C.P., F.R.S. · Medical Unit, St. Mary's Hospital, London, W2 1NY, England.

TABLE 1. Mechanisms Regulating Renin Release

Increase	Cause or source	Block or inhibition
Quick		
Sympathetic stimulation	Lowered blood pressure	Propranolol
Autoregulatory vasodilatation	and/or blood volume	Unknown
Beta stimulation	Isoproterenol	Propranolol
	Norepinephrine	Alpha stimulation
		Methoxamine
		Norepinephrine
Vasodilators	Glucagon	Vasoconstrictors
	Prostaglandins	Angiotensin
		Vasopressin
Diuretics	Frusemide	Unknown
Calcium efflux from juxtaglomerular cell	EDTA	Lanthanum
		Ionophore-mediated calcium influx
Slow		
Sodium deprivation or loss	Diet	Sodium load
	Gut	
	Skin	
	Thiazide diuretic	
	Adrenalectomy	Adrenal
		Conn's tumor
		Mineralocorticoids
		Aldosterone

often been difficult to analyze. It was for this reason that Davis and his collaborators went on to study the nonfiltering kidney preparation,[5,6] which, of course, does not exclude a function for the macula densa, but does show that many of the stimuli which we know to influence renin release can operate in the absence of urinary change. I think that the evidence for marked macula densa involvement in renin release is still debatable despite the elegant experiments of Thurau and his colleagues.[2-4] My assessment is that the state of the afferent arteriole will provide most of the answers.

Circadian Rhythms

It has become apparent that study of interrelated hormones can profit from determination of hormone levels over the 24-hour cycle with sampling carried out at quite short intervals. In many ways this is a more physiological approach to problems of interrelationships. It is often possible to interfere with the rhythm for one hormone without doing so for others, and

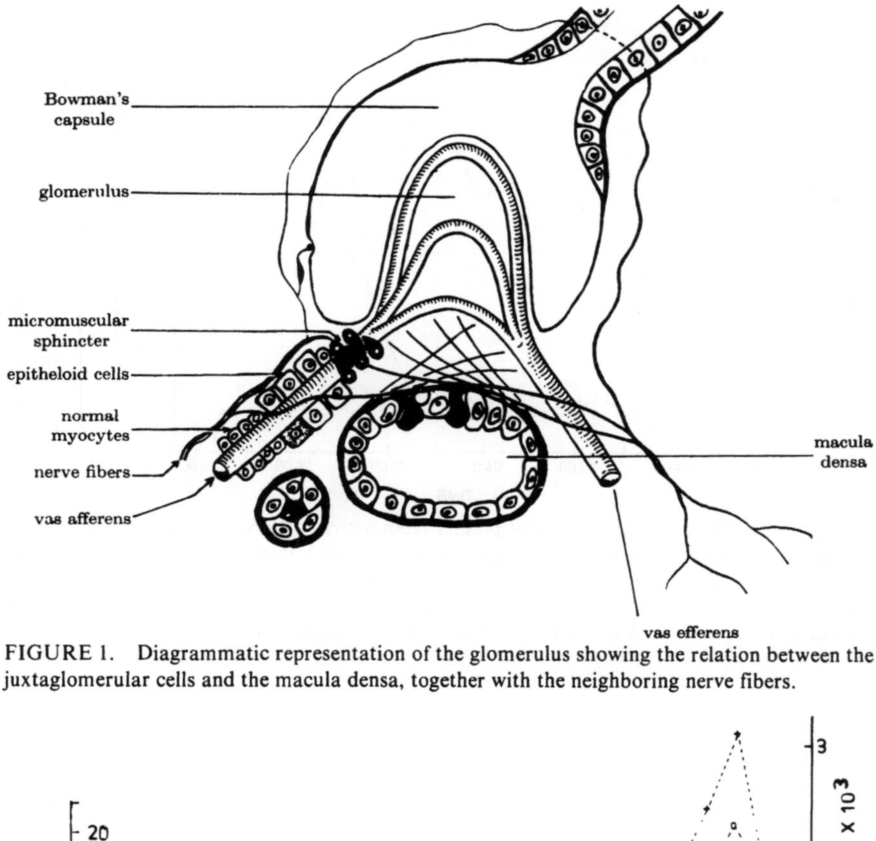

FIGURE 1. Diagrammatic representation of the glomerulus showing the relation between the juxtaglomerular cells and the macula densa, together with the neighboring nerve fibers.

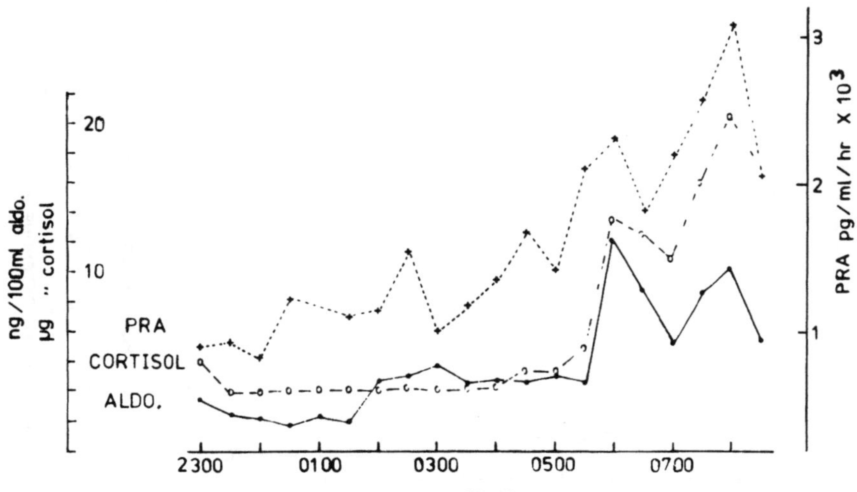

FIGURE 2. The circadian rhythm of plasma renin activity (PRA), cortisol, and aldosterone in a normal recumbent subject. There is a marked correlation of the peaks of the early morning rise in all values.

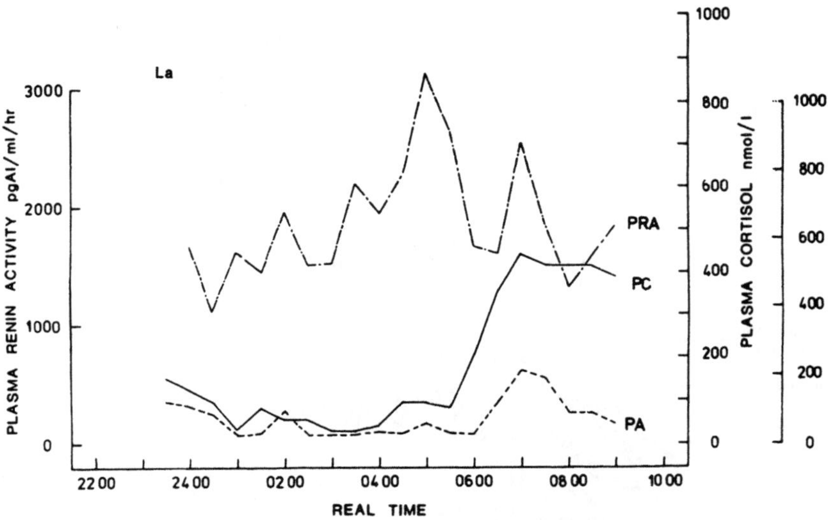

FIGURE 3. The circadian rhythm of plasma renin activity (PRA), cortisol and aldosterone in a normal recumbent subject. This subject, in contrast with that of Figure 2, shows a much higher level of renin activity with peaks which do not correlate very well with plasma aldosterone or cortisol. The early morning rise in cortisol is synchronous with that of aldosterone, as well as with a smaller peak of plasma renin activity. (Reprinted from James et al.[13])

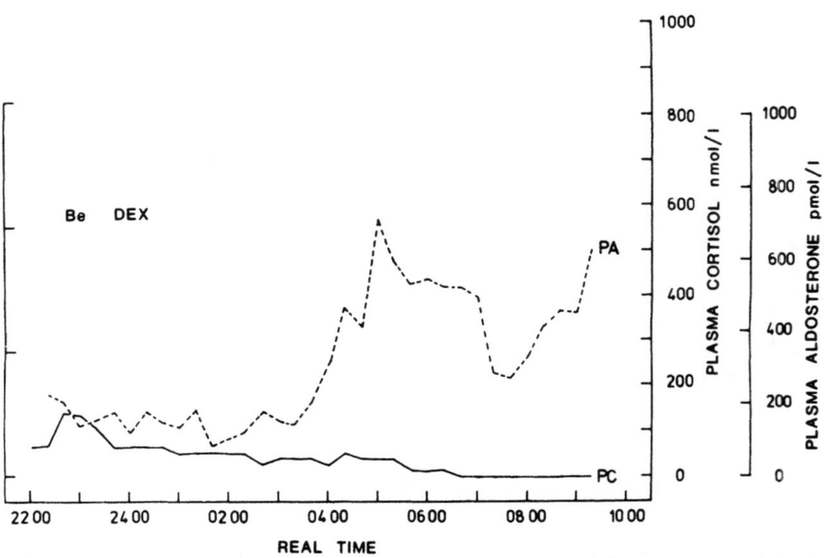

FIGURE 4. The circadian rhythm of cortisol and aldosterone in a normal recumbent subject. Dexamethasone (2 mg) was given orally at 2200. The cortisol rise in the early morning is suppressed, while that of aldosterone is unaffected. (Reprinted from James et al.[13])

this gives some clue as to common controlling mechanisms. This approach has been used in studying interrelationships among renin, aldosterone, and cortisol.[7-13] The conclusions are that in some normal subjects, asleep in the ordinary recumbent position for 12 hr overnight, there is a highly significant correlation among the changes in cortisol, aldosterone, and plasma renin activity (Figure 2). This suggests a common higher neural controlling factor. There are other individuals, however, in whom the correlation is not so clear-cut and, for example, renin and aldosterone are not necessarily closely correlated (Figure 3). There are a number of ways in which these correlations may be broken. It is easy to suppress ACTH and therefore plasma cortisol levels by use of dexamethasone (Figure 4). The cortisol rise in the early morning is abolished, while that for aldosterone persists. The same also was true of a further study where renin, aldosterone, and cortisol were studied simultaneously under dexamethasone suppression.[13] This implies that if there is a common controlling mechanism, it occurs before the release of ACTH and is not susceptible to dexamethasone.

Postural Change

On standing, plasma renin activity rises quickly.[14,15] In approaching the possible mechanisms, it was obvious to think that sympathetic activity in the renal nerves would be implicated[16,17]; in fact, it has been shown that propranolol, which experimentally is known to block the release of renin produced by stimulation of renal nerves,[18,19] will prevent this rise in plasma renin activity.[15] Advantage has therefore been taken of a group of unfortunate patients with complete transection of their cervical cord between C-3 and C-7 to study the responses of various hormones to changes of posture. Their hemodynamic changes have been the subject of much previous study,[20,21] which can be summarized by the statement that control of the circulation was grossly defective on tilting, so that the blood pressure falls to very low levels, often 50 to 60 mm Hg systolic, without loss of consciousness, and that as the tilt is continued, the blood pressure slowly rises but never to the starting pressure. The major sympathetic outflow from the cord is derived from fibers running down the cervical cord and leaving between T-1 and T-6 to reach the various viscera. Reduced sympathetic activity is strongly suggested by the low levels of plasma norepinephrine and epinephrine in the resting state.[22] This does not mean, however, that there are no other sympathetic invluences; the spinal reflexes which are still possible include venoconstriction in response to a deep breath or the application of cold to the trunk, and very marked rises of blood pressure from stimulation of the lower part of the trunk as by lower abdominal percussion leading to bladder contraction.[23-25] This is why the old observation on the severe hypertension occurring with a full bladder is of such great interest.[26] It is presumed that this is caused by a large sympathetic discharge and is a spinal sympathetic reflex. It has been shown that the plasma norepinephrine, but not epinephrine, rises with this stimulus,[27] and this is to be contrasted with the failure of either norepinephrine or epinephrine to rise on tilting in such patients.[28]

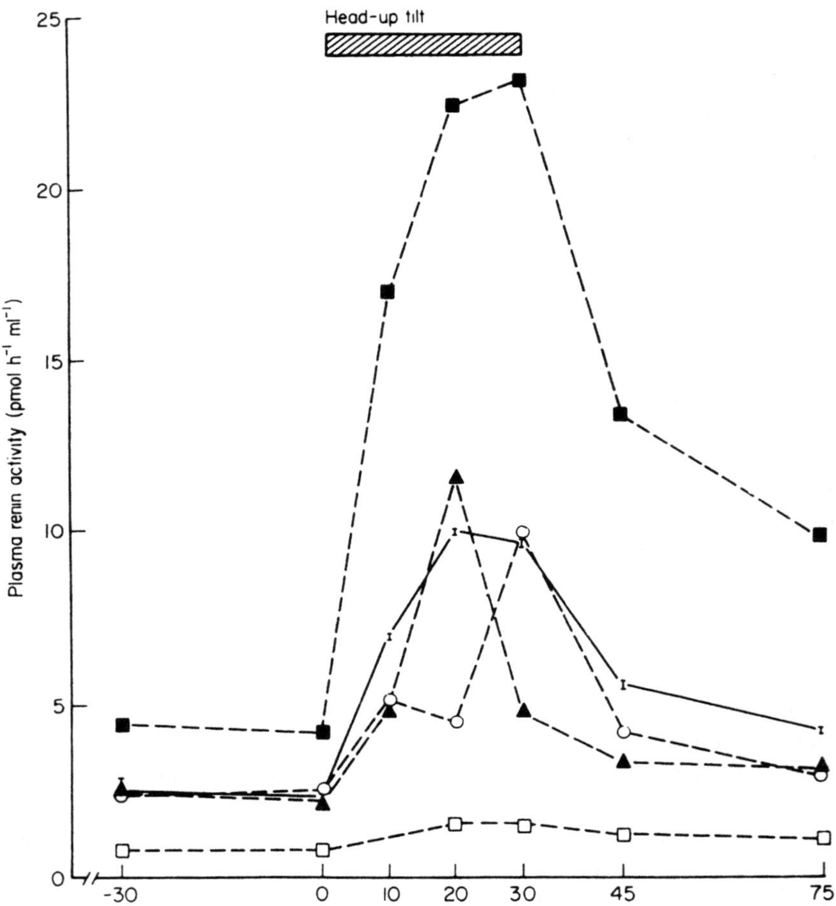

FIGURE 5. Plasma renin activity in 4 tetraplegic subjects (▲, ■, ○, □) 30 min before and 0, 10, 20, and 30 min after 45° head-up tilt, and 45 and 75 minutes after the start of head-up tilt when they had been horizontal again for 15 and 45 min. In calculating changes in plasma renin activity, the resting value is taken as the mean of the values 30 minutes (−30) before and immediately (0) before tilting. The unbroken line represents mean values for the four patients.

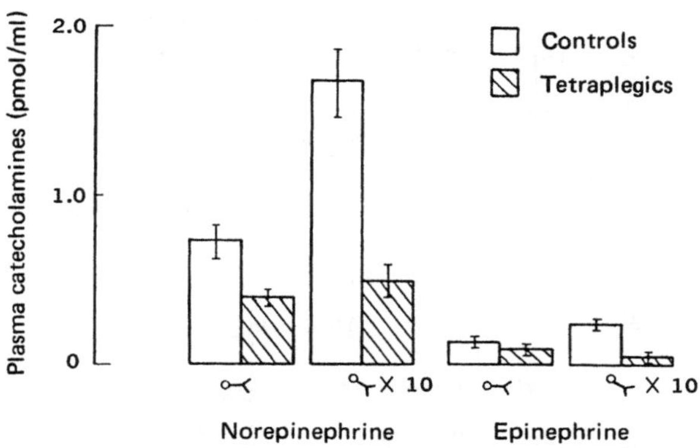

FIGURE 6. The changes in plasma norepinephrine and epinephrine on tilting in 10 normal subjects and 4 tetraplegics. The marked rise in the normals for both catecholamines is contrasted with the insignificant change in the tetraplegics.

Tilting

When patients with cervical cord transection were tilted, the plasma renin activity rose quickly from an already high resting level[28] (Figure 5). This resting level had previously been noted to be higher than normal in similar patients studied both here and elsewhere.[29,30] During this period of tilt only one of the five patients failed to show a fall in blood pressure. As a further measure of sympathetic activity, the plasma norepinephrine and epinephrine levels did not increase significantly in marked contrast to the changes observed in normal subjects (Figure 6). On the other hand, the plasma aldosterone level rose at about the same rate and with the same increase as the plasma renin activity. The effect of change of posture on plasma aldosterone level in normal subjects has previously been noted[31]; however, a rise of plasma level cannot be simply equated with an increased secretion rate, since the clearance of plasma aldosterone is largely through the liver, and tilting may well decrease splanchinc blood flow and thereby lead to decreased clearance. The conclusion from these studies could be either that renin release with tilting and lowering of blood pressure is independent of sympathetic innervation on the assumption that the kidney is truly denervated. or that there are some sympathetic fibers reaching the kidney from the cord that are reflexly excited on lowering pressure. It would perhaps be surprising if renin release were more marked than normal under these circumstances, but other factors influencing the amount of renin present in the kidney might have to be considered. Finally, an increase in hormones known to release renin from the kidney might be more important

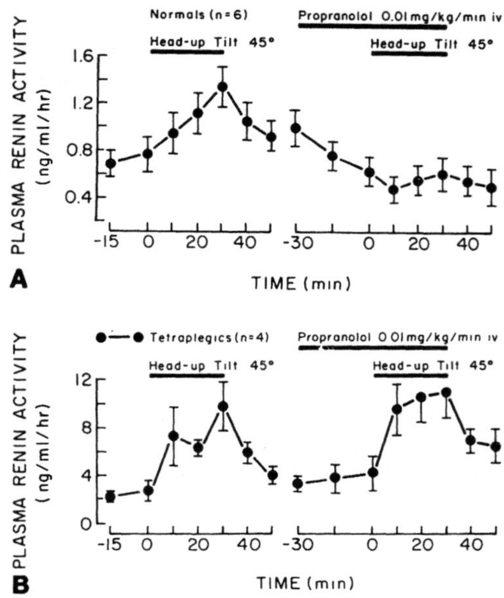

FIGURE 7. (A) The normal rise in plasma renin activity is abolished by propranolol. (B) The marked rise on tilting in tetraplegic subjects is not affected by propranolol Bars, SEM.

in the tetraplegic than in normal subjects. Obviously, norepinephrine and epinephrine would be the prime candidates, but it has already been shown that there is no significant change in their levels in tetraplegic subjects (Figure 6). Norepinephrine was given in doses sufficient to raise the blood pressure, and there was no significant rise in plasma renin activity in either the normal or tetraplegic subjects; thus, increased sensitivity to circulating norepinephrine is probably not the answer (C. J. Mathias, J. Dulieu, W. S. Peart, and R. D. G. Tunbridge, unpublished observations).

The problem called for another approach, and the effect of beta blockade with propranolol was investigated in tetraplegic and normal subjects. In the normals, the usual rise in renin on tilting was abolished by propranolol, whereas in the tetraplegics the rise was completely unchanged (Figure 7). It therefore seemed very unlikely that this rise in the tetraplegics is related to sympathetic discharge.

Bladder Percussion

It has already been mentioned that tetraplegic patients will raise their blood pressure very markedly under the influence of a full bladder or in response to percussion over the suprapubic region which causes contraction of the bladder.[26] This effect is almost certainly mediated by a spinal sympathetic discharge which is unmodified by the usual baroreceptor reflexes and is associated with a rise in the plasma norepinephrine.[27] In our tetraplegic subjects, when bladder percussion was carried out, the usual rise of presure occurred, but there was no rise in plasma renin, even after the blood pressure had returned to normal levels (C. J. Mathias, J. Dulieu, W. S. Peart, and R. D. G. Tunbridge, unpublished observations) (Figure 8). This again suggests that the kidney does not partake in this sympathetic discharge, or that if it does, then the marked rise of arterial pressure is capable of inhibiting renin release in some way.

The Shy–Drager Syndrome

The Shy-Drager Syndrome broadly encompasses the syndrome of postural hypotension where such conditions as diabetes and tabes dorsalis have been excluded.[32] The pathological basis of the condition seems to be

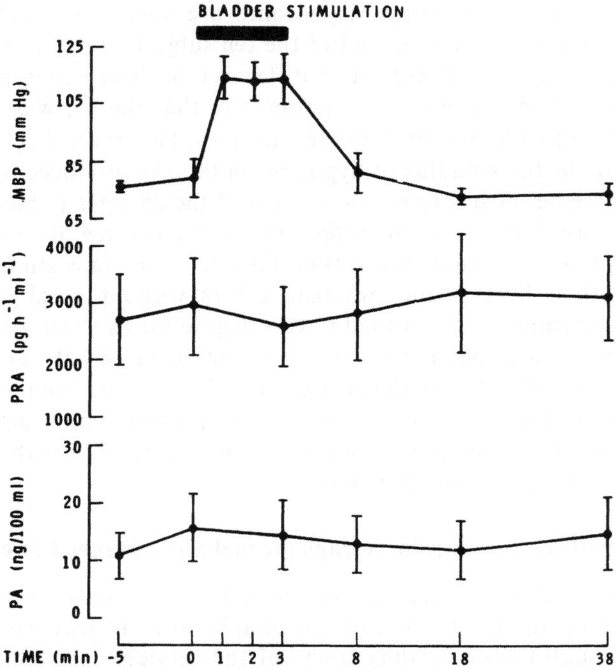

FIGURE 8. The effect of percussion over the bladder in four tetraplegic patients. There is a marked rise of blood pressure (MBP) with a failure of the plasma renin activity (PRA) and aldosterone (PA) to rise.

degeneration of the intermediolateral tracts in the cervical cord and similar degeneration further up the brain stem in the sympathetic pathways, particularly those associated with melanin producing cells.[33,34] There is probably also degeneration in the efferent pathways of the sympathetic nervous system and, in some cases, it has been suggested that the afferent pathways are also affected.[35,36] The main difficulty in analysis is the precise isolation of any one of these pathways, whether afferent, efferent, or central, by tests, some of which are much more specific than others.[35] With these reservations, study of such patients does provide data of interest in relation to the release of renin. Some recent studies provide the basis for the following analysis.[37]

Tilting

The blood pressure falls in the usual way, and concurrent measurements of plasma norepinephrine show that in most subjects there is very little change, and only in one out of ten subjects was there a significant increase despite the considerable fall in blood pressure produced. In these terms, patients with Shy–Drager syndrome are very like the tetraplegic patients. By contrast, only three out of the ten subjects failed to show a rise of plasma renin activity. There was a difference in these experiments from those carried out on the tetraplegic patients in that the tilt was only for 5 min as compared with 20 min in the tetraplegics. However, this is probably adequate time for the stimulus of hypotension to have produced its effect. It would of course be most interesting to know if the changes in blood flow to the kidneys were different in the different individuals since, if some of these subjects still preserved renal innervation, they could perhaps stimulate renin release over this short period, whereas others without renal innervation could not. In normal subjects tiltled to this degree for as short a period as 5 min, the rise of norepinephrine and of plasma renin activity are not very great. It may be that the patients with Shy–Drager syndrome who show very little response to tilting in terms of plasma renin activity and norepinephrine are behaving in a normal fashion compared with those who show a larger rise in plasma renin activity.

Interpretation of the Findings in Tetraplegic and Shy–Drager Patients

In the case of the tetraplegic patients, it seems most likely that the kidneys share in the denervation of the peripheral resistance vessels whose control is through the descending tracts of the cervical cord which emerge between T-1 and T-6. It seems unlikely that the kidney is involved very much in the spinal reflex system, as shown by the failure of plasma renin to

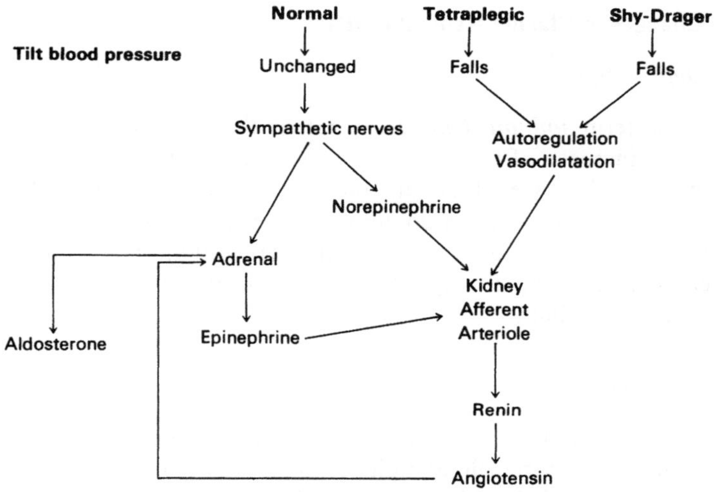

FIGURE 9. Diagrammatic representation of the events which occur on tilting normal, tetraplegic, and "Shy–Drager" subjects. In the normals the sympathetic nerves provided the main stimulus with an unchanged blood pressure, whereas in the other two groups autoregulatory vasodilatation occurs within the kidney as the pressure falls.

rise following bladder percussion. I think the most reasonable way of looking at the situation is to suggest that under normal circumstances the acute response controlling renin release is through the renal nerves. If this is overridden, or in the absence of proper sympathetic innervation as in the tetraplegics and in many patients with the Shy–Drager syndrome, autoregulatory adjustment is the major factor, and renin is released when afferent vasodilatation occurs within the kidney (Figure 9). This model is in general accord with the experimental observations that vasodilators, whether they be beta stimulators such as isoproterenol or hormones such as glucagon, will liberate renin,[38-40] and that vasoconstrictors such as methoxamine inhibit renin release.[41] Some excellent experiments on the dog carried out by Eide, Løyning, and Kiil[42] strongly support this view. They showed that renin release reached a maximum during the period of reduction of renal artery pressure where renal blood flow was maintained unchanged by autoregulatory vasodilatation and did not increase thereafter when autoregulation failed to prevent reduction in renal blood flow. If this emphasis on renin release triggered by local hemodynamic changes and on the action of the sympathetic nerves seems to neglect the macula densa and the influence of urinary composition, it is purely because of the difference in the quantity of evidence available.[6]

Chronic Changes in Plasma Renin Activity

Sodium Deprivation

I use the term *sodium deprivation* rather than *sodium depletion* since the signal for increase of plasma renin activity in man is usually perceived when a negative balance of about 100 to 150 mEq of sodium has been reached.[43,44] This is of course a common daily urinary loss of sodium in an adult. The source of the signal and its nature are still unknown, but I would like to emphasize its sensitivity. It is not associated with any significant change in plasma sodium.

Volume Changes

It has been thought that body fluid space changes, particularly of plasma volume and extracellular fluid volume, may play a part in stimulating renin production[45-48] and that this might explain some of the effects of chronic diuretic treatment.[49] In the case of diuretics of the thiazide group, such a correlation is unlikely to be true, since plasma renin activity may be chronically elevated after months of treatment, at which time plasma and extracellular fluid volume have returned to the starting value.[50] Certainly, the stimulating effect of a thiazide can overcome the suppression of a beta blocker, so its action is not through beta receptors or associated common factors.[51,52] However, propranolol will reduce the elevated plasma renin activity caused by a low sodium diet,[15] but this only proves that the sympathetic system is active and not necessarily overactive.

The pathological situation which sheds most light on inhibition of renin release in normal circumstances, hyperaldosteronism, is of great interest. At one time it was suggested that the increased plasma volume sometimes observed in hyperaldosteronism might initiate the changes leading to inhibition of renin.[53] However, volume increase is a very variable occurrence in such patients, yet the inhibition of renin activity is almost universal. The suppression is much more likely to result from some change in the membrane or metabolism of the juxtaglomerular cell produced by aldosterone. It can readily be reversed by spironolactone, and the difficulty of trying to interpret possible actions is shown in Figure 10 where administration of the drug to a patient with a Conn's tumor produced rapid change in the plasma potassium and sodium, a drop of blood pressure, a contraction of exchangeable sodium, and an increase of exchangeable potassium, all of which were associated with a slow rise of plasma renin activity.[54] In the ordinary experimental situation, there is no doubt that volume reduction has to be quite severe before plasma renin activity increases,[53] and the most likely explanation seems to be that the volume reduction, as by bleeding, has to be such as to lead to autoregulation in the kidney with or without activity of the sympathetic nerves.

Angiotensin

Since it has been shown that angiotensin is one of the most powerful inhibitors of renin release,[56-58] the renin–angiotensin system could be

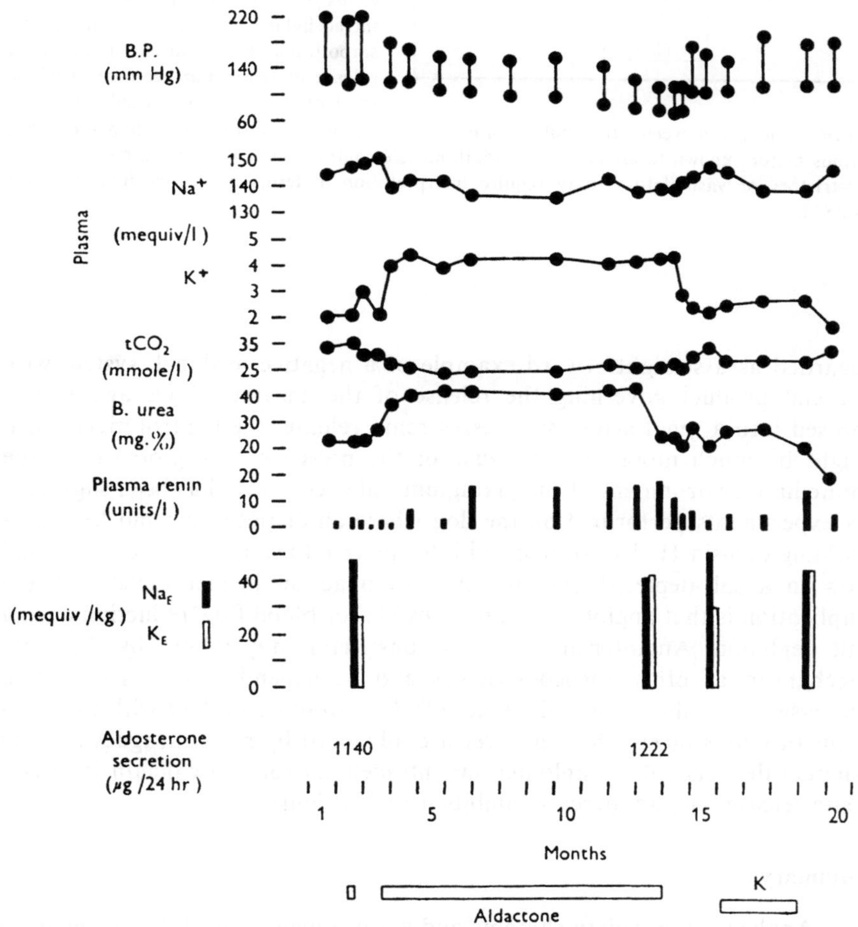

FIGURE 10. The changes produced by spironolactone, 300 mg daily, in a patient with Conn's syndrome who was subsequently cured by surgical removal of the tumor. The plasma renin activity is back within the normal range (10–20 units/liter) after 2 months, but there was a preceding rise in plasma potassium and blood urea and a fall in plasma sodium and bicarbonate levels. (Reprinted from Brown et al., 1965.[54])

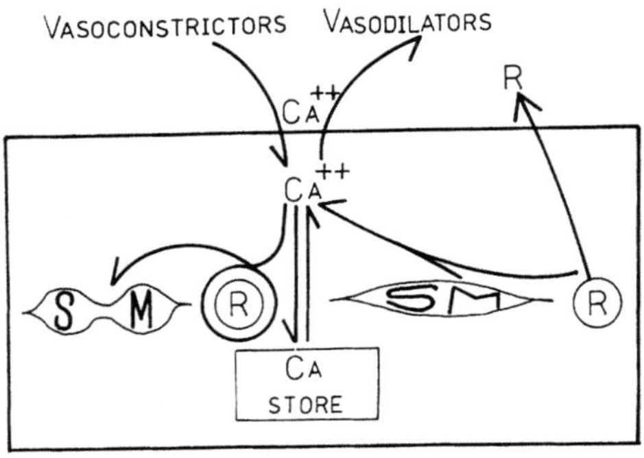

FIGURE 11. A diagrammatic representation of the calcium flux hypothesis relating renin release (R) and arteriolar smooth muscle contraction (SM). On the left, influx of calcium leading to increased intracellular ionized calcium (Ca^{2+}) causes, on the one hand, smooth muscle contraction, and on the other, inhibition of renin release. On the right, efflux of calcium leading to reduction of intracellular ionized calcium causes smooth muscle relaxation and increased release of renin. Further control of the level of intracellular ionized calcium is shown by the flux between intracellular storage sites (Ca store). According to this hypothesis, the various factors known to affect either smooth muscle contraction or renin release—e.g., vasoconstrictors or vasodilators—may require interpretation in terms of net calcium flux (see Table 1).

regarded as a straightforward example of a negative feedback system with the end product governing the release of the enzyme. Since angiotensin infused into a renal artery suppresses renin release, the control mechanism might be much more local because of the presence of angiotensin in the immediate environment of the juxtaglomerular cell. This has been suggested by experiments performed on the dog where an angiotension blocker, sar^1-ala^8-angiotensin II (P113), injected into the renal artery increases the blood flow in a salt-depleted animal but has no action in salt repletion[59]; the implication is that angiotensin is responsible for blood flow reduction during salt depletion. Angiotensin as a vasoconstrictor may inhibit by the same mechanism as other vasoconstrictors and be dependent on its ability to increase intracellular ionized calcium.[60] This would correlate with the "calcium flux hypothesis" for renin release advanced by my colleagues and me wherein decrease of juxtaglomerular intracellular ionized calcium increases renin release, and an increase inhibits it[41,61,62] (Figure 11).

Summary

Analysis of circadian rhythms and various neurological deficits helps to clarify the role of the nervous system in renin release: in the short term sympathetic stimulation and autoregulatory vasodilatation account for most of the release seen. Greater emphasis is accorded to the state of the afferent arteriole than to the macula densa. The longer term control with respect to dietary intake, particularly of sodium, and volume changes produced in a variety of ways, is much more complicated to analyze, as is seen in the case of primary hyperaldosteronism. The nature of the signal and its route to the kidney, either directly or indirectly, can only be a matter of speculation at the present time.

References

1. Tobian L: Interrelationship of electrolytes, juxtaglomerular cells and hypertension. *Physiol Rev* 40:280–312, 1960.
2. Thurau K, Schnermann J: Die Natriumkonzentration an den Macula densa-Zellen als regulierender Faktor für das Glomerulumfiltrat. *Klin Wochenschr* 43:410–413, 1965.
3. Thurau K, Dahlheim H. Grüner A, Mason J, Granger P: Activation of renin in the single juxtaglomerular apparatus by sodium chloride in the tubular fluid at the macula densa. *Circ Res* 30–31 (Suppl.II):182–186, 1972.
4. Schnermann J: Regulation of filtrate formation by feedback, in Giovanetti S, Bonomini V, D'Amico G (eds): *Proceedings of the Sixth International Congress on Nephrology*. Basel, Karger, 1976, pp 230–234.
5. Davis JO: The regulation of renin release, in Onesti G, Kim KE, Moyer JH (eds): *Hypertension: Mechanisms and Management*. New York, Grune & Stratton, 1973, pp 617–629.
6. Davis JO: The control of renin release. *Am J Med* 55:333–350, 1973.
7. Horton R: Stimulation and suppression of aldosterone in plasma of normal man and in primary aldosteronism. *J Clin Invest* 48:1230–1236, 1969.
8. Katz FH, Romfh P, Smith JA: Episodic secretion of aldosterone in supine man: Relationship to cortisol. *J Clin Endocrinol Metab* 35:178–181, 1972.
9. Vetter H, Berger M, Armbruster H, Siegenthaler W, Werning C, Vetter W: Episodic secretion of aldosterone in primary aldosteronism: Relationship to cortisol. *Clin Endocrinol* 3:41–48, 1974.
10. Katz FH, Romfh P, Smith JA: Diurnal variation of plasma aldosterone, cortisol and renin activity in supine man. *J Clin Endocrinol Metab* 40:125–134, 1975.
11. Weinberger MH, Kem DC, Gomez-Sanchez C, Kramer NJ, Martin BT, Nugent CA: The effect of dexamethasone on the control of plasma aldosterone concentration in normal recumbent man. *J Lab Clin Med* 85:957–967, 1975.
12. Armbruster H, Vetter W, Beckerhoff R, Nussberger J, Vetter H, Siegenthaler W: Dirunal variations of plasma aldosterone in supine man: Relationship to plasma renin activity and plasma cortisol. *Acta Endocrinol (Kbh)* 80:95–103, 1975.
13. James VHT, Tunbridge RDG, Wilson GA: Studies on the control of aldosterone secretion in man. *J Steroid Biochem* 7:941–948, 1976.
14. Gordon RD, Küchel O, Liddle GW, Island DP: Role of the sympathetic nervous system in regulating renin and aldosterone production in man. *J Clin Invest* 46:599–605, 1967.
15. Michelakis AM, McAllister RG: The effect of chronic adrenergic receptor blockage on plasma renin activity in man. *J Clin Endocrinol Metab* 34:386–394, 1972.
16. Vander AJ: Effect of catecholamines and the renal nerves on renin secretion in anesthetized dogs. *Am J Physiol* 209:659–661, 1965.
17. Ganong WF: Sympathetic effects on renin secretion. Mechanism and physiological role,

in Assaykeen TA (ed): *Control of Renin Secretion.* New York, Plenum Press, 1972, pp 17–32.
18. Johns EJ, Singer B: Specificity of blockage of renal renin release by propranolol in the cat. *Clin Sci Mol Med* 47:331–343, 1974.
19. Taher MS, McLain LG, McDonald KM, Schrier RW: Effect of beta adrenergic blockage on renin response to renal nerve stimulation. *J Clin Invest* 57:459–465, 1976.
20. Guttmann L, Munro AF, Robinson R, Walsh JJ: Effect of tilting on the cardiovascular responses and plasma catecholamine levels in spinal man. *Paraplegia* 1:4–18, 1963.
21. Corbett JL, Frankel HL, Harris PJ: Cardiovascular responses to tilting in tetraplegic man. *J Physiol* (*Lond*) 215:411–431, 1971.
22. Debarge O, Christensen NJ, Corbett JL, Eidelman BH, Frankel HL, Mathias CJ: Plasma catecholamines in tetraplegics. *Paraplegia* 12:44–49, 1974.
23. Corbett, JL, Frankel HL, Harris PJ: Cardiovascular changes associated with skeletal muscle spasm in tetraplegic man. *J Physiol* (*Lond*) 215:381–393, 1971.
24. Corbett JL, Frankel HL, Harris PJ: Cardiovascular reflex responses to cutaneous and visceral stimuli in spinal man. *J Physiol* (*Lond*) 215:395–409, 1971.
25. Corbett JL, Debarge O, Frankel HL, Mathias CJ: Cardiovascular responses in tetraplegic man to muscle spasm, bladder percussion and head-up tilt. *Clin Exp Pharmacol Physiol* suppl 2:189–193, 1975.
26. Guttmann, L Whitteridge D: Effects of bladder distension on autonomic mechanism after spinal cord injuries. *Brain* 70:361–404, 1947.
27. Mathias CJ, Christensen NJ, Corbett JL, Frankel HL, Spalding JMK: Plasma catecholamines during aproxysmal neurogenic hypertension in quadriplegic man. *Circ Res* 39:204–208, 1976.
28. Mathias CJ, Christensen NJ, Corbett JL, Frankel HL, Goodwin TJ, Peart WS: Plasma catecholamines, plasma renin activity and plasma aldosterone in tetraplegic man, horizontal and tilted. *Clin Sci Mol Med* 49:291–299, 1975.
29. Johnson RH, Park D, Frankel HL: Orthostatic hypotension and the renin-angiotensin system in paraplegia. *Paraplegia* 9:146–152, 1971.
30. Mendelsohn FA, Johnston CI: Renin release in chronic paraplegia. *Aust NZ J Med* 4:393–397, 1971.
31. Balikian HM, Brodie AH, Dale SL, Melby JC, Tait JF: Effect of posture on the metabolic clearance rate, plasma concentration and blood production rate of aldosterone in man. *J Clin Endocrinol Metab* 28:1630–1640, 1968.
32. Shy GM, Drager GA: A neurological syndrome associated with orthostatic hypotension. *Arch Neurol* 2:511–527, 1960.
33. Johnson RH, Lee G de J, Oppenheimer DR, Spalding JMK: Autonomic failure with orthostatic hypotension due to intermediolateral column degeneration. *Q J Med* 35:276–292, 1966.
34. Bannister R, Oppenheimer DR: Degenerative diseases of the nervous system associated with autonomic failure. *Brain* 95:457–474, 1972.
35. Bannister R, Ardill L, Fentem P: Defective autonomic control of blood vessels in idiopathic orthostatic hypotension. *Brain* 90:725–746, 1967
36. Bannister R: Degeneration of the autonomic nervous system. *Lancet* 2:175–179, 1971.
37. Bannister R, Sever PS, Gross M: Cardiovascular reflexes and biochemical responses in progressive autonomic failure. *Brain* 100:327–344, 1977.
38. Assaykeen TA, Clayton PL, Goldfien A, Ganong WF: Effect of alpha- and beta-adrenergic blocking agents on the renin response to hypoglycaemia and epinephrine in dogs. *Endocrinology* 87:1318–1322, 1970.

39. Ueda H, Yasuda H, Takabatake Y, Iizuka M, Iizuka T, Ihori M, Sakamoto Y: Observations on the mechanism of renin release by catecholamines. *Circ Res* 26 & 27(*suppl* II):195–200, 1970.
40. Vandongen R, Peart WS, Boyd GW: Adrenergic stimulation of renin secretion in the isolated perfused rat kidney. *Circ Res* 32:290–296, 1973.
41. Vandongen R, Peart WS: The inhibition of renin secretion by alpha-adrenergic stimulation of the isolated rat kidney. *Clni Sci Mol Med* 47:471–479, 1974.
42. Eide I, Løyning E, Kiil F: Evidence for hemodynamic autoregulation of renin release. *Circ Res* 32:237–245, 1973.
43. Brown JJ, Davies DL, Lever AF, Robertson JIS: Influence of sodium loading and sodium depletion on plasma-renin in man. *Lancet* 2:278–279, 1963.
44. Boyd GW, Adamson AR, Arnold M, James VHT, Peart WS: The role of angiotensin II in the control of aldosterone in man. *Clin Sci* 42:91–104, 1972.
45. Ledingham JM, Cohen RD: Changes in extracellular fluid volumes and cardiac output during the development of experimental renal hypertension. *Can Med Assoc J* 90:292–294, 1964.
46. Bianchi G, Tilde–Tenconi L, Lucca R: Effect in the conscious dog of constriction of the renal artery to a sole remaining kidney on haemodynamics, sodium balance, body fluid volumes, plasma renin concentration and pressor response to angiotensin. *Clin Sci* 38:741–766, 1970.
47. Liard J-F, Peters G: Role of the retention of water and sodium in two types of experimental renovascular hypertension in the rat. *Pflügers Arch* 344:93–108, 1973.
48. Liard J-F, Cowley AW Jr, McCaa RE, McCaa CS, Guyton AC: Renin, aldosterone, body fluid volumes, and the baroreceptor reflex in the development and reversal of Goldblatt hypertention in conscious dogs. *Circ Res* 34:549–560, 1974.
49. Vaughan ED Jr, Laragh JH, Gavras I, Bühler FR, Gavras H, Brunner HR, Baer, L: Volume factor in low and normal renin essential hypertension. Treatment with either spironolactone or chlorthalidone. *Am J Cardiol* 32:523–532, 1973.
50. Tarazi RC: Diuretic drugs: Mechanisms of antihypertensive action, in Onesti G, Kim KE, Moyer JH (eds): *Hypertension: Mechanisms and Management*. New York, Grune & Stratton, 1973, pp 251–260.
51. Bravo EL, Tarazi RC, Duston HP: β-adrenergic blockade in diuretic-treated patients with essential hypertension. *N Engl J Med* 292:66–70, 1975.
52. Lancaster R, Goodwin TJ, Peart WS: The effect of pindolol on plasma renin activity and blood pressure in hypertensive patients. *Br J Clin Pharmacol* 3:453–460, 1976.
53. Conn JW: An overall view of primary aldosteronism, Onesti G, Kim KE, Moyer JH (eds): Hypertension: Mechanisms and Management. New York, Grune & Stratton, 1973, pp 471–480.
54. Brown JJ, Davies DL, Lever AF, Peart WS, Robertson JIS: Plasma concentration of renin in a patient with Conn's syndrome with fibrinoid lesions of the renal arterioles: The effect of treatment with Spironolactone. *J Endocrinol* 33:279–293, 1965.
55. Brown JJ, Davies DL, Lever AF, Robertson JIS, Verniory A: The effect of acute haemorrhage in the dog and man on plasma-renin concentration. *J Physiol* (*Lond*) 182:649–663, 1966.
56. Vander AJ, Geelhoed GW: Inhibition of renin secretion by angiotensin II. *Proc Soc Exp Biol Med* 120–399–403, 1965.
57. Bunag RD, Page IH, McCubbin JW: Inhibition of renin release by vasopressin and angiotensin. *Cardiovasc Res* 1:67–73, 1967.

58. Vandongen R, Peart WS, Boyd GW: Effect of angiotensin II and its nonpressor derivatives on renin secretion. *Am J Physiol* 226:277:282, 1974.
59. Freeman RH, Davis JO, Vitale SJ, Johnson JA: Intrarenal role of angiotensin II. Homeostatic regulation of renal blood flow in the dog. *Circ Res* 32:692–698, 1973.
60. Vandongen R, Peart WS: Calcium dependence of the inhibitory effect of angiotensin on renin secretion in the isolated perfused kidney of the rat. *Br J Pharmacol* 50:125–129, 1974.
61. Peart WS, Quesada T, Tenyi I: The effects of EDTA and EGTA on renin secretion. *Br J Pharmacol* 59:247–252, 1977.
62. Fynn M, Onomakpome N, Peart WS: The effects of ionophores (A23187 and R02-2985) on renin secretion and renal vasoconstriction. *Proc R Soc Lond B* 199:199–212 (1977).

Chapter 5

Angiotensin as a Determinant of Renal Perfusion and Function

Norman K. Hollenberg

Introduction

Investigation of the renin–angiotensin system has focused primarily on control of blood pressure and hypertension on the one hand, and sodium homeostasis via angiotensin's control of aldosterone release on the other. A number of lines of evidence have accumulated over the last decade which point to a central role for angiotensin in the normal control of the renal circulation[19,49,90,96] and in the pathogenesis of a variety of diseases that involve the kidney. Indeed, a compelling argument can be made for assigning a primal function of renin and angiotensin II to control of renal circulation early during phylogeny, with the other influences of angiotensin on blood pressure and on the adrenal gland arising later.

Evidence from Phylogeny

Homer Smith[95] emphasized that the evolution of the kidney is essentially the response to a series of challenges involving salt and water regulation and the control of the tonicity and volume of the body fluids (Figure 1). Viewed from this perspective, the phylogeny of the renin–angiotensin–aldosterone system can provide insight into the roles of these substances in the body economy and in the control of renal function. Sokabe et al.[97] demonstrated in eurhyaline fish and eels that exposure to fresh water resulted in a striking increase in urine flow and glomerular filtration rate that was associated with an increase in the renin activity of the kidney; conversely, adaptation to the salinity of sea water was associated with a decrease in urine flow, glomerular filtration rate, and intrarenal renin activity. Malvin and Vander[74] were unable to demonstrate changes in

NORMAN K. HOLLENBERG, M.D., Ph.D. Department of Radiology, Harvard Medical School, and Renal Division, Peter Bent Brigham Hospital, Boston, Massachusetts 02115.

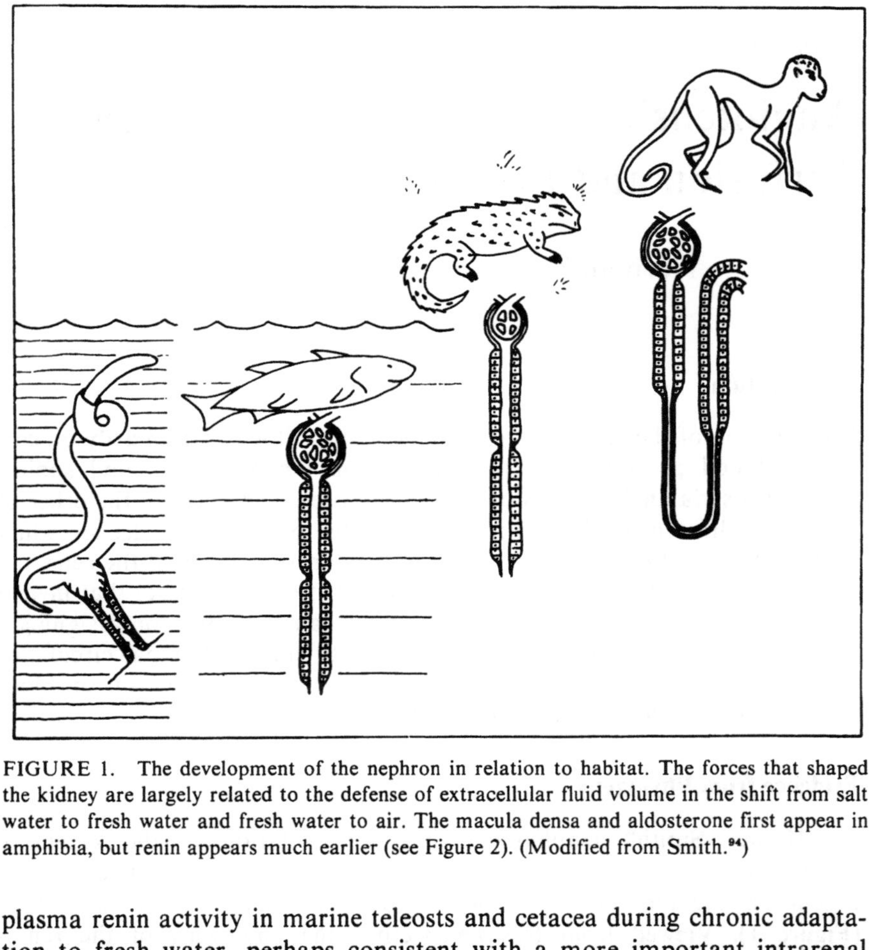

FIGURE 1. The development of the nephron in relation to habitat. The forces that shaped the kidney are largely related to the defense of extracellular fluid volume in the shift from salt water to fresh water and fresh water to air. The macula densa and aldosterone first appear in amphibia, but renin appears much earlier (see Figure 2). (Modified from Smith.[94])

plasma renin activity in marine teleosts and cetacea during chronic adaptation to fresh water, perhaps consistent with a more important intrarenal than systemic role of renin in these organisms.[22] Sokabe et al. concluded from their data that the renin–angiotensin system may regulate glomerular filtration rate in teleosts: they argue that renin secreted from the granular cells into the afferent artery formed angiotensin, which in turn constricted the efferent arteriole and thus increased glomerular filtration rate. The fine structure of the glomerulus is in accord with this possibility.[18]

Renin activity and juxtaglomerular granules were not found in the kidneys of the most primitively living vertebrates, the cyclostomes and elasmobranchs by Nishimura et al.[83] who did confirm their presence in teleosts and tetrapods. Sokabe[96] pointed out that the renin–angiotensin system probably first appeared in bony fishes (Figure 2). A macula densa has not been visualized in these fishes. Little is known concerning blood pressure control in these primitive organisms, but the lungfish as a representative example has an arterial pressure of about 15 mm Hg and at this level would appear to be effectively unregulated.[89] There is no evidence of a role played by renin or angiotensin in blood pressure control in these primitive species.

The amphibian, phylogenetically, represents the first vertebrate to venture from the protective environment of water to air, where defense of extracellular fluid volume took on a new challenge. Capelli et al.[26] pointed out that the appearance of the recurrent nephron and the macula densa in the amphibian may "represent the beginnings of a structural element within the nephron to aid electrolyte and volume homeostasis by sampling fluids reaching the distal segments of the nephron." Whereas there is little doubt that the renin–angiotensin system plays an important role in electrolyte homeostasis by way of control of mineralocorticoid secretion in the mammal, Bern[13] concluded that aldosterone may be "an invention of land-living vertebrates," appearing late in phylogeny. A possible interpretation of this overview is that the renin–angiotensin system initially evolved as a control mechanism for the kidney, especially the glomerular circulation, and that its role broadened with increasingly more ambitious ventures into new and more hostile environments.[96] In view of the remarkable amount of attention focused on the role of the renin–angiotensin system and the control of aldosterone secretion, it is surprising that so little attention has been paid to a probable primary role of angiotensin as a local renal hormone controlling glomerular perfusion and function.

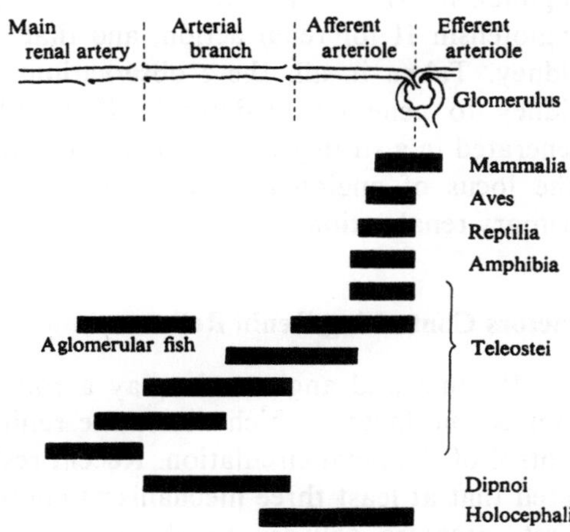

FIGURE 2. Distribution of juxtaglomerular (JG) cells in vertebrate kidneys. In general, where JG cells are demonstrable, renin has been demonstrated in the kidneys. Not shown are elasmobranchs and cyclostomes in which neither JG cells nor renin have been demonstrated. (From Sokabe,[96] by permission.)

Where Is Angiotensin II Generated?

The answer to this question can also provide insight into angiotensin's action. Renin is produced primarily in the renal cortex, arising in the uterus, placenta, salivary glands, brain, and some blood vessels.[93] Renal synthesis occurs in specialized cells in the juxtaglomerular apparatus which have intimate contact with the vascular pole of the glomerulus; thus, secretion occurs immediately adjacent to the afferent and efferent arterioles. Renin acts on an α-globulin that serves as substrate to split off an inactive precursor decapeptide, angiotensin I. A specific converting enzyme splits two amino acids off the decapeptide to form the active moiety, angiotensin II. Because the largest concentration of converting enzyme is found in the lung, it was believed until recently that conversion occurred only there.[82] On this basis the function of angiotension II was considered to be primarily systemic rather than intrarenal.

Three unrelated lines of evidence have evolved in the last 5 years which suggest, conversely, that there is a critical intrarenal focus for conversion and that angiotensin II is indeed a local renal vascular hormone. First, while the total amount of converting enzyme in the kidney is considerably smaller than that in the lung, the available converting-enzyme activity in the kidney is sharply localized to the juxtaglomerular apparatus, the area in which renin is released.[45,70] Second, lymph draining the kidney contains considerably higher concentrations of angiotensin II than are found in either arterial or renal venous blood; it must have been generated within the kidney.[6,7] Third, specific competitive antagonists to converting enzyme infused into the renal artery blocks the local action of angiotensin I but not angiotensin II.[32] Angiotensin I, therefore, must require conversion to angiotensin II for renal action, and that conversion must occur within the kidney. Taken in all, these observations demonstrate the capacity of the kidney to generate angiotensin II locally and the likelihood that it is generated in a strategic locus adjacent to the afferent and efferent arterioles. The locus of angiotensin generation supports phylogeny in suggesting a primary renal action.

Factors Controlling Renin Release

If renin and angiotensin play a role in the control of renal hemodynamics, the factors which determine renin release must be relevant to the control of the renal circulation. Recent reviews of the subject[29,103] have indicated that at least three mechanisms control renin release from the kidney. First, pressure delivery to the juxtaglomerular apparatus represents an important determinant of renin release. Second, sodium delivery to or transport within the macula densa region of the distal tubule represents a major contributing factor. Third, sympathetic activity operating upon β-receptors in the juxtaglomerular apparatus also promotes renin release. Conversely, the angiotensin concentration in the region of the juxtaglomerular apparatus blunts renin release, providing a homeostatic feedback control mechanism.

While there has been considerable debate concerning which factor has primacy, it is important to recognize that changes in pressure delivery to the region of the juxtaglomerular apparatus, sympathetic activity, and sodium reaching the distal tubule are not mutually exclusive phenomena, but rather might be expected to act in concert. When a volume deficit is perceived, all three factors are likely to play a role in promoting renin release. A parallel reduction in renal blood flow is a consequence as well as a cause of the activation of the renin–angiotensin system.

The states in which an abnormality of volume, either actual or perceived, results in renin release include trauma, shock, hemorrhage, congestive heart failure, hepatic cirrhosis, the hepatorenal syndrome, acute renal failure, and, in some patients, hypertension.[9,35,78,85,103] In all of these states some combination of decreased perfusion pressure, increased sympathetic nerve activity, and activation of the macula densa results in renin release and reduced renal blood flow and filtration.

On the one hand, maneuvers that modify intrarenal renin levels influence renal blood flow.[63] On the other, a number of observations of the autoregulatory response are not in accord with this hypothesis. Dilatation of the afferent arteriole which occurs with decreasing perfusion pressure is associated with renin release[64,102] and an increase in the interstitial concentration of angiotensin II.[6] Thus vasodilatation is associated with an increase in the local generation and concentration of angiotensin II. Moreover, a number of agents which interrupt the renin–angiotensin axis, such as antibody specific for angiotensin II,[33] converting enzyme inhibitors,[41] β-adrenergic blocking agents, and angiotensin antagonists,[2,27] do not influence the autoregulatory process. While it could be argued that these agents did not achieve effective concentrations at the angiotensin receptor, Eide et al.[33] demonstrated effective arteriolar concentrations of even the large and polar antibody molecules. Certainly the pharmacological agents, which are much smaller and very diffusable, must have reached arteriolar concentrations within the kidney. Perhaps when arterial pressure falls, as the major mechanisms promoting renin release, the direct autoregulatory dilator influence on the renal vasculature is dominant, overcoming the constrictor effects of angiotensin.

Sensitivity of Renal Vasculature to Angiotensin

Angiotensin II is among the most active endogenous vasoconstrictor agents identified to date, with an especially marked influence on the renal vasculature: a striking reduction in blood flow to the kidney occurs with doses that are well below those required to induce a pressor response[2,4,30,53,56,57,75,90] (see Figure 3).

The amount of angiotensin required to reduce renal blood flow can be astonishingly minute: as little as 0.1 ng/kg per min infused intravenously in normal subjects on a high sodium intake—a dose which is about 3% of that required to raise blood pressure—provides the threshold reduction in renal blood flow.[57] The consequent change in plasma angiotensin II concentration, in the range of 3–10 pg/ml, is well within the range of physiological fluctuation. Given the probability of local generation in high concentration within the kidney, as reviewed above, it would be astonishing if angiotensin did not exert an important influence on the renal vasculature.

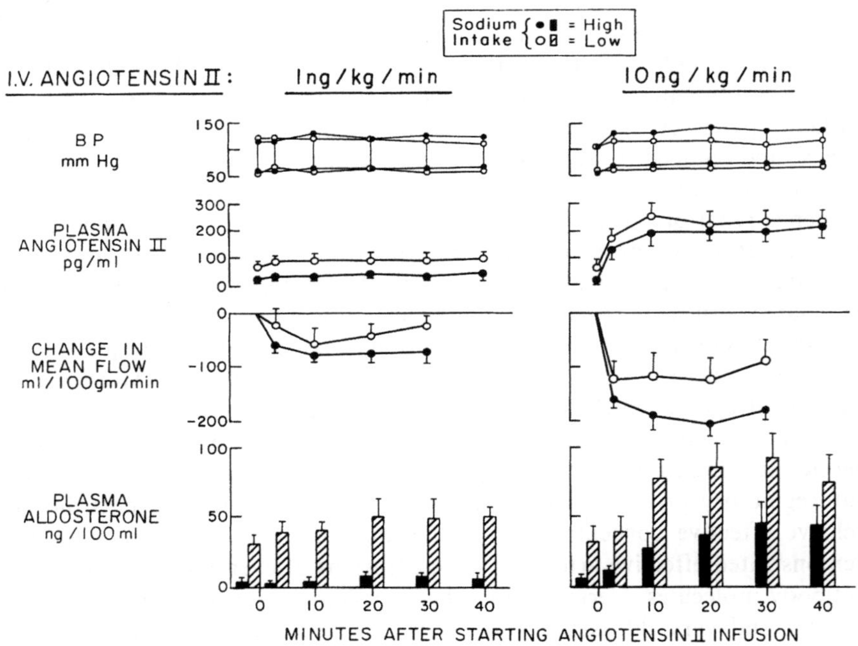

FIGURE 3. Time course of the response to angiotensin II at a subpressor and pressor dose. Note that the renal vascular and adrenal response occur with changes in the plasma angiotensin II concentration well within the physiological range and well below the pressor dose. Sodium intake exerts a profound and reciprocal influence on the sensitivity of the vascular smooth muscle and the adrenal. (From Hollenberg et al.[51])

Renal vascular responses to angiotensin II are reduced strikingly during the continuous exposure to large amounts of angiotensin, either exogenous[24,40,65] or endogenous, when the renin–angiotensin system is activated by restriction of sodium intake,[53,56] restriction of potassium intake,[56] oral contraceptive agents in the presence of any diet,[55] or ischemia.[78] A similar phenomenon has been seen in the dog,[23] where induction of anesthesia with barbiturate activated the renin–angiotensin system and reduced both renal blood flow and the renal vascular response to angiotensin II strikingly. The blunting of the renal vascular response probably reflects occupation of receptors by angiotensin, thus reducing the response to additional administered agents.[21,23,101] Thus a blunted renal vascular response to angiotensin, especially in a setting in which the renin–angiotensin system is activated, provides an indication that angiotensin is occupying and activating renal vascular receptors—this may be responsible for the state of the renal vasculature. The possibility also exists that angiotensin-induced prostaglandin release contributes to the blunted renal response to angiotensin.[1,76] Studies on renal responses to angiotensin in patients with either cirrhosis or hypertension are reviewed below.

Angiotensin's Actions on the Normal Kidney

Angiotensin II induces a larger reduction in blood flow than in glomerular filtration rate in the isolated, perfused kidney[67,86] and in the intact kidney in animals[40,81] and in man.[17,36,57]

These studies performed on the kidney of the rabbit, cat, dog, and man suggest an increase in the filtration fraction which has been attributed to a predominant efferent arteriolar action, as was suggested in more primitive species by Sokabe et al.[97] Also as pointed out by Sokabe,[96] the juxtaglomerular apparatus extends to the efferent arteriole only in mammals. A number of other factors which could determine the filtration fraction as an alternative to a predominant efferent action require examination, however, since the precise locus of angiotensin's action may have important therapeutic implications. If angiotensin has a predominant efferent action, then the pharmacological antagonists, as they increase renal blood flow, will do so at the price of a reduction of glomerular capillary pressure and filtration rate.

What additional actions induced by angiotensin may be relevant to the relationship between renal blood flow and filtration rate? There are several. First, angiotensin increases blood pressure, and, as discussed below, the relative influence on pressure and renal function may be a major determinant of the resultant renal response.[71] Second, angiotensin exerts a larger influence on the outer than the inner cortical blood supply.[28,59,79] To the extent that outer cortical nephrons have a higher blood flow and lower filtration rate,[62] a preferential outer cortical vasoconstrictor will result in an increase in the filtration fraction. Finally, evidence is accumulating which suggests a prominent intraglomerular action of angiotensin II; this has been reviewed in detail.[49] In brief, multiple observations from embryogenesis,[47,72] from morphological examination,[10,73] and from physiological considerations[11,15,16,42,43,49] suggest a potential for variation in intraglomerular perfusion which could modify the surface area available for filtration.

There is also evidence for an intraglomerular control system. Goormaghtigh[44] first pointed out the fibrillar structure of mesangial cells 3 decades ago and clearly indicated that this could provide a contractile function. Supporting morphological evidence came from Hornych et al.[59] who demonstrated by scanning electron microscopy that glomerular capillaries constricted in response to angiotensin, especially in the superficial cortex. Bernik[14] demonstrated spontaneous contractile activity in elements of human glomeruli grown in tissue culture, activity which was attributed to mesangial cells. Becker[12] demonstrated that highly specific antiserum to human smooth muscle actomyosin showed great affinity for the mesangial contractile elements, providing an immunochemical link between the contractile elements of smooth muscle and mesangium: he suggested that "contraction of mesangium may play a significant role in regulating glomerular blood flow." Sraer et al.[98] and Osborne et al.[84] demonstrated specific, high affinity receptors for angiotensin in glomeruli, which Osborne localized to mesangial cells. Moreover, Sraer et al. demonstrated that angiotensin would reduce the volume of glomeruli in vitro. Blantz et al.[16] demonstrated a striking influence of angiotensin on the ultrafiltration coefficient (i.e., the product of capillary surface area and intrinsic permeability of the glomerular capillaries) in Munich–Wistar rats which have glomeruli available for direct micropuncture in the superficial cortex. This was denied by Myers et al.[80] but Blantz's study was performed in volume-expanded rats, which created an enhanced and more consistent sensitivity to angiotensin. Taken in all, these observations suggest that beyond angiotensin's actions on afferent and efferent arterioles, a potentially important influence on events within the glomerulus may occur and play an important role in angiotensin's ultimate action on the kidney.

McGiff and Fasy[77] concluded that the renal vascular response to angiotensin involved the sympathetic nervous system, since the responsiveness was reduced by guanethidine, which prevents neural release of norepinephrine, and by denervation. The mechanisms was not straightforward, however, since neither ganglionic nor α-adrenergic blocking agents modified the response to angiotensin II. DiSalvo and Fell[31] could find no influence of acute or chronic denervation or chronic reserpine treatment on the renal vascular response to angiotensin and suggested, therefore, that the renal vasoconstrictor action was largely independent of the renal vasomotor innervation. α-Adrenergic blockade also did not influence the response to angiotensin in normal man.[56]

In the normal animal and man,[20,69,81] a reduction in blood flow is accompanied by a reduction in urine flow rate and electrolyte excretion, with a striking reduction in urine sodium. This response is evident with even the smallest angiotensin II dose required to influence the renal vasculature.[57] There is, in general, a good correlation between the reductions in renal blood flow, glomerular filtration rate, and urine flow in animals[81,91] and in man.[4,17,57]

Angiotensin's actions thus include reductions in renal blood flow, glomerular filtration rate, and sodium excretion—a triad that characterizes a wide variety of renal insults which occur in animal models and in patients in whom the renin–angiotensin system is activated.

Angiotensin's Actions on the Kidney in Patients with Relevant Disease

Sensitivity of the renal vasculature normally falls strikingly in settings in which the renin–angiotensin system is activated (see *Sensitivity of Renal Vasculature to Angiotensin*, above) and where multiple lines of evidence suggest that the reduction in sensitivity reflects not only occupation of receptors by angiotensin but also their activation. This approach in man has identified patients in whom an identical phenomenon has been apparent.

In a number of circumstances, including some patients with essential hypertension[20,104] or hepatic cirrhosis,[46,69] angiotensin induced an unanticipated diuresis and natriuresis, a response which only occurred with doses which raise blood pressure strikingly.[71] Villarreal et al.[103] found that some patients with essential hypertension responded to angiotensin with a striking diuresis. In these patients filtration rate tended to rise with little or no blood flow reduction. In other patients in whom an antidiuresis occured, both blood flow and filtration rate fell strikingly. Gutman et al.[46] also demonstrated that renal blood flow fell and filtration fraction rose in nearly all patients with cirrhosis who did not respond to angiotensin with a natriuresis, but changed little in those who did. Both observations are consistent with findings in the dog.[25,91]

Pharmacological Interruption of the Renin–Angiotensin System and the Kidney

The recent development of pharmacological agents which interrupt the renin–angiotensin axis has made it possible to define further the role of

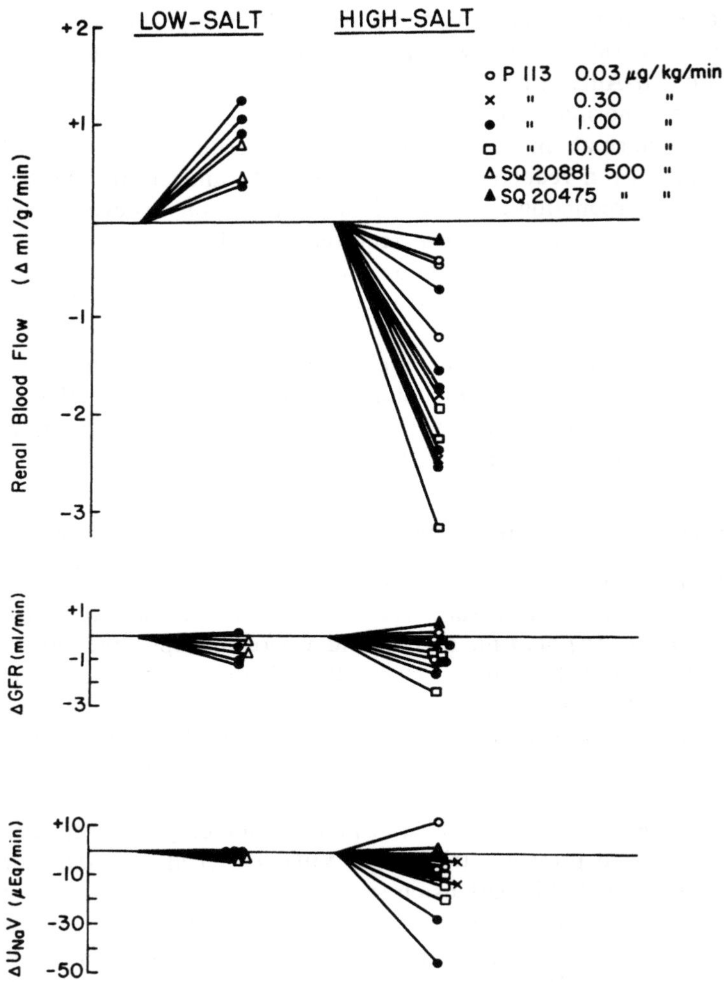

FIGURE 4. Both competitive antagonists to angiotensin II and converting enzyme inhibition increase renal blood flow in the rabbit in balance on a low-salt diet but not in rabbits on a high-salt diet. Failure of glomerular filtration rate and sodium excretion to change may reflect a 10–20 mm Hg blood pressure fall in rabbits on a low–salt diet (not shown). (From Mimran et al.[79])

angiotensin as a determinant of the state of the renal vasculature. When renal blood flow is reduced by restriction of sodium intake in the dog[23,38] or in the rabbit,[79,104] the administration of an agent such as propranolol (which prevents renin release), SQ 20,881 (which prevents conversion of angiotensin I to angiotensin II), or a structural analogue of angiotensin II (which acts as a competitive antagonist), all increase renal blood flow. None of these agents do so when the renin–angiotensin system is suppressed by a high salt intake (Figure 4). We have made similar observations in man (Figure 5).

In animal models, the renal vascular responses in anesthesia and trauma,[23] in thoracic inferior vena cava obstruction[38,100] in experimental heart failure,[37] in hemorrhagic shock,[61,68] in impaired reflow following hemorrhagic hypertension,[39] in renal hypertension,[88,106] and in acute renal

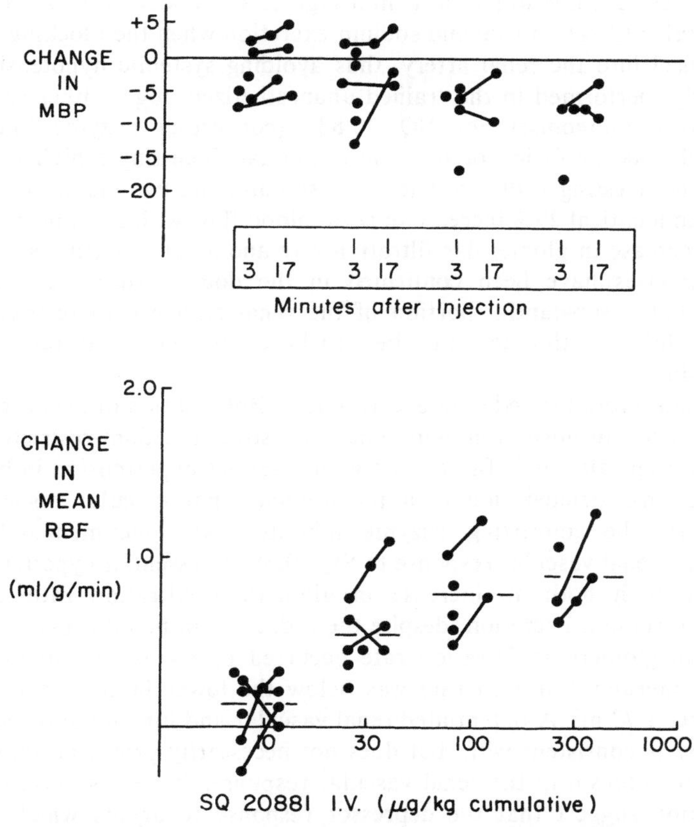

FIGURE 5. Converting enzyme blockade reduces arterial blood pressure (MBP) and increases mean renal blood flow (RBF) in normal man in whom the renin–angiotensin system (RAS) has been activated by restriction of sodium intake. These changes do not occur when the RAS is suppressed by a high salt intake, and effectively identical changes occur with angiotensin analogues which act as competitive antagonists. The increase in blood flow was associated with a parallel, dose-related reduction in plasma angiotensin II concentration despite a rise in plasma renin activity and no change in plasma bradykinin concentration (From Hollenberg et al. [58]).

failure,[60] have all been reversed in part or completely by pharmacological interruption of the renin–angiotensin system. Where assessed, glomerular filtration rate did not increase in parallel with the increase in renal blood flow.[5,37,38,60,79] While this may reflect a predominant action of the blockers on the efferent arteriole—an interpretation which would certainly be consistent with the available evidence on the primary locus of angiotensin's action—most studies were complicated by a striking fall in blood pressure, which may have blunted the influence on glomerular filtration rate, and by the intrinsic activity of the partial agonists in use.[57,79]

In an elegant investigation, Kimbrough et al.[66] documented an increase in glomerular filtration rate and sodium excretion when the blocking agents were infused into the renal artery, thus avoiding systemic hypotension. In their study, performed in the trained unanesthetized dog, neither saralasin (angiotensin antagonist) nor SQ 20,881 (converting enzyme inhibitor) influenced renal perfusion or function in animals ingesting a high-salt diet. In animals ingesting a diet restricted in sodium, the two classes of agents induced an identical 29% increase in renal blood flow with an approximately parallel increase in glomerular filtration rate and a brisk natriuresis. All of these responses have been confirmed in the dog.[48] From these data it appears that a substantial portion of the renal response to restriction of sodium intake in the dog can be attributed to the renal response to angiotensin.

In man, more limited data are available. Both classes of agent increase renal perfusion in normal human beings ingesting a sodium-restricted diet, but not a high-salt one.[58] In patients with essential hypertension in balance on a sodium-restricted intake, a potentiated renal vascular response to SQ 20,881, the converting enzyme inhibitor, was documented.[105] The potentiated renal vascular response to SQ 20,881 in essential hypertension is associated with both an increase in glomerular filtration rate and an increase in sodium excretion, despite the reduction in blood pressure.[54] The increase in glomerular filtration rate occurred primarily in individuals in whom glomerular filtration rate was below the lower limit of normal, 90 ml/min per 1.73 m^2. A potentiated renal vascular and functional response to SQ 20,881 is consistent with, but does not necessarily prove, an important role for angiotensin in the renal vascular response. Indeed, several lines of investigation suggest that the depressor response to agents which inhibit converting enzyme involves factors other than reduced angiotensin formation,[99] and identical logic applies to the renal response. The parallel renal vascular response to SQ 20,881 and saralasin in normal man when on a sodium-restricted intake suggests that angiotensin is involved in that response in man as it is in animals. Similar evidence will be required before a parallel conclusion can be drawn concerning the potentiated response to converting enzyme inhibition in the patient with essential hypertension.

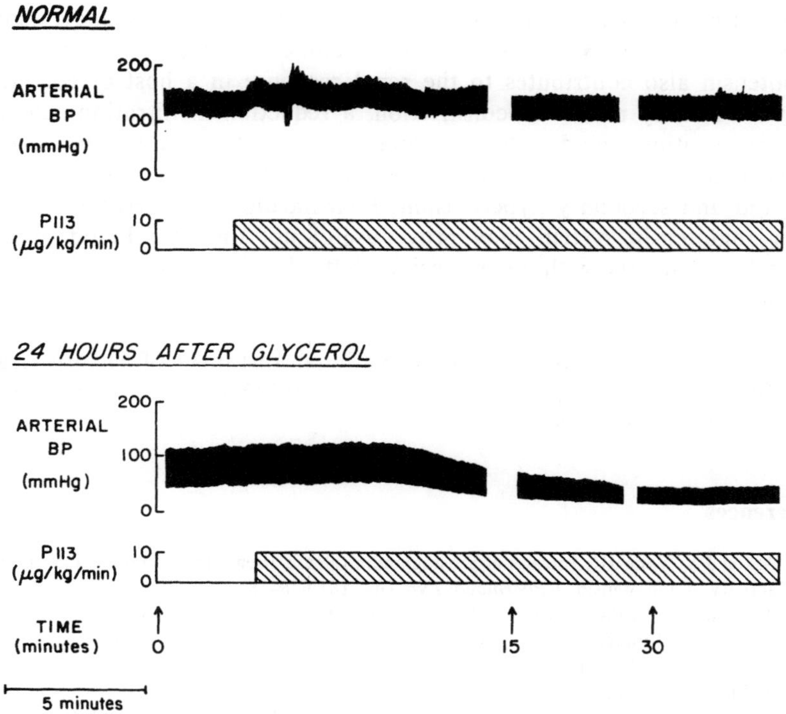

FIGURE 6. Effect of an angiotensin antagonist (P113; Sar-1-Ala-8-angiotensin II) on blood pressure in a normal rat (*above*) and in a rat with myohemoglobinuric acute renal failure induced by glycerol (*below*). As in other states not characterized by hypertension but associated with activation of the renin–angiotensin system, pharmacologic interruption of the system results in hypotension which can, by itself, limit the renal functional response. (From Ishikawa and Hollenberg.[60])

The blood pressure reduction during pharmacological interruption of the renin–angiotensin system occurs not only in patients with secondary hypertension in whom the renin–angiotensin system is activated, but also in animals with activation of the renin–angiotensin system and a normal or reduced blood pressure[37,38,60,79] and in patients with cirrhosis of the liver,[92] Bartter's syndrome[87] and congestive heart failure (unpublished observations). The resultant hypotension represents a limiting factor in the therapeutic potential of the angiotensin antagonists (Figure 6).

Taken in all, the available evidence suggests that angiotensin plays an important role in the control of the renal circulation—and perhaps that this is its original, primitive function. Through its vascular action, angiotensin has an important action on filtration and tubular reabsorption. The possibility that angiotensin has an additional, intraglomerular action was reviewed earlier (see *Angiotensin's Actions on the Normal Kidney*, above). Even more circumstantial but certainly compelling evidence suggests that angiotensin also contributes to the renal response in a host of conditions characterized by renal vasoconstriction, a reduction in filtration rate, and sodium retention including heart failure, cirrhosis of the liver, complications of pregnancy, the renal response to trauma and shock, and selected cases of essential and secondary hypertension. Pharmacological interruption of the renin–angiotensin system may prove useful not only for blood pressure control in patients with hypertension, but also in some or all of these conditions.

ACKNOWLEDGMENTS. Supported by National Institutes of Health Grants HL–14944, GM–18674, HL–11668, and HE–05832 and a contract from the National Aerospace Agency.

References

1. Aiken JW, Vane JR: Intrarenal prostaglandin release attenuates the renal vasoconstrictor activity of angiotensin. *J Pharmacol Exp Ther* 181:678–687, 1973.
2. Anderson RJ, Taher S, Cronin RE, McDonald KM, Schrier RW: Effect of β-adrenergic blockade and inhibitors of angiotensin II and prostaglandins on renal autoregulation. *Am J Physiol* 229:731–736, 1975.
3. Aukland K: Effect of adrenaline, noreadrenaline, angiotensin and renal nerve stimulation on intrarenal distribution of blood flow in dogs. *Acta Physiol Scand* 72:498, 1968.
4. Aurell M: Renal response in man to plasma volume expansion and angiotensin. *Scand J Clin Lab Invest* 24(suppl 112):1–59, 1969.
5. Bailie MD Barbour JA: Effect of inhibition of peptidase activity on distribution of intrarenal blood flow. *Am J Physiol* 228:850–853, 1975.
6. Bailie MD, Loutzenhiser R, Moyer S: Relation of renal hemodynamics to angiotensin II in renal hilar lymph of the dog. *Am J Physiol* 222:1075–1078, 1972.
7. Bailie MD, Rector FC Jr., Seldin DW: Angiotensin II in arterial and renal venous plasma and renal lymph in the dog. *J Clin Invest* 50:119–126, 1971.
8. Barajas L: Anatomical considerations in the control of renal secretion, in Assaykeen TA (ed): *Control of Renin Secretion*. New York, Plenum Press, 1972, pp 1–16.
9. Barger AC: Renal hemodynamic factors in congestive heart failure. *Ann NY Acad Sci* 139:273–284, 1966.
10. Barger AC, Herd JA: The renal circulation. *N Engl J Med* 284:482–490, 1971.
11. Baylis C, Shinagawa L, Wilson CB, Brenner BM: A relationship between systemic protein concentration and glomerular capillary ultrafiltration coefficient. *Fed Proc* 35:542, 1976.
12. Becker CG: Demonstration of actomyosin in mesangial cells of the renal glomerulus. *Circulation* 14:II–66, 1971.
13. Bern HA: Hormones and endocrine glands of fishes. *Science* 158:455–462, 1967.
14. Bernik MB: Contractile activity of human glomeruli in culture. *Nephron* 6:1, 1969.
15. Blantz RC: Effect of manitol on glomerular ultrafiltration in the hydropenic rat. *J Clin Invest* 54:1135–1143, 1974.

16. Blantz RC, Konnen KS, Tucker BJ: Angiotensin II effects upon the glomerular microcirculation and ultrafiltration coefficient of the rat. *J Clin Invest* 57:419–434, 1976.
17. Bock KD, Krecke HJ: Die Wirkung von synthetischem Hypertensin II auf die PAH-und Inulin-clearance, die renale Hamodynamik und die Diurese beim Menschen. *Klin Wochnschr* 36:69, 1958.
18. Boyer CS: The vascular pattern of the renal glomerulus as revealed by plastic reconstruction from serial sections. *Anat Rec* 125:443–440, 1956.
19. Brown JJ, Chinn RH, Gavras H, Leckie B, Lever AF, McGregor J, Morton J, Robertson JIS: Renin and renal function, in Genest J, Koiw E (eds) *Hypertension '72*, Berlin, Springer-Verlag, 1972, pp 81–97.
20. Brown JJ, Peart WS: The effect of angiotensin on urine flow and electrolyte excretion in hypertensive patients. *Clin Sci* 22:1–17, 1962.
21. Brunner HR, Chang P, Wallach R, Sealey JE, Laragh JH: Angiotensin II vascular receptors: Their avidity in relationship to sodium balance, the autonomic nervous system, and hypertension. *J Clin Invest* 51:58–67, 1972.
22. Bulger RE, Trump BF: Ultrastructure of granulated arteriolar cells (juxtaglomerular cells) in kidney of a fresh and a salt water teleost. *Am J Anat* 124:77–88, 1969.
23. Burger BM, Hopkins T, Tulloch A, Hollenberg NK: The role of angiotensin in the canine renal vascular response to barbiturate anesthesia. *Circ Res* 38:196–202, 1976.
24. Caldicott WJH, Hollenberg NK, Abrams HL: Characteristics of the response of the renal vascular bed to contrast media: Evidence of vasoconstriction induced by the renin–angiotensin system. *Invest Radiol* 5:539–547, 1970.
25. Cannon PJ, Ames RP, Laragh JH: Indirect action of angiotensin infusion to inhibit tubular sodium reabsorption in dogs. *Am J Physiol* 211:1021–1030, 1966.
26. Capelli JP, Wesson LG Jr, Aponte GE: A phylogenetic study of the renin–angiotensin system. *Am J Physiol* 218:1171, 1970.
27. Carlson DE, Schramm LP: Renal autoregulation in the cat: Effects of angiotensin II blockade and indomethacin. *Fed Proc* 35:705, 1976.
28. Carriere S: Effect of norepinephrine, isoproterenol and adrenergic blockers upon the intrarenal distribution of blood flow. *Can J Physiol Pharmacol* 47:199–208, 1969.
29. Davis JD, Freeman RH: Mechanisms regulating renin release. *Physiol Rev* 56:1–56, 1976.
30. DeBono E, Lee GdeJ, Mottram FR, Pickering GW, Brown JJ, Keen H, Peart WS, Sanderson PH: The action of angiotensin in man. *Clin Sci* 25:123–157, 1963.
31. DiSalvo J, Fell C: Effects of angiotensin on canine renal blood flow. *Proc Soc Exp Biol Med* 133:1432, 1970.
32. DiSalvo J, Peterson A, Montefusco C, Menta M: Intrarenal conversion of angiotensin I to angiotensin II in the dog. *Circ Res* 29:398–406, 1971.
33. Eide I, Loyning E, Aars H, Akre S: Autoregulation of renal blood flow in rabbits immunized with angiotensin II. *Scand J Clin Lab Invest* 31:123–127, 1973.
34. Eide I, Loyning E, Kiil F: Evidence for hemodynamic autoregulation of renin release. *Circ Res* 32:237–245, 1973.
35. Epstein M, Berke DP, Hollenberg NK, Adams DF, Chalmers TC, Abrams HL, Merrill JP: Renal failure in the patient with cirrhosis: The role of active vasoconstriction. *Am J Med* 49:175–185, 1970.
36. Finnerty FA: Hemodynamics of angiotensin in man. *Circulation* 25:255–258, 1962.
37. Freeman RH, Davis JO, Spielman WS, Lohmeier TE: High-output heart failure in the dog: Systemic and intrarenal role of angiotensin II. *Am J Physiol* 229:474–478, 1975.
38. Freeman RH, Davis JO, Vitale SJ, Johnson JA: Intrarenal role of angiotensin II. *Circ Res* 32:692–698, 1973.

39. Frega N, Guerther B, Dibona D, Leaf A: The role of angiotensin II in the impaired reflow following hemorrhagic hypotension. *Am Soc Nephrol* 6:37, 1973.
40. Furuyama T, Suzuki C, Shioji R, Saito H, Maebashi M, Aida M: Effect of angiotensin on renal function of the dog. *Tohoku J Exp Med* 92:73–81, 1967.
41. Gagnon JC, Rice MK, Flamenbaum W: Effect of angiotensin converting enzyme inhibition on renal autoregulation. *Proc Soc Exp Biol Med* 146:414–418, 1974.
42. Gassee JP, Decoodt P, Verniory A, Lambert PP: Autoregulation of effective glomerular filtration pressure. *J Physiol* (*Lond*) 226:616–623, 1974.
43. Gertz KH, Mangos JA, Braun G, Pagel HD: Pressure in the glomerular capillaries of the rat kidney and its relation to arterial pressure. *Pflügers Arch* 288:369, 1966.
44. Goormaghtigh N: La doctrine de la cellule musculaire affibrillaire endocrine en pathologie humaine. Le rein de l'eclampsie puerpuale. *Bull Acad R Med Belg* 7:194, 1942.
45. Granger P, Dahlheim H, Thurau K: Enzyme activities of the single juxtaglomerular apparatus in the rat kidney. *Kidney Internat* 1:78–88, 1972.
46. Gutman RA, Forrey AW, Fleet WP, Cutler RE: Vasopressor–induced natriuresis and altered intrarenal haemodynamics in cirrhotic man. *Clin Sci Mol Med* 45:19–34, 1973.
47. Hall BV, Roth LE: Preliminary studies on the development and differentiation of cells and structures of the renal corpuscle. *Proc Stockholm Conference on Electron Microscopy,* pp 176–179, 1956.
48. Hall JE, Guyton AC, Trippodo NC, Lohmeier TE, McCaa RE, Cowley AW: Intrarenal control of electrolyte excretion by angiotensin II. *Am J Physiol* 232:F538–F544, 1977.
49. Hollenberg NK: The physiology of the renal circulation, in *Renal Disease*, Fourth Edition (Black, D, Jones NF, eds) Oxford, Blackwell Scientific Publications, chap 2.
50. Hollenberg NK, Adams DF, Rashid A, Epstein M, Abrams HL, Merrill JP: The renal vascular response to salt restriction in norman man: Evidence against adrenergic mediation. *Circulation* 43:845–851, 1971.
51. Hollenberg NK, Chenitz WR, Adams DF, Williams GH: Reciprocal influence of salt intake on adrenal glomerulosa and renal vascular responses to angiotensin II in normal man. *J Clin Invest* 54:34–42, 1974.
52. Hollenberg NK, Epstein M, Basch RI, Merrill JP, Hickler RB: Renin secretion in the patient with hypertension: Relationship to intrarenal blood flow distribution. *Circ Res* 14:113–122, 1969.
53. Hollenberg NK, Solomon HS, Adams DF, Abrams HL, Merrill JP: Renal vascular response to angiotensin and norepinephrine in normal man: The effect of salt intake. *Circ Res* 31:750–757, 1972.
54. Hollenberg NK, Swartz SL, Passan DR, Williams GH: Increased glomerular filtration rate following converting enzyme inhibition in essential hypertension. *N Engl J Med* 301:9–12, 1979.
55. Hollenberg NK, Williams GH, Burger B, Chenitz WR, Hooshmand I, Adams DF: Renal blood flow and its response to angiotensin II: An interaction between oral contraceptive agents, sodium intake and the renin–angiotensin system in healthy young women. *Circ Res* 38:35–40, 1976.
56. Hollenberg NK, Williams GH, Burger BM, Hooshmand I: Potassium's influence on the renal vasculature, the adrenal and their responsiveness to angiotensin II in normal man. *Clin Sci Mol Med* 49:527–534, 1975.
57. Hollenberg NK, Williams GH, Burger BM, Ishikawa I, Adams DF: Blockade and stimulation of renal, adrenal and vascular receptors for angiotensin II with 1-Sar, 8-Ala angiotensin II in normal man. *J Clin Invest* 57:39–46, 1976.

58. Hollenberg NK, Williams GH, Taub KJ, Ishikawa I, Brown C, Adams DF: Renal vascular response to interruption of the renin–angiotensin system in normal man. *Kidney Int* 12:285–293, 1977.
59. Hornych H, Beaufils M, Richet G: The effect of exogenous angiotensin on superficial and deep glomeruli in the rat kidney. *Kidney Int* 2:336–343, 1972.
60. Ishikawa I, Hollenberg NK: Pharmacologic interruption of the renin–angiotensin system in myohemoglobinuric acute renal failure. *Kidney Int* 10:S183–S190, 1976.
61. Jakschik BA, McKnight RC, Marshall GR, Feldhaus RA, Needleman P: Renal vascular changes during hemorrhagic shock. *Circ Shock* 1:231–237, 1974.
62. Jamison RL: Micropunture study of superficial and juxtamedullary nephrons in the rat. *Am J Physiol* 218:46–55, 1970.
63. Kaloyanides GJ, Bastron RD, DiBona GF: Impaired autoregulation of blood flow and glomerular filtration rate in the isolated dog kidney depleted of renin. *Circ Res* 35:400–412, 1974.
64. Kiil F: Influence of autoregulation on renin release and sodium excretion. *Kidney Int* 8:S208–S218, 1975.
65. Kiil F, Kjekshus J, Loyning E: Renal autoregulation during infusion of noradrenaline, angiotensin and acetylcholine. *Acta Physiol Scand* 76:10–23, 1969.
66. Kimbrough HM Jr, Vaughan ED Jr, Carey RM, Ayers CR: Effect of intrarenal AII blockade on renal function in dogs. *Cir Res* 40:174–178, 1977.
67. Krahe P, Hofbauer KG, Gross F: Effects of endogenous renin on the function of the isolated kidney. *Life Sci* 9:1317–1320, 1970.
68. Lachance JG, Arnoux E, Brunette MG, Carriere SC: Factors responsible for the outer cortical ischemia observed during hemorrhagic hypotension in dogs. *Circ Shock* 1:131–144, 1974.
69. Laragh JH, Cannon PG, Bentzel CJ, Sicinski AM, Meltzer JI: Angiotensin II, norepinephrine and renal transport of electrolytes and water in normal man in cirrhosis with ascites. *J Clin Invest* 42:1179, 1963.
70. Leckie B, Gavras H, McGregor J, McElwee G: The conversion of angiotensin I to angiotensin II by rabbit glomeruli. *J Endocrinol* 55:229–230, 1972.
71. Lever AF: The vasa recta and countercurrent multiplication. *Acta Med Scand* 178:434, 1965.
72. Lewis OH: The vascular arrangement of the mammalian renal glomerulus as revealed by a study of its development. *J Anat* 92:433–440, 1958.
73. Ljungqvist A: Ultrastructural demonstration of a connection between afferent and efferent juxtamedullary glomerular arterioles. *Kidney Int* 8:239–244, 1975.
74. Malvin RL, Vander AJ: Plasma renin activity in marine teleosts and cetacea. *Am J Physiol* 213:1582–1584, 1967.
75. Mandel MJ, Sapirstein LA: Effect of angiotensin infusion on regional blood flow and regional vascular resistance in the rat. *Circ Res* 10:807–816, 1962.
76. McGiff JC, Crowshaw K, Terragno NA, Lonigro AJ: Release of a prostaglandin-like substance into renal venous blood in response to angiotensin II. *Circ Res* 26–27(suppl 1):I121–I130, 1970.
77. McGiff JCM, Fasy TM: The relationship of the renal vascular activity of angiotensin II to the autonomic nervous system. *J Clin Invest* 44:1911, 1965.
78. McGiff JC, Itskovitz HD: Loss of the renal vasoconstrictor activity of angiotensin II during renal ischemia. *J Clin Invest* 43:2359–2367, 1964.
79. Mimran A, Guiod L, Hollenberg NK: Angiotensin's role in the cardiovascular and renal response to salt restriction. *Kidney Int* 5:348–355, 1974.

80. Myers BD, Deen WM, Breener BM: Effects of norepinephrine and angiotensin II on the determinants of glomerular ultrafiltration and proximal tubule fluid reabsorption in the rat. *Circ Res* 37:101–110, 1975.
81. Navar LG, Langford HG: Effects of angiotensin on the renal circulation. *Angiotensin: Handbook of Experimental Pharmacology* 37:455–474, 1974.
82. Ng KKF, Vane JR: Conversion of angiotensin I to angiotensin II. *Nature* 216:762–766, 1967.
83. Nishimura H, Ogawa M, Sawyer WH: Renin–angiotensin system in primitive bony fishes and a holocephalian. *Am J Physiol* 224:950–956, 1973.
84. Osborne MJ, Drox B, Meyer P, Morel F: Angiotensin II: Renal localization in glomerular mesangial cells by autoradiography. *Kidney Int* 8:245–254, 1975.
85. Peart WS, Brown JJ: Effect of angiotensin (hypertensin or angiotonin) on urine flow and electrolyte excretion in hypertensive patients. *Lancet* 1:28–29, 1961.
86. Regoli D, Gauthier R: Site of action of angiotensin and other vasoconstrictors on the kidney. *Can J Physiol Pharmacol* 49:608–612, 1971.
87. Sasaki H, Okomura H, Ikeda H, Kawasaki I, Fukiyama K: Hypotensive response to angiotensin II analog in Bartter's syndrome. *N Engl J Med* 294:611–612, 1976.
88. Satoh S, Zimmerman BG: Effect of (Sar^1–Ala^8)angiotensin II on renal vascular resistance. *Am J Physiol* 229:640–645, 1975.
89. Sawyer WH, Blair-West JR, Simpson PA, Sawyer MK: Renal responses of Australian lungfish to vasotocin, angiotensin II, and NaCl infusion. *Am J Physiol* 231:593–602, 1976.
90. Schmid HE Jr: Renin, a physiologic regulator of renal hemodynamics. *Circ Res* 11:185–193, 1962.
91. Schmid HE Jr: Action of angiotensin in normal, adrenalectomized, and renal hypertensive trained dogs. *Nephron* 5:265–281, 1968.
92. Schroeder ET, Anderson GH, Goldman SH, Streeten DHP: Effects of angiotensin II (AII) blockade with 1-Sar-8-Ala AII (Saralasin) in patients with cirrhosis and ascites. *Kidney Int* 9:511–519, 1976.
93. Smeby RR, Bumpus FM: Renin, in Page IH, McCubbins JW (eds) *Renal Hypertension*, Chicago, Year Book Medical Publishers, 1968, pp 14–61.
94. Smith HW: *Lectures on the Kidney*, Lawrence, University of Kansas Press, 1943.
95. Smith HW: *The Kidney: Structure and Function in Health and Disease*. New York, Oxford University Press, 1951.
96. Sokabe H: Phylogeny of the renal effects of angiotensin. *Kidney Int* 6:263–271, 1974.
97. Sokabe H, Mizogame S, Sato A: Role of renin in adaptation to sea water in eruyhaline fishes. *Jpn J Pharmacol* 18:332–343, 1968.
98. Sraer JD, Sraer J, Adraillou R, Mimoune O: Evidence for renal glomerular receptors for angiotensin II. *Kidney Int* 6:241–246, 1974.
99. Swartz SL, Williams GH, Hollenberg NK, Moore TJ, Dluhy RG: Converting enzyme inhibition in essential hypertension: The hypotensive response does not reflect only reduced angiotensin II formation. *Hypertension* 1:106–111, 1979.
100. Kaub KH, Caldicott WJH, Hollenberg NK: Identity of renal vascular receptors for angiotensin II (AII) and the 2–8 heptapeptide (AIII). *Am Soc Nephrol* 8:48, 1975.
101. Thurston H, Laragh JH: Prior receptor occupancy as a determinant of the pressor activity of infused angiotensin II in the rat. *Circ Res* 36:113–117, 1975.
102. Vander AJ: Control of renin release. *Physiol Rev* 47:359, 1967.
103. Villarreal H, Arcila H, Diaz J, Sierra P: Effect of angiotensin on the renal transport of sodium in essential hypertension. *Circulation* 35:889, 1967.

104. Warren DJ, Ledingham JGG: Effects of beta adrenergic receptor blockade on the renal vascular response to a low sodium diet in the rabbit. *Clin Sci Mol Med* 48:533–535, 1975.
105. Williams GH, Hollenberg NK: Accentuated vascular and endocrine response to SQ 20,881 in hypertension. *N Engl J Med* 297:184–188, 1977.
106. Zimmerman BG: Involvement of angiotensin-mediated renal vasoconstriction in renal hypertension. *Life Sci* 13:507–515, 1973.

Chapter 6

Systemic Vascular Resistance

Regulation and Effect on Left Ventricular Function

Jay N. Cohn

Introduction

The height of the systemic vascular resistance is largely dependent on the total cross-sectional area of the arterioles in the peripheral vasculature. The smooth muscle tone of these vessels is influenced by neural, humoral, and local environmental factors. In addition, changes in the caliber of these vessels may result from structural alterations, including the accumulation of water and electrolytes in the walls. The tone of these vessels also may be altered by so-called autoregulatory adjustments which tend, through several possible mechanisms, to keep flow relatively constant despite changes in perfusion pressure. The systemic vascular resistance cannot be measured directly but rather is calculated as the ratio of mean arterial pressure to cardiac output. Resistance calculated in this way is a mean value which disregards the pulsatile nature of flow and also disregards the marked regional differences in resistance which may exist in the various parallel circuits that make up the total vascular resistance.

The level of the systemic vascular resistance has been considered in most detail in hypertension. It is generally agreed that in most forms of experimental and clinical hypertension the primary hemodynamic abnormality is an elevated vascular resistance.[1] The mechanism of this resistance increase has been the subject of extensive investigation over a long period of time. Abnormalities of neural control have been implicated, including the possibility of heightened central nervous system stimulation,[2] increased sensitivity to released catecholamines,[3] and altered neural feedback control of blood pressure changes.[4] Altered humoral control has been considered in extensive studies of activity of the renin–angiotensin system[5] and in the study of various vasoactive circulating substances such as prostaglandin,

JAY N. COHN, M.D. · Department of Medicine, Cardiovascular Division, University of Minnesota Medical School, Minneapolis, Minnesota 55455.

kinins, and other polypeptide hormones.[6,7] Alterations in the sodium and potassium concentrations of extracellular and intracellular compartments have also been demonstrated to have an effect on systemic vascular resistance and have been implicated as possible mechanisms of the heightened resistance in hypertension.[8] Similarly, the water logging of arteries in various forms of experimental hypertension may play a role in the heightened resistance in this syndrome.[9] Autoregulation as a factor in the high resistance has been popularized by Guyton and his associates who have suggested that an early increase in flow tends to overperfuse tissues which respond with vasoconstriction in order to restore flow to normal.[10] In this proposed sequence of events, the high resistance may be viewed as an autoregulatory mechanism to control perfusion of tissues. Any or all of these mechanisms may be operative in individual patients with essential hypertension and in experimental models of the disease.

Therapy for hypertension over the years has largely been empirical and has involved administration of drugs which have in common only that they lower blood pressure. Most of the drugs employed do indeed result in a long-term reduction in systemic vascular resistance. However, the mechanism by which some of these drugs lower resistance is not well understood. In recent years attempts to attack more specifically the elevated resistance of hypertension have been spearheaded by Laragh and his associates.[11] These investigators have focused particularly on the renin–angiotensin system and have suggested that in the presence of high renin activity, β-adrenergic blockers, which lower renin activity, may be specific therapy for hypertension. The controversy over the appropriateness of this approach to the treatment of hypertension is well known.

Systemic Vascular Resistance in Heart Failure

The hallmark of congestive heart failure is a reduced cardiac output either at rest or, especially, during exercise. Since arterial pressure is normal or sometimes even elevated, the calculated systemic vascular resistance in congestive heart failure tends to be elevated. The mechanism of this elevated resistance has received less attention than that associated with hypertension. Activation of the sympathetic nervous system with increased circulating norepinephrine has been demonstrated in heart failure,[12] and the renin–angiotensin system also appears to be stimulated.[13] An increase in the water content of vascular walls also has been suspected. The relative importance of each of these potential factors and the possible interplay of other factors have not been extensively studied.

Teleologically, an increased resistance when the cardiac output falls would appear to be appropriate. A fall in cardiac output would result in a fall in blood pressure were it not for adjustment of the systemic arterial bed.

The cardiovascular system is well endowed with mechanisms to prevent a reduction in arterial pressure, and these are therefore called into action when the cardiac output falls. (Indeed, the high incidence of hypertension in our adult society indicates that the body is far more likely to adjust with a high blood pressure than with a low blood pressure in response to physiological stresses.) A breakdown in the homeostatic system comes about when the fall in cardiac output results from heart failure and not from volume depletion. The primary role of these primitive cardiovascular reflexes probably is to adjust to loss of circulating volume. When the heart is normal, a mild "overshoot" in which the blood pressure rises to hypertensive levels should be well tolerated. However, when cardiac dysfunction precipitates the fall in output, the rise in resistance may become self-defeating by further reducing output.

Therapeutic interventions aimed at altering the systemic vascular resistance in the management of heart failure have not been widely employed in the past. The reason for this is that the nonhypertensive patient who develops heart failure does not usually manifest a significantly elevated blood pressure even though his systemic vascular resistance may be high. With the blood pressure as a guide, physicians have not been cognizant of the elevation of systemic vascular resistance. Therefore, therapy has been directed toward improving the contractile function of the heart and relieving the edema resulting from secondary salt and water retention.

Effect of Systemic Vascular Resistance on Left Ventricular Function

The left ventricle is normally endowed with considerable reserve capacity which allows it to generate considerably more wall tension than is usually required under physiological conditions. Sudden rises of systemic vascular resistance when the heart is normal do not significantly impair left ventricular output because the left ventricle is able to generate a high pressure and maintain normal shortening. Some of this enhanced performance probably results from a modest increase in end-diastolic fiber length (preload). When heart failure supervenes in the patient with longstanding hypertension, it can usually be attributed either to an increase in resistance above the level to which the normal left ventricle can adjust or, more commonly, to an impairment of left ventricular function which reduces its ability to maintain stroke volume against even a moderately heightened resistance.

When the left ventricular myocardium is damaged, the ability of the heart to adjust to heightened work loads is impaired. Under these circumstances stroke volume becomes inversely related to the height of the systemic resistance or impedance (Figure 1). Consequently, an increase in resistance may result in a reduction in stroke volume and cardiac output.

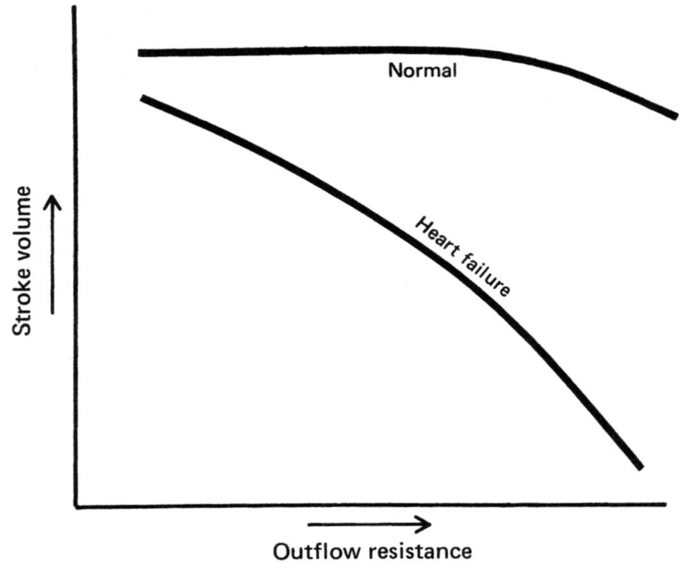

FIGURE 1. Relationship between systemic outflow resistance and stroke volume when the left ventricle is normal and when function is impaired (heart failure). In the presence of normal function, left ventricular stroke volume falls only when resistance is at very high levels. When the left ventricle is abnormal, stroke volume increases relative to resistance.

Since this fall in stroke volume may be the stimulus to a rise in resistance through reflex neurohumoral mechanisms, it can be appreciated that a rise in resistance in the failing heart may lead to a further rise in resistance and thus a vicious cycle of progressive cardiac impairment.

In considering the response of the left ventricle to alterations in systemic vascular resistance, the metabolic as well as the mechanical effects of resistance change must be considered. A rise in wall tension resulting from an increase in outflow resistance increases myocardial oxygen consumption.[14] When the coronary arterial system is normal, such an increase in metabolic demand can easily be met by augmentation of coronary blood flow. When coronary disease accompanies left ventricular dysfunction, however, the metabolic demand of the heightened outflow resistance may precipitate myocardial ischemia which may further impair the performance of the left ventricle.

Response to Vasodilator Drugs in Heart Failure

The aptness of the above thesis regarding the relationship between outflow resistance and left ventricular output can be demonstrated by observing the response of the left ventricle as outflow resistance is reduced.[15] A number of vasodilator drugs have been demonstrated to increase stroke volume, increase ejection fraction, reduce left ventricular filling pressure, and reduce left ventricular volume in patients with heart failure of a variety of causes.[16] This response appears not to be transient but is sustained as long as the vasodilator agent is administered.

The effectiveness of the vasodilator drugs in improving left ventricular output in heart failure is directly dependent upon the arterial and/or arteriolar vasodilating properties of the drug employed. All of the drugs share an effect on the arterial bed, although the mechanism of this action appears to be quite variable. Some drugs appear to have at least some effect on the large arteries to increase compliance, whereas others probably have an effect confined to the smaller resistance vessels.

The variable effect of vasodilating drugs on arterial pressure has led to some confusion about the use of these agents in the treatment of heart failure. In the hypertensive patient, systemic vascular resistance and blood pressure are usually directly related; therefore any agent which reduces vascular resistance usually reduces blood pressure. This relationship has become so accepted that physicians tend to equate resistance with blood pressure. In the setting of heart failure, however, resistance and blood pressure may vary independently. The reason for this variability is that a fall in resistance may result in a rise in output such that the blood pressure may be supported at unchanged levels while the resistance is drastically reduced. On the other hand, an increase in resistance may result in a fall in cardiac output so that significant rises in resistance may be accompanied by no change in blood pressure or even a fall in blood pressure if left ventricular function is severely impaired. Consequently, the therapeutic goal in the use of vasodilators in managing heart failure is reduction of systemic vascular resistance, not necessarily reduction in arterial pressure.

The total circulatory response to vasodilator drugs, however, is in large part dependent upon other actions of individual drugs. One must consider in this response the effect of the drugs on the venous circulation, the pulmonary vascular bed, and on the intensity of reflex neurohumoral stimulation (Table 1).

Venous Effect

Vasodilator drugs which have a potent effect on the venous bed not only reduce the outflow resistance—which should improve left ventricular output—but also reduce the preload of the left ventricle—which might otherwise tend to reduce output. Therefore, the net effect of such drugs on cardiac output would depend not only on the relative action of the drugs on the venous and arterial bed but on the state of the left ventricle at the time the drug is administered. The normal ventricle operates on a fairly steep

TABLE 1. Actions of Vasodilators

Systemic arterioles
Reduced systemic vascular resistance
Large arteries
Increased compliance
Systemic veins
Venous pooling
Pulmonary vessels
Reduced pulmonary vascular resistance
Pulmonary venous pooling
Reflex adrenergic stimulation
Increased heart rate
Increased myocardial contractility
Arterial constriction
Venoconstriction
Renin release

Frank–Starling curve so that changes in filling, or preload, have a considerable effect on stroke volume.[17] This normal left ventricle is relatively insensitive to changes in outflow resistance (Figure 1), and therefore a drug with both arterial and venous dilating properties would tend to reduce cardiac output when the heart is normal. On the other hand, the damaged left ventricle operates on a relatively flat Frank–Starling curve and is relatively insensitive to changes in preload but is very sensitive to alterations in outflow resistance.[18] Therefore, a drug with both arterial and venous dilating properties administered to a patient with a damaged left ventricle would be likely to raise the stroke volume and cardiac output. Sodium nitroprusside, the most potent vasodilating drug available for the treatment of heart failure, exerts both venous and arterial effects and therefore behaves in this way.[19] Nitrates, on the other hand, have somewhat more venous than arterial effects, and therefore a rise in cardiac output occurs only when left ventricular function is markedly impaired.[20] Hydralazine and phentolamine exert relatively pure arterial effects, and therefore changes in preload are slight and result primarily from the improved emptying of the ventricle resulting from the reduced outflow resistance and not from reduced filling because of venous pooling.[19] The relative venodilating properties of many of the vasodilator drugs is not known. Since angiotensin has little direct effect on veins,[21] it is likely that angiotensin inhibitors would not exert much venous effect.

Pulmonary Vascular Effects

The direct effect of vasodilator drugs on the pulmonary circulation has not been well studied. Agents such as nitroprusside and nitroglycerin appear to have some pulmonary arterial effect because pulmonary artery pressure falls during their administration, the pulmonary arteriolar resistance is reduced, and arterial oxygen saturation often falls modestly indicating the opening up of pulmonary arteriovenous shunts.[16] In contrast, drugs such as hydralazine do not appear to exert much pulmonary vasodilating properties, since pulmonary artery pressure falls less if at all, and arterial oxygen saturation is not reduced.[22] Indeed, minoxidil, a potent arterial dilating agent used in the treatment of hypertension, has been noted to produce pulmonary hypertension in some individuals presumably because the pulmonary vascular bed does not share in the systemic vasodilating properties of the drug.

Sympathetic Reflex Response

The variability in reflex tachycardia in response to various vasodilator drugs used both in the treatment of hypertension and in heart failure indicates that we do not thoroughly understand the mechanisms by which the sympathetic nervous system is activated. Drugs such as minoxidil and hydralazine are usually associated with prominent reflex tachycardia, whereas agents such as sodium nitroprusside and nitroglycerin appear to produce considerably less. Intravenous phentolamine also is frequently accompanied by a tachycardia greater than that observed with similar blood pressure reductions induced by intravenous sodium nitroprusside.[23]

Although the mechanism of this variation in reflex response is not understood, changes in heart rate may be of importance in the therapeutic response to the drugs. Heart rate is one of the most critical determinants of myocardial oxygen consumption.[24] In clinical situations in which increases in oxygen consumption may be deleterious, such as unstable coronary artery disease, avoidance of tachycardia is important. Fortunately, however, patients with heart failure tend to demonstrate cardiac slowing rather than tachycardia in response to vasodilator drugs. This response appears to relate to a paradoxical decrease in sympathetic nervous system activity consequent to the increase in stroke volume despite a fall in arterial pressure.[25] Therefore, vasodilator drugs are safer than they might otherwise be expected to be in the treatment of heart failure associated with coronary artery disease.

Regional Sites of Action of Vasodilator Drugs

The mechanism of action of vasodilator drugs on the arterial vascular bed is poorly understood. β-Adrenergic agonists such as isoproterenol interact with a specific receptor mechanism which subserves vasodilation. The distribution of the vascular effects of the β-agonists would depend upon the distribution of β-receptors in the various vascular tissues. Since skeletal muscle is richly endowed with β-receptors, β-agonists would be expected to redistribute blood flow toward the skeletal muscle and often away from the visceral bed which is relatively poorly supplied with β-receptors. α-Adrenergic receptors have a very different peripheral distribution favoring the renal, cutaneous, and splanchnic vascular beds. Therefore, α-blocking agents might be expected to redistribute blood flow to these areas. Drugs which inhibit the renin–angiotensin system, such as the converting enzyme inhibitors, would be expected to exert their vasodilating effect primarily on vascular beds which are under the tonic influence of angiotensin. Since angiotensin appears to exert rather uniform effects throughout the arterial bed, an angiotensin inhibitor might be expected not to alter markedly the distribution of blood flow but to exert an effect in direct proportion to the height of circulating angiotensin levels. The effects of other directly acting vasodilator drugs, such as nitroprusside, nitroglycerin, and hydralazine, on the regional distribution of blood flow has not been well established. The mechanism of action of these drugs is also not understood. It is likely that the common denominator of their action is a reduction of available calcium for smooth muscle contraction, and this effect may be exerted by stimulation of smooth muscle sodium potassium ATPase.[26] Since these vasodilator drugs are so dissimilar in structure and effect, it is likely that each of these drugs exerts different effects on various vascular beds and might uniquely alter the distribution of blood flow.

The Future of Vasodilator Therapy

Drugs which relax vascular smooth muscle have an exciting potential for the management of hypertension and heart failure. The synthesis of a variety of new agents with differing structures suggests that an almost infinite variety of compounds with unique hemodynamic effects may eventually be available for therapeutic use. Since these agents do not disturb neural reflex control of the circulation, they provide what should be a more physiological approach to the management of hypertension. Since they relax the heightened resistance of heart failure and thus improve left ventricular function without increasing myocardial work, they provide an exciting alternative or supplement to conventional therapy for the failing heart.

Up to the present time most studies of vasodilator agents in heart failure have been limited to acute interventions with demonstration of hemodynamic efficacy. Long-term controlled studies of the therapeutic response to vasodilator drugs either alone or in addition to digitalis and diuretics will represent the next important step in the evaluation of this therapeutic approach. The introduction of new drugs with more specific vascular sites of action and further elucidation of the precise mechanism by which systemic vascular resistance is increased in heart failure should lead the way to more effective and rational therapy.

References

1. Freis ED: Hemodynamics of hypertension. *Physiol Rev* 40:27, 1960.
2. Zanchetti A, Bartorelli C: Central nervous mechanisms in arterial hypertension: Experimental and clinical evidence, in Genest J, Koiw E, Kuchel O (eds): *Hypertension*. New York, McGraw-Hill, 1977, p 59.
3. Mendlowitz M: Vascular reactivity in systemic arterial hypertension. *Am Heart J* 85:252, 1973.
4. McCubbin JW, Green JH, Page IH: Baroreceptor function in chronic renal hypertension. *Circ Res* 4:205, 1956.
5. Davis JO: The control of renin release. *Am J Med* 55:333, 1973.
6. McGiff JC, Itskovitz HD: Prostaglandins and the kidney. *Circ Res* 33:479, 1973.
7. Margolius HS, Geller R, Pisano JJ, Sjoerdsma A: Altered urinary kallikrein excretion in human hypertension. *Lancet* 2:1063, 1971.
8. Haddy FJ: Local control of vascular resistance as related to hypertension *Arch Intern Med* 133:916, 1974.
9. Tobian L: Interrelationship of electrolytes, juxtaglomerular cells and hypertension. *Physiol Rev* 40:280, 1960.
10. Guyton AC, Coleman TG, Cowley AW Jr, Manning RD Jr, Norman RA Jr: Arterial pressure regulation: Overriding dominance of the kidneys in long-term regulation and in hypertension. *Am J Med* 52:584, 1972.
11. Laragh JH: Vasoconstriction–volume analysis for understanding and treating hypertension: The use of renin and aldosterone profiles. *Am J Med* 55:261, 1973.
12. Chidsey CA, Braunwald E, Morrow AG: Catecholamine excretion and cardiac stores of norepinephrine in congestive heart failure. *Am J Med* 39:442, 1965.
13. Johnston CI, Davis JO, Robb CA, Mackenzie JW: Plasma renin in chronic experimental heart failure and during renal sodium "escape" from mineralocorteriods. *Circ Res* 22:113, 1968.
14. Rodbard S, Williams CB, Rodbard D, Berglund E: Myocardial tension and oxygen uptake. *Circ Res* 14:139, 1964.
15. Cohn JN: Vasodilator therapy for heart failure: The influence of impedance on left ventricular performance (editorial). *Circulation* 48:5, 1973.
16. Guiha NH, Cohn JN, Mikulic E, Franciosa JA, Limas CJ: Treatment of refractory heart failure with infusion of nitroprusside. *N Engl J Med* 291:587, 1974.
17. Sarnoff SJ, Berglund E: Ventricular function. I. Starling's law of the heart studied by simultaneous right and left ventricular function curves in the dog. *Circulation* 9:706, 1954.
18. Ross J Jr, Braunwald E: The study of left ventricular function by increasing resistance to ventricular ejection with angiotensin. *Circulation* 29:739, 1964.
19. Franciosa JA, Pierpont G, Cohn JN: Hemodynamic improvement after oral hydralazine in left ventricular failure: A comparison with nitroprusside infusion in 16 patients. *Ann Intern Med* 86:388, 1977.
20. Franciosa JA, Blank RC, Cohn JN: Nitrate effects on cardiac output and left ventricular outflow resistance in chronic congestive heart failure. *Am J Med* 64:207, 1978.
21. Cohn JN: Relationship of plasma volume changes to resistance and capacitance vessel effects of sympathomimetic amines and angiotensin in man. *Clin Sci* 30:267, 1966.

22. Pierpont GL, Hale KA, Franciosa JA, Cohn JN: Effects of vasodilators on pulmonary hemodynamics and gas exchange in left ventricular failure. *Am Heart J* (in press).
23. Kelly DT, Delgado CE, Taylor DR: Use of phentolamine in acute myocardial infarction associated with hypertension and left ventricular failure. *Circulation* 47:729, 1973.
24. Sonnenblick EH, Skelton CL: Myocardial energetics: Basic principles and clinical implications. *N Engl J Med* 285:668, 1971.
25. Cohn JN, Taylor N, Vrobel T, Moskowitz R: Contrasting effect of vasodilators on heart rate and plasma catecholamines in patients with hypertension and heart failure. *Clin Res* 26:547A, 1978.
26. Limas CJ, Cohn JN: Stimulation of vascular smooth muscle sodium, potassium-adenosinetriphosphatase by vasodilators. *Circ Res* 35:601, 1974.

Part II · Angiotensin–Converting Enzyme

Its Role and Development of Inhibitors

Chapter 7

Physiological, Biochemical, and Immunologic Aspects of Angiotensin-Converting Enzyme

Richard L. Soffer and Edmund H. Sonnenblick

Introduction

Angiotensin-converting enzyme (EC.3.4.15.1) is an exopeptidase that catalyzes cleavage of dipeptidyl residues from the COOH termini of peptide substrates.[1] It was first detected by Skeggs et al.[2] who found that the product of the action of porcine renin on crude equine angiotensinogen could be resolved into two compounds, provided the incubation was carried out in the presence of chloride ions. Subsequently,[3] they established that this was due to a contaminating activity in their angiotensinogen preparation that released His-Leu from the COOH terminus of angiotensin I to yield angiotensin II, an octapeptide. Although both angiotensins were found to be vasopressor after intravenous infusion, angiotensin II was identified as the biologically active component of the renin–angiotensin system, since only it induced contraction of rabbit aortic strips in vitro[4] and increased the perfusion pressure of isolated rat kidneys.[5] The vasopressor response to angiotensin I was therefore assumed to be due to its conversion to angiotensin II, mediated by the plasma-converting enzyme, until 1967, when Ng and Vane[6] recognized that this enzyme activity was insufficient to account for the rapidity of conversion in vivo. They found that intravenously administered angiotensin I was much more potent than the same dose given intraarterially and that substantial conversion to angiotensin II

Reprinted from *Progress in Cardiovascular Diseases* 21(3):167–175, 1978, by permission of the authors and the publisher, Grune & Stratton.

RICHARD L. SOFFER, M.D. · Departments of Medicine and Biochemistry, Cornell University Medical College, New York, New York 10021. EDMUND H. SONNENBLICK, M.D. · Division of Cardiology, Albert Einstein College of Medicine, Bronx, New York 10461.

occurred during a single passage through the pulmonary circulation.[6,7] Their results suggested that physiological conversion was catalyzed by a pulmonary enzyme located in close approximation to the circulating blood. It has since become clear that converting enzyme is a vascular endothelial component of many tissues,[8-10] and electron microscopic studies with microperoxidase-labeled antibody have localized it on the lumenal surface of the plasma membrane.[11] The importance of the lung in angiotensin conversion is due to its large vascular bed, its strategic anatomic location, and the fact that enzymatically generated angiotensin II is not extensively metabolized within the pulmonary vascular bed but is delivered intact into the systemic circulation.[7,12]

Ng and Vane[7] first suggested that the same pulmonary enzyme might catalyze angiotensin conversion and bradykinin inactivation, since Ferreira and Vane[13] had previously found that the biologic activity of bradykinin disappeared during transit through the pulmonary circulation. In 1968, Bakhle made the important discovery that bradykinin-potentiating factor, a mixture of peptides from the venom of *Bothrops jararaca*, inhibited conversion of angiotensin catalyzed by canine pulmonary particles.[14] Ferreira had originally demonstrated that this peptide mixture potentiated the action of bradykinin on smooth muscle by inhibiting its degradation.[15] It was soon shown that pure peptides isolated from the mixture could inhibit both angiotensin-converting and bradykininase activities in pulmonary extracts,[16] and it was later established that pure pulmonary-converting enzymes from rabbit[17] and hog lung[18] could catalyze sequential release of Phe-Arg and Ser-Pro from the COOH terminus of bradykinin. The action of this enzyme on its two currently recognized physiological substrates may thus be considered vasopressor, i.e., removal of His-Leu from angiotensin I yields a potent pressor molecule, and hydrolytic cleavage of bradykinin inactivates a powerful vasodepressor agent.

The snake venom (*Bothrops*) peptide inhibitors of angiotensin-converting enzyme provided an important tool for examining the contribution of the renin–angiotensin system to the maintenance of blood pressure. The first of these to be sequenced[19] and synthesized[20] was a pentapeptide that was shown to inhibit the vasopressor response to angiotensin, I,[20] to augment the vasodepressor effect of bradykinin,[20] and to reverse experimental renovascular hypertension in the rat.[21] A number of other venom inhibitors were also characterized, synthesized,[22,23] and shown to possess similar pharmacological properties.[24-27] The determinants responsible for the inhibitory action of these compounds were carefully delineated using a large number of synthetic peptides.[28] A nonapeptide, SQ 20,881,[29] was the first converting-enzyme inhibitor to be tested in man. It was shown to block the vasopressor action of angiotensin I,[30] and early clinical studies with it provided the initial evidence that inhibition of the renin–angiotensin system might be beneficial in most human hypertensive disease.[31] Because angiotensin-converting enzyme is also a bradykininase, studies with agents that inhibit it cannot distinguish whether salutory physiological effects are due to suppressed formation of angiotensin II or enhanced endogenous bradykinin activity. In addition, use of the venom peptides is restricted to relatively acute experiments, since they are effective only after intravenous infusion and exhibit a short-lived duration of action. It is also unlikely that these peptides are completely specific in their site of action, since they have been reported,[32,33] to potentiate the biologic activity of certain bradykinin analogues that are not substrates of converting enzyme. Such results suggest that the venom derivatives may inhibit at least one other enzyme with bradykininase activity. SQ 14,225, the orally effective, highly potent, and apparently specific inhibitor of the enzyme,[34,35] whose properties are described in the accompanying chapters, appears to be the reagent with which to establish whether chronic blockade of converting enzyme is a safe and useful approach to regulating blood pressure. This compound is also a powerful inhibitor of bacterial COOH-terminal dipeptidyl peptidase activity,[36] and its use in bacterial systems may disclose some previously unrecognized functions served by this type of enzyme.

Biochemical Properties of Angiotensin-Converting Enzyme

Since angiotensin I is a peptide that is susceptible to the action of many enzymes present in crude extracts, serious characterization of converting enzyme required the development of artificial substrates. This requirement was met by model tripeptides protected at their NH_2 termini.[37,38] The simple assay procedures using such reagents have been useful for the detection of elevated converting-enzyme-like activity in pathological states, such as sarcoidosis,[39] and Gaucher's disease,[40] and in facilitating studies on the regulation of enzyme activity in cultured vascular endothelial cells[41] and in pulmonary alveolar macrophages[42] where steroid hormones are thought to induce de novo synthesis. These assay techniques have also greatly expedited the development of purification procedures for the enzyme. However, certain reservations apply to the use of model substrates. When they are employed, it is absolutely mandatory to establish that angiotensin I can actually function as substrate for the same enzyme whose activity their cleavage reflects. Furthermore, artificial substrates cannot be used to compare converting-enzyme activities in material from different species, since evolutionary conservation of the unnatural hydrolytic activity does not parallel that observed for cleavage of angiotensin I. Thus, pure dog and rabbit enzymes exhibit virtually identical kinetic parameters with angiotensin I as substrates, whereas the canine pulmonary enzyme is much less effective than that of the rabbit in catalyzing hydrolysis of Hip-His-Leu.[43]

Within recent years, emerging attention to the renin–angiotensin system has been reflected in the isolation of pure converting enzyme from a number of species and tissues. These include pig,[44,45] rabbit,[17,29,46] rat,[47] and dog[43] lung; pig[48] and bovine[49] kidney; and rabbit[50] as well as human[51] serum. The biochemical characteristics of the enzyme are of particular interest because it is a plasma membrane component that can be isolated in pure water-soluble form and may, therefore, be useful as a probe for examining membrane–enzyme interaction. The most extensively characterized of the pure preparations is that obtained from rabbit pulmonary membranes after solubilization with a nonionic detergent.[17,46] The molecular weight of the native enzyme, estimated by gradient centrifugation or equilibrium sedimentation analysis, was 130,000–140,000, and a similar figure for that of the reduced, denatured protein was obtained by gel electrophoresis and equilibrium sedimentation. This correspondence indicates that the enzyme contains a single polypeptide chain. Converting enzyme from a number of mammalian sources[17,43,50,52] has been found to elute paradoxically early during gel filtration, which leads to an erroneously high estimate of molecular weight. This discrepancy provided the first clue[17] that the enzyme contained covalently bound oligosaccharide, since the molecular weight of glycoproteins is often overestimated by the Sephadex technique. It is now known that carbohydrate accounts for 25–30% of the total weight of rabbit pulmonary angiotensin-converting enzyme.[46,50] Recent data[53] suggest that more than 90% of this carbohydrate is present in a unit of the average composition $(Fuc)_1(Man)_4(Gal)_4(GlcNAc)_4(S.A.)_1$ and that there are 12–14 such units attached via asparagine residues to each enzyme molecule. Pure rabbit[46] and dog[43] pulmonary enzymes display high absorption coefficient at 280 nm due to their large content of tryptophanyl residues. It has long been known that EDTA inhibits converting activity,[2] and the presence of a molar equivalent of zinc has been demonstrated in the rabbit and canine enzymes.[43,46]

As noted previously, the use of pure preparations has established that converting enzyme catalyzes sequential release of Phe-Arg and Ser-Pro from the COOH terminus of bradykinin.[17,18,43,50,54] In addition to acting on angiotensin I, the pure enzyme also cleaves successive dipeptidyl residues from the COOH terminus of renin tetradecapeptide substrate to yield angiotensin II as the limit product,[55] and it acts on des-Asp^1-angiotensin I to generate angiotensin III.[56] It exhibits decreasing activity with bradykinin analogues extended at their NH_2 terminus[57] and does not act on peptides containing a blocked COOH terminus (e.g., amides) or on peptide bonds containing the imino group of a prolyl residue.[54] Activity is inhibited by virtually all peptides including nonsubstrates such as saralasin[56] and unsubstituted tripeptides and dipeptides.[46] Certain of the venom peptides are distinguished by a particularly high affinity for the enzyme, and most contain Pro-Pro at their COOH terminus and are therefore not cleaved by its action.[29] Converting activity is also inhibited by various chelating agents and sulfhydryl-containing compounds but not by serine esterase inhibitors.[38] At least one enzyme has been characterized that can catalyze the conversion of angiotensin I to angiotensin II but that appears to function as an endopeptidase.[58] This enzyme, tonin, is of unknown physiological function and has been obtained in pure form from rat salivary glands and shown to possess characteristics completely different from those described above. It is interesting that a COOH-terminal dipeptidyl exopeptidase resembling converting enzyme in its catalytic properties has been obtained in homogeneous form from *Escherichia coli*.[59] A mutant defective in this enzyme has recently been isolated[36] and thus far found to differ from the parental strain only in its inability to grow using Acetyl-Ala-Ala-Ala as a sole source of nitrogen.

Immunobiology of Converting Enzyme

We become interested in angiotensin-converting enzyme in late 1971, by which time there was already good evidence that its active site was directly accessible to the circulation and that it represented a potentially important therapeutic target for controlling renovascular hypertension. We reasoned that if anticatalytic antibodies against the pure enzyme could be obtained, they might effectively inhibit enzyme activity in vivo, since after introduction into the circulation, they would not have to penetrate permeability barriers to reach their site of action. To examine the feasibility of this immunologic approach, we developed a procedure for isolating substantial amounts of the pure enzyme from rabbit pulmonary membranes[17,46] and elicited antienzyme antibodies in goats.[60] These antibodies inhibited enzyme activity, and a quantitative formulation for their anticatalytic action was devised. Specific antiholoenzyme antibodies were isolated from affinity columns containing pure enzyme as ligand covalently bonded to an insoluble matrix. Use of the antiholoenzyme antibodies enabled us to determine that each antibody molecule could bind two molecules of enzyme and that at least 18% of the antibody population was directed against determinants that influence catalysis. It was also established that inhibition of activity by antibody was essentially identical regardless of whether Hip-His-Leu, angiotensin I, or bradykinin was employed as substrate. A critical observation was that comparable antibody inhibition dose–response curves were obtained with the anti-lung enzyme antibody and equivalent amounts of activity from various rabbit organs and body fluids. This result indicated immunologic homology of the determinants influencing catalysis in the molecules from different anatomic locations and suggested that antibody against the lung enzyme could inhibit activity throughout the body, provided it had direct access from the circulation to the responsible enzymes at the various sites.

We were curious whether immunologic homology extended to parts of the enzyme molecule unrelated to its catalytic action. The degree of homology between protein molecules ultimately reflects the extent of identity of their amino acid sequences. We therefore determined the ratio of catalytic activity to competing antigen in physiological fluids and extracts from different organs.[60] Competing antigen was measured by its ability to displace radioiodinated pure pulmonary enzyme from an immune complex with anti-lung enzyme antibody. Our rationale was that if converting activity in an extract were due to a molecule identical to the pulmonary enzyme, then the ratio of catalytic activity to competing antigen in that extract should equal the specific activity of the pure lung enzyme (90–100 U/mg), provided the latter is used as the reference antigen. The competition radioimmunoassay represents a much more general measure of immunologic homology than does the anticatalytic assay, since it encompasses all antigenic determinants rather than only those associated with enzyme activity. As shown in Table 1, by this criterion, converting activity in kidney, brain, and serum is due to a molecule immunologically identical to the pure lung enzyme. Interestingly, the enzyme responsible for seminal fluid activity could be distinguished by this technique, although its inhibition by antibody had been found to be similar to that of the other enzyme

TABLE 1. Catalytic Activity and Immunoreactivity of Converting Enzyme from Various Rabbit Tissue Extracts and Fluids[a,b]

Tissue extract or fluid	Catalytic activity (mU/mg protein)	Competing antigen (μg/mg protein)	U/mg
Lung nonidet P-40 extract	545	5.89	93
Kidney nonidet P-40 extract	59	0.617	95
Brain nonidet P-40 extract	4.6	0.049	94
Serum	1.8	0.0174	103
Seminal plasma	219	0.676	324

[a] Data are from reference 60.

[b] Catalytic activity was measured using Hip-His-Leu as substrate. A unit of activity is the amount required to generate 1.0 μmole hippuric acid/min at 37°C.[38] Competing antigen was estimated using pure radioiodinated pulmonary enzyme as the displaceable antigen, pure unlabled enzyme as the reference antigen, and goat antibodies directed against the enzyme. The last column is the ratio of catalytic activity to competing antigen.

TABLE 2. Carbohydrate Composition of Angiotensin-Converting Enzyme from Rabbit Lung and Serum[a]

Carbohydrate	Lung enzyme[b]	Serum enzyme[b]	Lung enzyme[c]	Serum enzyme[c]
Fucose	10.2	7.6	8	6
Mannose	76.8	51.7	56	38
Galactose	75.0	67.0	55	49
N-acetylglucosamine	92.6	85.7	54	50
N-acetylneuraminic acid	35.4	110	14	45
Total	290	322	187	188

[a] Data are from reference 50.
[b] Measured in μg/mg of protein.
[c] Measured in residues/mole of protein.

activities. The lack of homology between the seminal plasma enzyme, which increases dramatically during sexual maturation,[27] and the pulmonary enzyme thus appears to be associated with determinants unrelated to catalysis. It should be emphasized, however, that even immunologic identity by the criterion described above does not necessarily imply complete chemical identity. This was established by comparing the properties of pure serum and pulmonary converting enzymes.[50] Since these exhibited immunologic identity, it was possible to develop an immunoaffinity technique using anti-lung enzyme antibody to select out serum enzyme molecules. This step, in conjunction with more conventional procedures, allowed us to achieve the 60,000-fold purification required to obtain the serum glycoprotein in pure form. Although the lung and serum enzymes exhibited many identical physicochemical, catalytic, and immunologic properties, the serum glycoprotein was found to be markedly enriched with respect to sialic acid (Table 2). This result is consistent with the possibility that the serum enzyme is derived from the tissue glycoprotein but represents a population from which those molecules containing a terminal, nonreducing galactosyl residue have been selectively extracted by a specific hepatic lectin,[61] which spares the fully sialylated molecules. Also consistent with this interpretation is the observation that an average molecule of the major oligosaccharide unit in the rabbit pulmonary enzyme contains at least one and possibly two exposed galactosyl residues and that this unit is heterogenous with respect to its content of sialic acid.[53] It is not surprising that immunologic identity fails to reflect the oligosaccharide moiety, since the major glycopeptide fraction obtained after pronase digestion, although accounting for about one-quarter of the weight of the enzyme, does not compete with the intact glycoprotein for binding to goat antienzyme antibodies.[53]

In order to assess the possibility that anti-lung enzyme antibodies might be effective in vivo, it was necessary not only to define their ability to inhibit activity throughout the body but also to determine whether they might be expected to reach the responsible enzymes after intravenous administration. Since Ryan et al.[11] had already demonstrated that the pulmonary enzyme was localized on the luminal surface of vascular endothelial cells, we examined the distribution of extrapulmonary enzyme using fluorescein-labeled anti-lung enzyme antibody.[10] In general, the enzyme was found to be a specific component of vascular endothelial cells, and this observation, coupled with the subcellular localization studies of Ryan et al.,[11] suggested that most enzyme would be directly accessible to circulating macromolecules. It is interesting that we found enzyme in the brush border of proximal tubular cells as well as in vascular endothelial cells of the kidney. While converting enzyme may conceivably play an important role in renal physiology, it is noteworthy that there is enormous variation with respect to its concentration in the kidneys of different species. For example, the enzyme is abundant in rabbit renal tissue and almost undetectable in that of the rat.[27]

The evidence that converting enzyme throughout the body was susceptible to inhibition by anti-lung enzyme antibodies and was directly accessible to the blood stream suggested that its activity could be regulated by antibodies introduced into the circulation and that an immunologic approach was feasible for suppressing angiotensin conversion and potentiating the action of bradykinin. The first direct experimental tests on this possibility were carried out in the homologous recipient animal, i.e., the rabbit.[62] It was found that the goat antibodies yielded an immediate immune-specific lethal reaction even in amounts insufficient to profoundly inhibit enzyme activity. Although small immune-dependent effects on the metabolism of exogenous angiotensin I and bradykinin were discerned, it was not possible to administer sufficient antibody to anticipate important alterations in the biological responses to these vasoactive peptides. Recently, the toxic process in rabbits associated with these anti-rabbit enzyme antibodies has been investigated in some detail.[63] The precipitating lethal hemodynamic event is acute pulmonary hypertension, which is consistent with an anaphylactoid reaction conceivably resulting from an antigen-adherent form of anaphylaxis.[64] Fab fragments prepared from the holoantibodies were found to induce the same deleterious consequences, indicating that the responsible immunologic mechanism is probably not mediated by complement.

In order to circumvent this lethal reaction, we used anti-rabbit enzyme antibody to probe immunologic homology among converting enzymes in crude pulmonary extracts of other species.[65] Using these antibodies, it was possible to demonstrate homology to the rabbit enzyme in preparations from rat, guinea pig, and dog lungs by immunodiffusion, competition radioimmunoassay, and cross-anticatalytic action. A surprising finding[65] was that antisera from different goats varied markedly in their spectrum of inhibitory action on the heterologous activities, although they exhibited comparable inhibitory effects on homologous enzyme and yielded similar estimates of homology in the various extracts by immunodiffusion and radioimmunoassay. Presumably, this reflects the fact that the small number of catalytic determinants need not be representative of those comprised by the entire enzyme molecule. Another unanticipated result was that holoantibodies and Fab fragments were equally effective as inhibitors of the homologous enzyme, whereas the Fab fragments were much less effective than the holoantibodies in their cross-anticatalytic action.[43]

The rat was selected to examine the effect in vivo of anti-rabbit enzyme antibodies on the metabolism of vasoactive peptides. This animal tolerated the intravenous infusion of the heterologous antibodies without ill effect,[65] and it was possible to administer at least nine times the amount of immune globulin required to completely inhibit the converting activity of a pair of rat lungs as extrapolated from the linear portion of an antibody inhibition dose–response curve. Immunologic blockade of converting enzyme in vivo was readily demonstrable in this heterologous system,[65] although there was considerable variation in the amounts of different antibody preparations required to achieve it. The immunologic suppression occurred almost immediately after the globulin infusion and persisted several days, i.e., much longer than the inhibition associated with chemical agents. Table 3 summarizes the immune-specific effect on vasoactive peptide metabolism induced by these anti-rabbit enzyme antibodies in the rat. The vasopressor response to angiotensin I and the vasodepressor action of bradykinin were respectively inhibited and potentiated by approximately an order of mag-

TABLE 3. Effect of Immune Globulin on Rat Response to Vasoactive Peptides[a]

		Relative dose required to elicit standard test response		
Animals	Globulin	Angiotensin I	Angiotensin II	Bradykinin
7	Immune	8.8 (3.5–13.6)	2.9 (1.8–3.9)	0.077 (0.040–0.25)
2	Preimmune	0.85 (0.80–0.90)	0.95 (0.70–1.2)	1.1 (1.1–1.1)
4	Nonimmune	0.96 (0.74–1.1)	0.74 (0.60–0.95)	0.94 (0.86–1.0)

[a] The amount of peptide required to elicit a change in blood pressure of 25 mm Hg was determined before and 1 hr after infusion of globulin. The data are expressed as ratios with the preinfusion dose normalized to 1.0. Mean and extreme values are shown for each group. For further details see reference 65.

TABLE 4. Vasodepressor Effect of Antirabbit Enzyme Antibody in the Rat

			Mean arterial pressure (mm Hg)[a]		
Animal	Globulin	*n*	Preinfusion	Postinfusion	Decrease
Hypertensive	Immune	5	152 (130–177)	104 (97–118)	48 (31–75)
	Nonimmune	5	142 (120–159)	140 (118–156)	2 (1–5)
Normotensive	Immune	5	108 (105–110)	84 (73–93)	24 (14–34)
	Nonimmune	2	111 (110–112)	107 (107–107)	4 (3–5)

[a] Mean arterial pressures were determined before and 24 hr after infusion of globulins. Average and extreme values are shown for each experimental group. For further details see reference 66.

nitude. Biological specificity was indicated by the fact that there was no immune alteration of the vascular response to norepinephrine. A small but definite inhibition of the vasopressor response to angiotensin II was unexpected. One possible explanation for this result is that it may reflect a functional association of converting enzyme and the angiotensin II receptor such that antibody bound to the enzyme may, by steric hinderance, prevent access of angiotensin II to its effector site.

The effect of the anti-rabbit enzyme antibodies on the blood pressure of rats with renovascular hypertension and on that of normotensive animals (Table 4) was also examined.[66] In the two-kidney Goldblatt hypertensive model, there was a dramatic immune-dependent reduction of mean arterial pressure to a normal level that persisted for as long as 72 hr. Curiously, the pressure nadir was not reached until 24 hr after the antibody infusion, although inhibition of the vasopressor response to angiotensin I is already maximal within 1 hr. This result may reflect the partial-dependence of hypertension in this model on secondary pressor influences of angiotensin II, such as increased elaboration of aldosterone by the adrenal cortex.[67] An important immune-specific decrease of mean arterial pressure (22%) was also noted in normotensive animals, although it was considerably less than that (32%) found in the hypertensive group. Previous investigations with chemical inhibitors of converting enzyme in conscious, unrestrained rats have suggested that the contribution of the renin–angiotensin system to the maintenance of normal blood pressure is relatively small.[34] The vasodepressor effect of antienzyme antibodies observed by us in normotensive animals may indicate that this system plays a role in the long-term support of arterial blood pressure that could not be discerned in acute studies.

Conclusions

Angiotensin-converting enzyme is a COOH terminal dipeptidyl exopeptidase. Its two most important currently recognized substrates are the vasoactive peptides angiotensin I and bradykinin, and its action on each is physiologically vasopressor. It consists of a single glycopolypeptide chain with a molecular weight of approximately 140,000 and a molar equivalent of associated zinc. Although the lung plays a particularly prominent role in generating angiotensin II destined for the systemic circulation, the responsible enzyme is found in most organs and is a relatively specific component of vascular endothelial cells where it is localized on the luminal surface of the plasma membrane. Circulating molecules probably derive from sloughing or secretion of the tissue glycoprotein. Inhibition of the enzyme reduces the vasopressor response to angiotensin I and potentiates the vasodepressor effect of bradykinin. Chemical inhibitors appear to be therapeutically useful for eliminating the renin-dependent component of human hypertensive disease. Since the enzyme is directly exposed to the circulation, specific antienzyme antibodies may provide a biologically cognitive immunologic probe to complement the chemical inhibitors in studies directed at delineating the contribution of the renin–angiotensin system to normal and pathological processes.

ACKNOWLEDGMENTS. Research reported herein was supported in part by Grants HL 21394 and HL 07071 from the National Heart, Lung and Blood Institute, Bethesda, Maryland.

References

1. Soffer RL: Angiotensin-converting enzyme and the regulation of vasoactive peptides. *Ann Rev Biochem* 45:73–94, 1976.
2. Skeggs LT, Marsh WM, Kahn JR, et al: Existence of two forms of hypertensin. *J Exp Med* 99:275–282, 1954.
3. Lentz KE, Skeggs LT, Wood KR, et al: The amino acid composition of hypertensin II and its biochemical relationship to hypertensin I. *J Exp Med* 104:183–191, 1956.
4. Helmer OM: Differentiation between two forms of angiotonin by means of spirally cut strips of rabbit aorta. *Am J Physiol* 188:571–577, 1957.
5. Skeggs LT, Kahn JR, Shumway NP: The preparation and function of the hypertensin-converting enzyme. *J Exp Med* 103:295–299, 1956.
6. Ng KKF, Vane JR: Conversion of angiotensin I to angiotensin II. *Nature* 215:762–766, 1967.
7. Ng KKF, Vane JR: Fate of angiotensin I in the circulation. *Nature* 218:144–150, 1968.
8. Roth M, Wietzman AF, Piquilloud Y: Converting enzyme content of different tissues of the rat. *Experientia* 25:1257, 1969.
9. Cushman DW, Cheung HS: Concentration of angiotensin-converting enzyme in tissues of the rat. *Biochim Biophys Acta* 250:261–265, 1971.
10. Caldwell PRB, Seegal BC, Hsu KC, et al: Angiotensin-converting enzyme. Vascular endothelial localization. *Science* 191:1050–1051, 1976.
11. Ryan JW, Ryan VS, Schultz DR, et al: Subcellular localization of pulmonary angiotensin-converting enzyme. *Biochem J* 146:497–499, 1975.
12. Hodge RL, Ng KKF, Vane JR: Disappearance of angiotensin from the circulation of the dog. *Nature* 215:138–141, 1967.

13. Ferreira SH, Vane JR: The disappearance of bradykinin and eledoisin in the circulation and vascular beds of the cat. *Br J Pharmacol Chemother* 30:417–424, 1967.
14. Bakhle YS: Conversion of angiotensin I to angiotensin II by cell-free extracts of dog lung. *Nature* 220:919–920, 1968.
15. Ferreira SH: A bradykinin-potentiating factor (BPF) present in the venom of *Bothrops jararaca*. *Br J Pharmacol Chemother* 24:163–169, 1965.
16. Ferreira SH, Greene LJ, Alabaster VA, et al: Activity of various fractions of bradykinin-potentiating factor against angiotensin I-converting enzyme. *Nature* 225:379–380, 1970.
17. Soffer RL, Reza R, Caldwell PRB: Angiotensin-converting enzyme from rabbit pulmonary particles. *Proc Natl Acad Sci USA* 71:1720–1724, 1974.
18. Dorer FE, Kahn JR, Lentz KE, et al: Hydrolysis of bradykinin by angiotensin-converting enzyme. *Circ Res* 34:824–827, 1974.
19. Ferreira SH, Bartelt DC, Greene LJ: Isolation of bradykinin-potentiating peptides from *Bothrops jararaca* venom. *Biochemistry* 9:2583–2593, 1970.
20. Stewart JM, Ferreira SH, Greene LJ: Bradykinin-potentiating peptide PCA-Lys-Trp-Ala-Pro. *Biochem Pharmacol* 20:1557–1567, 1971.
21. Krieger EM, Salgado HC, Assan CJ, et al: Potential screening test for detection of overactivity of renin–angiotensin system. *Lancet* 1:269–271, 1971.
22. Ondetti MA, Williams NJ, Sabo EF, et al: Angiotensin-converting inhibitors from the venom of *Bothrops jararaca:* Isolation, elucidation of structure and synthesis. *Biochemistry* 10:4033–4039, 1971.
23. Kato H, Suzuki T: Bradykinin-potentiating peptides from the venom of *Agkistrodon halys blomhoffi*. Isolation of five bradykinin potentiators and amino acid sequences of two of them, potentiators B and C. *Biochemistry* 10:972–980, 1971.
24. Greene LJ, Camargo ACM, Krieger EM, et al: Inhibition of the conversion of angiotensin I to angiotensin II and potentiation of bradykinin by small peptides present in *Bothrops jararaca* venom. *Circ Res* 31(suppl II):62–71, 1972.
25. Miller ED, Samuels AL, Haber E, et al: Inhibition of angiotensin conversion in experimental renovascular hypertension. *Science* 177:1108–1109, 1972.
26. Engel SL, Schaeffer TR, Waugh MH, et al: Effects of the nonapeptide SQ 20,881 on blood pressure of rats with experimental renovascular hypertension. *Proc Soc Exp Biol Med* 143:483–487, 1973.
27. Cushman DW, Cheung HS: Studies in vitro of angiotensin-converting enzyme of lung and other tissues, in Genest J, Koiw E (eds): *Hypertension 1972*. Berlin, Springer–Verlag, 1972, pp 532–541.
28. Cushman DW, Pluscek J, Williams NJ, et al: Inhibition of angiotensin-converting enzyme by analogs of peptides from *Bothrops jararaca* venom. *Experientia* 29:1032–1035, 1973.
29. Cheung HS, Cushman DW: Inhibition of homogenous angiotensin-converting enzyme of rabbit lung by synthetic venom peptides of *Bothrops jararaca*. *Biochim Biophys Acta* 293:451–463, 1973.
30. Collier JG, Robinson BV, Vane JR: Reduction of pressor effects of angiotensin I in man by snythetic nonapeptide (BPP_{9a} or SQ 20,881) which inhibits converting enzyme. *Lancet* 1:72–74, 1973.
31. Case DB, Wallace JM, Keim HJ, et al: Possible role or renin in hypertension as suggested by renin–sodium profiling and inhibition of converting enzyme. *N Engl J Med 296*:641–646, 1977.
32. Ondetti MA, Engel SE: Bradykinin analogs containing β-homoaminoacids. *J Med Chem* 18:761–763, 1975.

33. LeDuc LE, Marshall GR, Needleman P: Differentiation of bradykinin receptors and of kininases with conformation analogs of bradykinin. *Mol Pharmacol* 14:413–421, 1978.
34. Ondetti MA, Rubin B, Cushman DW: Design of specific inhibitors of angiotensin-converting enzyme: New class of orally effective antihypertensive agents. *Science* 196:441–444, 1977.
35. Cushman DW, Cheung HS, Sabo EF, et al: Design of potent competitive inhibitors of angiotensin-converting enzyme. Carboxyalkanoyl and mercaptoalkanoyl amino acids. *Biochemistry* 16:5484–5491, 1977.
36. Deutch CE, Soffer RL: *Escherichia coli* mutants deficient in dipeptidyl carboxypeptidase. *Proc Natl Acad Sci USA* 75:5998–6001, 1978.
37. Piquilloud Y, Reinharz A, Roth M: Studies on the angiotensin-converting enzyme with different substrates. *Biochim Biopys Acta* 206:136–142, 1970.
38. Cushman DW, Cheung HS: Spectrophotometric assay and properties of angiotensin-converting enzyme of rabbit lung. *Biochem Pharmacol* 20:1637–1648, 1971.
39. Lieberman J: Elevation of serum angiotensin-converting enzyme (ACE) level in sarcoidosis. *Am J Med* 59:365–372, 1975.
40. Lieberman J, Beutler E: Elevation of serum angiotensin-converting enzyme in Gaucher's disease. *N Engl J Med* 294:1442–1444, 1976.
41. Ryan US, Ryan JW, Chiu AT: Kininase II (angiotensin-converting enzyme) and endothelial cells in culture. *Adv Exp Med Biol* 70:217–227, 1976.
42. Friedland J, Setton C, Silverstein E: Angiotensin-converting enzyme: Induction by steroids in rabbit alveolar macrophages in culture. *Science* 197:64–65, 1977.
43. Conroy JM, Hartley JL, Soffer RL: Canine pulmonary angiotensin-converting enzyme. Physicochemical, catalytic and immunological properties. *Biochim Biophys Acta* 524: 403–412, 1978.
44. Dorer FE, Kahn JR, Lentz KE, et al: Purification and properties of angiotensin-converting enzyme from hog lung. *Circ Res* 31:356–366, 1972.
45. Nakajima T, Oshima G, Yeh HSJ, et al: Purification of the angiotensin I converting enzyme of the lung. *Biochim Biophys Acta* 315:430–438, 1973.
46. Das M, Soffer RL: Pulmonary angiotensin-converting enzyme: Structural and catalytic properties. *J Biol Chem* 250:6762–6768, 1975.
47. Lanzillo JJ, Fanburg BL: Membrane-bound angiotensin-converting enzyme from rat lung. *J Biol Chem* 249:2312–2318, 1974.
48. Oshima G, Gecse A, Erdös EG: Angiotensin I converting enzyme of the kidney cortex. *Biochim Biophys Acta* 350:26–37, 1974.
49. Eliseeva YE, Pavlikhina LV, Orekhovich VN: Isolation of carboxycathepsin (peptidyl dipeptidase 3.4.15.1) from beef kidneys. *Dokl Adad Nauk SSSR* 217:953–956, 1974.
50. Das M, Hartley JL, Soffer RL: Serum angiotensin-converting enzyme. Isolation and relationship to the pulmonary enzyme. *J Biol Chem* 252:1316–1319, 1977.
51. Lanzillo JJ, Fanburg BL: Angiotensin I converting enzyme from human plasma. *Biochemistry* 16:5491–5495, 1977.
52. Lanzillo JJ, Fanburg BL: The estimation and comparison of molecular weight of angiotensin I converting enzyme by sodium dodecyl sulfate-polyacrylamide gel electrophoresis. *Biochim Biophys Acta* 439:125–132, 1976.
53. Hartley JL, Soffer RL: On the oligosaccharide moiety of angiotensin-converting enzyme. *Biochem Biophys Res Commun* 83:1545–1552, 1978.
54. Eliseeva YE, Orekhovich VN, Pavlikhina LV, et al: Carboxycathepsin. A key regulatory component of two physiologic systems involved in regulation of blood pressure. *Clin Chim Acta* 31:413–419, 1971.

55. Dorer FE, Kahn JR, Lentz KE, et al: Formation of angiotensin II from tetradecapeptide renin substrate by angiotensin-converting enzyme. *Biochem Pharmacol* 24:1137–1139, 1975.
56. Chin AT, Ryan JW, Stewart JM, et al: Formation of angiotensin III by angiotensin-converting enzyme. *Biochem J* 155:189–192, 1976.
57. Dorer FE, Ryan JW, Stewart JM: Hydrolysis of bradykinin and its higher homologues by angiotensin-converting enzyme. *Biochem J* 141:915–917, 1974.
58. Demassieux S, Boucher R, Grisé C, et al: Purification and characterization of tonin. *Can J Biochem* 54:788–795, 1976.
59. Yaron A, Mlynar D, Berger A: A dipeptidocarboxypeptidase from *E. coli Biochem Biophys Res Commun* 47:897–902, 1972.
60. Das M, Soffer RL: Pulmonary angiotensin-converting enzyme antienzyme antibody. *Biochemistry* 15:5088–5094, 1976.
61. Ashwell G, Morell AG: The role of surface carbohydrates in the hepatic recognition and transport of circulating glycoproteins. *Adv Enzymol Relat Areas Mol Biol* 41:91–128, 1974.
62. Caldwell PRB, Wigger HJ, Das M et al: Angiotensin-converting enzyme. Effect of antienzyme antibody in vivo. *FEBS Lett* 63:82–84, 1976.
63. Dickerson DD, Murthy VS: Anaphylactoid reaction after intravenous injection of antibodies against angiotensin-converting enzyme (ACE) in anaesthetized rabbits. *Fed Proc* 37:590A, 1978.
64. Becker EL, Austin KF: Anaphylaxis, in Miescher PA, Muller-Eberhard HJ (eds): *Textbook of Immunopathology*, vol I. New York, Grune & Stratton, 1976, pp 117–135.
65. Conroy JM, Hoffman H, Kirk ES, et al: Pulmonary angiotensin-converting enzyme. Interspecies homology and inhibition by heterologous antibody *in vivo*. *J Biol Chem* 251:4828–4832, 1976.
66. Markle RA, Sonnenblick EH, Conroy JM, et al: Reversal of renovascular hypertension by antibodies specific for angiotensin-converting enzyme. *Proc Natl Acad Sci USA* 75:5702–5705, 1978.
67. Laragh JH, Angers M, Kelly WG, et al: Hypotensive agents and pressor substances. The effect of epinephrine, norepinephrine, angiotensin II and others on the secretory rate of aldosterone in man. *JAMA* 174:234–240, 1960.

Chapter 8

Design of New Antihypertensive Drugs

Potent and Specific Inhibitors of Angiotensin-Converting Enzyme

David W. Cushman, Hong Son Cheung,
Emily F. Sabo, and Miguel A. Ondetti

Introduction

Angiotensin-converting enzyme is one of the enzyme components of the renin–angiotensin system (Figure 1), the products of which play physiologically important roles in maintenance of cardiovascular homeostasis and contribute to the elevation of arterial blood pressure in various hypertensive disease states.[1-4] The immediate product of the action of angiotensin-converting enzyme is the octapeptide, angiotensin II, the most potent naturally occurring pressor substance known. Angiotensin III, a heptapeptide derived from a further enzymatic cleavage of angiotensin II, is a potent stimulator of secretion of aldosterone by the adrenal cortex.[5] Angiotensin-converting enzyme also plays a biologically important role in the inactivation of the potent vasodepressor peptide bradykinin.[6]

Peptide Inhibitors of Angiotensin-Converting Enzyme

Until recently, the only pharmacologically characterized inhibitors of angiotensin-converting enzyme have been the nonapeptide, SQ 20,881 (< Glu-Trp-Pro-Arg-Pro-Gln-Ile-Pro-Pro), and several related peptides isolated from snake venom.[7,8] SQ 20,881 abolishes the pressor activity of angiotensin I, augments the vasodepressor activity of bradykinin, and

Reprinted from *Progress in Cardiovascular Diseases* 21(3):176–182, 1978, by permission of the authors and the publisher, Grune & Stratton.

DAVID W. CUSHMAN, Ph.D, HONG SON CHEUNG, M.S., EMILY F. SABO, B.S., and MIGUEL A. ONDETTI, Ph.D. • The Squibb Institute for Medical Research, Princeton, New Jersey 08540.

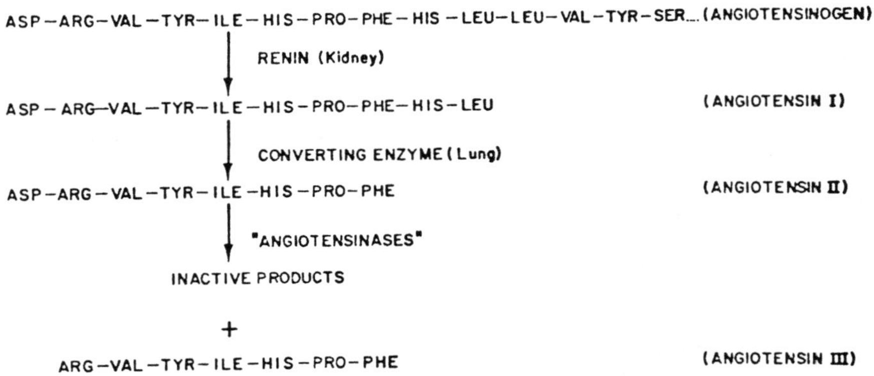

FIGURE 1. The renin–angiotensin system. Angiotensin-converting enzyme cleaves the dipeptide residue His-Leu from the carboxyl terminal end of the inactive decapeptide angiotensin I to form the potent vasopressor octapeptide angiotensin II.

lowers blood pressure in some animal models of renovascular hypertension.[9,10] Clinical studies with this nonapeptide have given a preliminary indication of the potential therapeutic utility of inhibitors of angiotensin-converting enzyme. At intravenous doses of 1 mg/kg or lower, SQ 20,881 produced a pronounced lowering of blood pressure in patients with renovascular and malignant hypertension. [11-15] A significant, but less dramatic, antihypertensive effect was observed in many patients whose condition had been diagnosed as essential hypertension.[11,12] In patients from all three classes of hypertension, a greater decrease in blood pressure was obtained when SQ 20,881 was administered after sodium depletion. The observed antihypertensive activity of SQ 20,881 could be due to any combination of its inhibition of vasoconstriction (angiotensin II), inhibition of aldosterone secretion (angiotensin III), or prolongation of the hypotensive effect of bradykinin.[16]

Although SQ 20,881 is a nontoxic antihypertensive agent of novel mechanism, its therapeutic utility is limited by its lack of oral activity. However, studies with SQ 20,881 and our knowledge or the properties of homogeneous angiotensin-converting enzyme of rabbit lung permitted the design of nonpeptidic compounds capable of interacting specifically with the active site of angiotensin-converting enzyme. These studies have led to a series of increasingly more potent and specific orally active inhibitors of angiotensin-converting enzyme.

Hypothetical Model of the Active Site of Angiotensin-Converting Enzyme

Early studies with substrates and inhibitors of angiotensin-converting enzyme[8,17] had indicated that this peptidase was a carboxypeptidase similar to pancreatic carboxypeptidase A, except that it releases dipeptides rather than single amino acids from the carboxylic acid end of peptide substrates. Other studies[18] had suggested that angiotensin-converting enzyme, like carboxypeptidase A, was a zinc-containing metalloprotein, an observation that has been verified by other investigators.[19] It thus seemed reasonable to assume that the mechanism of action and, therefore, the active site of angiotensin-converting enzyme would be similar to that of carboxypeptidase A.

The important substrate-binding groups at the active site of carboxypeptidase A,[20] and, in our hypothetical model, of the active site of angiotensin-converting enzyme, are depicted in Figure 2. Positively charged groups at both sites (arginine residue 145 in the case of carboxypeptidase A) form ionic bonds with the negatively charged terminal carboxyl groups of the substrates. An adjacent "hydrophobic pocket" with great affinity for aromatic rings is responsible for the specificity of carboxypeptidase A toward substrates containing carboxyl-terminal aromatic amino acids. No such hydrophobic pocket is expected to be present at the active site of angiotensin-converting enzyme, since its substrate specificity is very broad; but we felt that this enzyme might have a group, probably a hydrogen bond donor, that could bind the terminal nonscissile peptide bond of its substrate. The zinc ions are suitably located at the active sites of both enzymes to polarize the carbonyl groups of the scissile peptide bonds of substrates, making them more susceptible to hydrolytic cleavage.

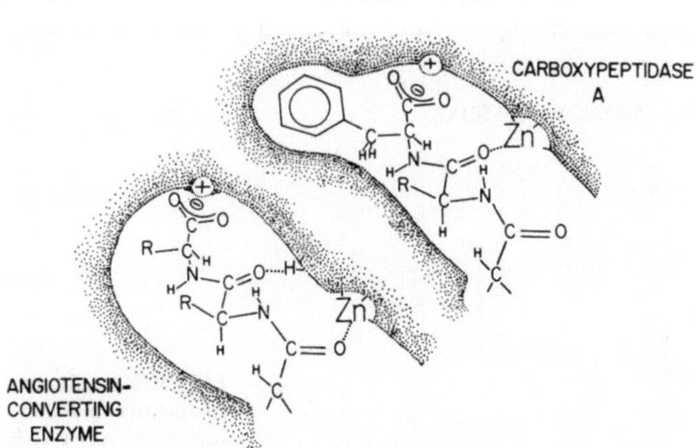

FIGURE 2. Model of the active site of angiotensin-converting enzyme compared to that of carboxypeptidase A. Postively charged groups on both enzymes bind the negatively charged carboxyl groups of the peptide substrates, and the enzyme-bound zinc ions polarize the carbonyl groups of the peptide bonds to be broken. The active site of carboxypeptidase A has a hydrophobic pocket (left in the figure) that has great affinity for an aromatic side-chain of the terminal amino acid residue of a substrate. Angiotensin-converting enzyme is proposed to have a hydrogen-bonding residue with affinity for the terminal peptide bond of a substrate.

Design of Inhibitors of Angiotensin-Converting Enzyme

In 1973, Byers and Wolfenden[21] reported that D-2-benzylsuccinic acid was a potent competitive inhibitor of carboxypeptidase A (enzyme inhibitor dissociation constant $K_i = 4.5 \times 10^{-7}$M). One of the most plausible explanations for this high inhibitory potency would be the simultaneous and stereospecific interaction of the inhibitor molecule with three substrate-binding groups at the active site of carboxypeptidase A (Figure 3). This observation, along with our previous speculations about the nature of the active site of angiotensin-converting enzyme, led us to pursue the design of specific inhibitors of this peptidase.[22,23]

The most distinctive feature of the hypothetical active site of angiotensin-converting enzyme (Figure 2) is that the distance between the cationic carboxyl-binding site and the zinc atom is greater than that present in carboxypeptidase A, probably by about the length of one amino acid unit. Therefore, we postulated that a succinyl amino acid rather than a succinic acid should be the prototype for inhibitors of angiotensin-converting enzyme. To test this hypothesis, we synthesized succinyl-L-proline (Figure 4; R_3 = H). The choice of proline was made on the basis of our structure–activity studies with peptidic inhibitors of this enzyme.[17] Succinyl-L-proline (SQ 13,745; Table 1) was only a moderately potent inhibitor of angiotensin-converting enzyme of rabbit lung; but, in an assay system[22,24] employing excised guinea pig ileum contracting in response to various agonists (Table 1), it showed the characteristic profile of a specific inhibitor of angiotensin-converting enzyme: inhibition of the contractile response to

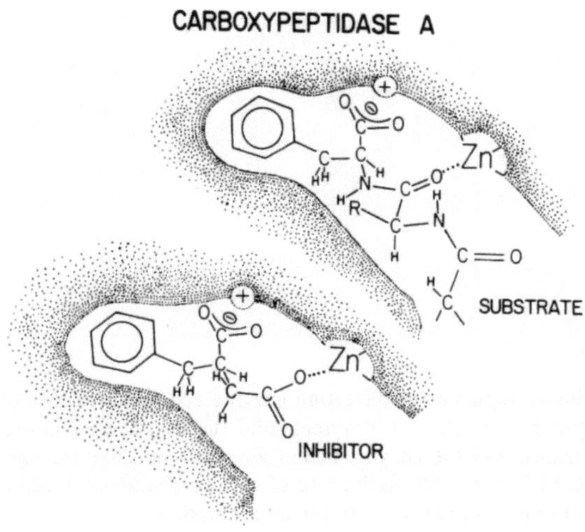

FIGURE 3. Binding of a potent competitive inhibitor of carboxypeptidase A. D-2-Benzylsuccinic acid binds as shown to the hydrophobic pocket, positively charged residue, and zinc ion of carboxypeptidase A and competes with the substrate for these binding sites on the enzyme.

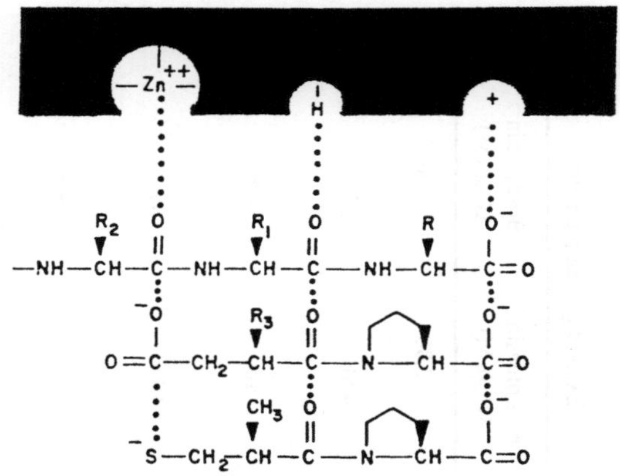

FIGURE 4. Proposed binding in inhibitors of angiotensin-converting enzyme. Peptide substrates, carboxylalkanoyl amino acid inhibitors, and mercaptoalkanoyl amino acid inhibitors are all proposed to bind, as shown, to the zinc ion, hydrogen-bonding group, and positively charged group at the active site of angiotensin-converting enzyme.

angiotensin I, augmentation of the contractile response to bradykinin, and no effect on responses to angiotensin II, acetylcholine, or other agonists. These results indicated that we had found a new lead in the search for inhibitors of the renin–angiotensin system.

A large number of compounds were synthesized with the aim of improving on the intrinsic inhibitory potency of succinyl-L-proline. These studies, which culminated in the synthesis of SQ 13,297 and SQ 14,102 (Table 1), can be summarized as follows: (1) Of several succinyl-L-amino acids tested, L-proline yielded the most active inhibitor; succinyl derivatives of D-amino acids were very weak inhibitors. (2) The optimal distance between the carboxyls of the dicarboxylic acid moiety was that of glutaric acid. (3) Substituents on the dicarboxylic acid group only led to increased inhibitory activity when positioned alpha to the amide bond, and in the D configuration (SQ 13,297 and SQ 14,102; Table 1); analogous compounds with L-substituents (SQ 13,493 and SQ 14,116) were at least 100 times less active. This positional and stereospecificity is consistent with our hypothetical model (Figure 4).

Even though SQ 13,297 and SQ 14,102 were 10–20 times more active than the prototype succinyl-L-proline (Table 1) and inhibited angiotensin-converting enzyme in vivo after oral administration, it was felt that their potency was not sufficient to yield a useful orally active antihypertensive drug. Once again, a careful consideration of the tentative model for the binding of these inhibitors to the active site of angiotensin-converting enzyme provided a clue for further development. If the carboxyl group of the carboxyalkanoyl moiety of these compounds was serving as a ligand of the enzyme-bound zinc ion as proposed in Figure 4, it was possible that replacement of this carboxyl group with a better ligand than the anionic

TABLE 1. Activities of Inhibitors of Angiotensin-Converting Enzyme

Compound number	Structure	Angiotensin-converting enzyme of rabbit lung[a]		Excised guinea pig ileum[b]	
		IC_{50}(μM)	K_i(μM)	Angiotensin I IC_{50}(μM)	Bradykinin AC_{50}(μM)
SQ 20,881	<Glu-Trp-Pro-Arg-Pro-Gln-Ile-Pro-Pro	0.55	0.10	0.06	0.0015
SQ 13,745	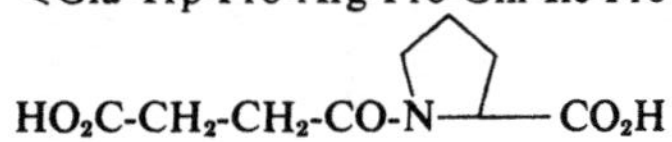	330	—	440	37
SQ 13,297	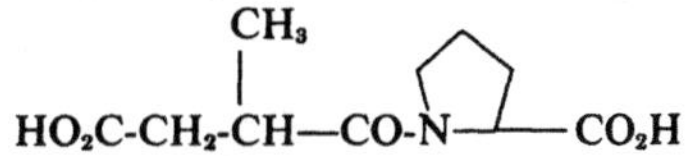	22	2.5	18	0.87
SQ 13,493	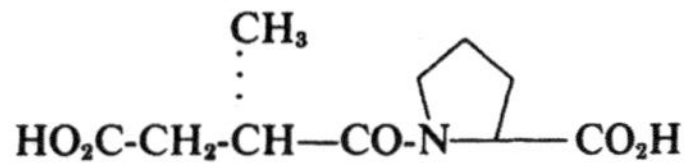	1480	—	>400	65
SQ 14,102	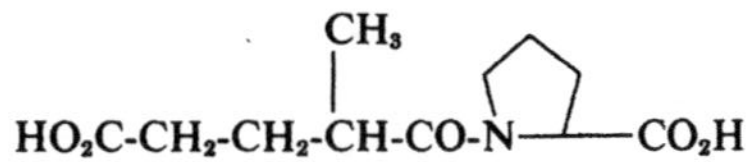	4.9	0.8	23	4.9
SQ 14,116	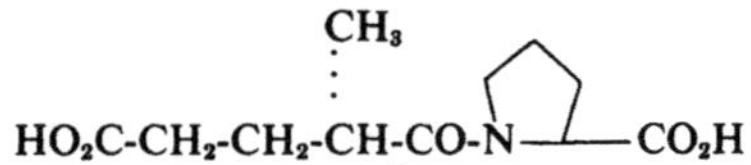	950	—	>400	19
SQ 13,863	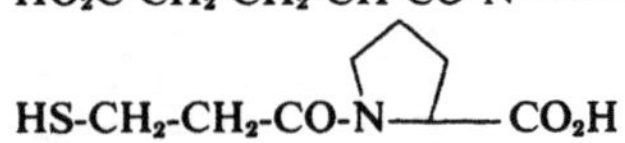	0.20	0.012	0.30	0.025
SQ 14,225	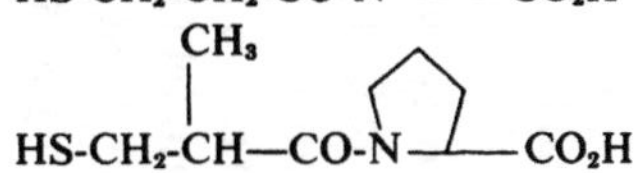	0.023	0.0017	0.023	0.0032
SQ 14,534	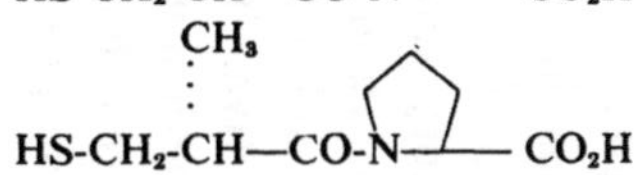	2.4	—	8.2	15

[a] The assay for inhibition of angiotensin-converting enzyme of rabbit lung is described by Cushman and Cheung.[18]

[b] The in vitro test for inhibition (IC_{50}) or augmentation (AC_{50}) of contractile responses of guinea pig ileum to various agonists is described by Ondetti et al.[22]; none of the compounds had any effect, at concentrations of 500 μM, on the contractile responses due to angiotensin II or acetylcholine.

oxygen would give a rise to a better inhibitor. Nitrogen and sulfur functionalities would be expected to meet this requirement. Several nitrogen-containing derivatives were synthesized, but none had significantly increased inhibitory potency. On the other hand, the replacement of the carboxyl with a sulfhydryl group led to the synthesis of SQ 13,863 (Table 1), an inhibitor that was more than 1000 times more inhibitory than succinyl-L-proline.

The outstanding activity of SQ 13,863 prompted a thorough study of the structural specificity of such mercaptoalkanoyl amino acids. Proline was again found to be the amino acid of choice, and the L configuration was an almost absolute requirement for activity. The optimal separation between the sulfhydryl and carboxyl residues of the mercaptoalkanoyl moiety was that of 3-mercaptopropionic acid (SQ 13,863), although 2-mercaptoacetyl amino acids are also quite active. It is important to point out that a sulfhydryl and a carboxyl group separated by an aliphatic chain do not per se yield potent inhibitors, an observation that supports the contention that a hydrogen-bonding region might be present in the active site of angiotensin-converting enzyme as postulated in the model (Figures 2–4). The introduction of a methyl group alpha to the amide bond of SQ 13,863 again led to a significant improvement of the inhibitory activity. The requirement for a substituent of the proper optical configuration is again strikingly apparent when one compares SQ 14,225 and SQ 14,534 (Table 1). The remarkable potency and specificity of the inhibitors developed so far lend considerable support to the hypothetical model with which we started our investigations (Figures 2–4).

Enzymatic Studies with SQ 14,225

Determinations of IC_{50} values for structure–activity correlations were performed with a spectrophotometric assay employing hippuryl-L-histidyl-L-leucine (Hip-His-Leu) as the substrate.[18] For kinetic experiments or other studies of the mechanism of action of SQ 14,225, angiotensin-converting enzyme was employed that had been purified to homogeneity.[8] For experiments in which increased sensitivity was required, cleavage of Hip-His-Leu was assayed by fluorometric determination of the amount of His-Leu released.[8]

Compounds such as SQ 13,863 and SQ 14,225, which were designed for multifunctional interaction at the active site of angiotensin-converting enzyme, might be expected to be reasonably specific for inhibition of this enzyme. Although these mercaptoalkanoyl amino acids have been tested for inhibition of only a few other enzymes, they have been evaluated as inhibitors of the similar zinc-containing peptidase, carboxypeptidase A. As shown in Table 2, SQ 13,863 and SQ 14,225 inhibit carboxypeptidase A only at concentrations that are 10,000–50,000 times higher than those required for their inhibition of angiotensin-converting enzyme. Benzylsuccinic acid, the potent inhibitor of carboxypeptidase A that we have used as a model for development of our own inhibitors of angiotensin-converting enzyme, does not inhibit angiotensin-converting enzyme. These comparisons not only strengthen our hypothetical model for interaction of compounds such as SQ 13,863 and SQ 14,225 with the active site of angiotensin-converting enzyme, but also provide evidence for the specificity of these mercaptoalkanoyl amino acids as inhibitors of angiotensin-converting enzyme.

Kinetic studies of the effect of substrate concentration on inhibition of an enzyme such as angiotensin-converting enzyme may be used to determine both the absolute binding affinity of the inhibitor and to provide evidence as to its mechanism of action. Double reciprocal plots, such as that shown in Figure 5, indicate that both carboxyalkanoyl amino acids (SQ 13,297 and SQ 14,102) and mercaptoalkanoyl amino acids (SQ 13,863 and SQ 14,225) are purely competitive inhibitors. The plots shown in Figure 5 indicate that SQ 14,225 is a competitive inhibitor with a K_i value (enzyme-inhibitor dissociation constant) of 1.7×10^{-9} M.

Thus, using a simple hypothetical model for the active site of angiotensin-converting enzyme, we have been able to design compounds of quite simple molecular structure that are unusually potent and specific as inhibitors of this biologically important enzyme. SQ 14,225 is an orally active inhibitor of angiotensin-converting enzyme in rats and an orally effective antihypertensive agent in animal models.[22,24,25] It thus appears to have great potential as a tool for studying the role of the renin–angiotensin system in different physiological and pathological situations and for use in the therapy of human hypertensive disease.

TABLE 2. Inhibition of Angiotensin-Converting Enzyme and Carboxypeptidase A

Compound	Angiotensin-converting enzyme $IC_{50}(\mu M)$	Carboxypeptidase A $IC_{50}(\mu M)$
Carboxypeptidase inhibitor		
D-2-Benzylsuccinic acid	>5000	1.1
Converting-enzyme inhibitors		
SQ 20,881	0.55	1800
SQ 13,297	22	1500
SQ 13,863	0.20	1500
SQ 14,225	0.023	1500

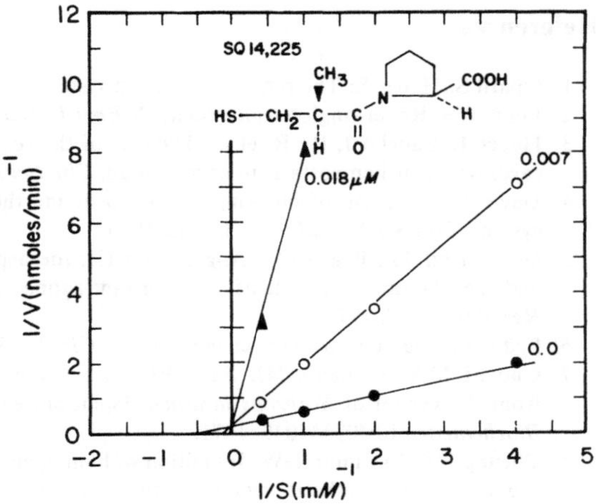

FIGURE 5. Competitive inhibition of angiotensin-converting enzyme by SQ 14,225. The double reciprocal plots of activity of angiotensin-converting enzyme versus substrate concentration at 0, 0.07, and 0.2 μM concentrations of the inhibitor SQ 14,225 indicates a competitive mechanism of inhibition. The enzyme-inhibitor dissociation constant (K_i value) for SQ 14,225 calculated from these plots is 1.7×10^{-9}M.

Summary

The similarity of the biologically important enzyme angiotensin-converting enzyme to the structurally characterized digestive enzyme carboxypeptidase A has led us to develop a hypothetical model of the mechanism of binding of substrates to its active site. In this model, a positively charged group on the enzyme forms an ionic bond with the negatively charged carboxyl group of the substrate; a hydrogen-bonding group of the enzyme binds with the terminal peptide bond of the substrate, and the tightly bound zinc ion of the enzyme binds to the penultimate (scissile) peptide bond of the substrate. Succinyl-L-proline (SQ 13,745) was synthesized as a potential inhibitor of angiotensin-converting enzyme by analogy to D-2-benzylsuccinic acid, an inhibitor of carboxypeptidase A; it was a moderately potent but specific inhibitor of the enzyme. Structure–activity studies carried out using the hypothetical model as a guide led to the synthesis of D-2-methylsuccinyl-L-proline (SQ 13,297) and D-2-methylglutaryl-L-proline (SQ 14,102), more potent inhibitors of the enzyme that were shown to be orally active in rats. Attempts to replace the zinc-binding carboxyl group of these compounds with groups with greater affinity for zinc have led to the synthesis of extremely potent inhibitors such as 3-mercaptopropanoyl-L-proline (SQ 13,863) and D-3-mercapto-2-methylpropanoyl-L-proline (SQ 14,225). The most active compound, SQ 14,225, is a purely competitive inhibitor of angiotensin-converting enzyme with an enzyme-inhibitor dissociation constant (K_i) of 1.7×10^{-9} M. It is an extremely potent and specific inhibitor of angiotensin-converting enzyme and appears to have great potential for the treatment of hypertensive disease.

References

1. Oparil S, Haber E: The renin–angiotensin system. *N Engl J Med* 291:389–401, 1974.
2. Peart WS: Renin–angiotensin system. *N Engl J Med* 292:302–306, 1975.
3. Haber E, Sancho J, Re R, et al: The role of the renin–angiotensin-aldosterone system in cardiovascular homeostasis in normal man. *Clin Sci Mol Med* 48:49s–52s, 1975.
4. Davis JO: The use of blocking agents to define the functions of the renin–angiotensin system. *Clin Sci Mol Med* 48:3s–14s, 1975.
5. Goodfriend TL, Peach MJ: Angiotensin III: (desaspartic acid[1])-angiotensin II: Evidence and speculation for its role as an important agonist in the renin–angiotensin system. *Circ Res* 37:I38–I48, 1975.
6. Erdös E: Angiotensin I converting enzyme. *Cir Res* 36:247–255, 1975.
7. Ondetti MA, Williams NJ, Sabo EF, et al: Angiotensin-converting enzyme inhibitors from the venom of *Bothrops jararaca.* Isolation, elucidation of structure, and synthesis. *Biochemistry* 10:4033–4039, 1971.
8. Cheung HS, Cushman DW: Inhibition of homogeneous angiotensin-converting enzyme of rabbit lung by synthetic venom peptides of *Bothrops jararaca. Biochim Biophys Acta* 293:451–463, 1973.
9. Engel SL, Schaeffer TR, Gold BI, et al: Inhibition of pressor effects of angiotensin I and augmentation of depressor effects of bradykinin by synthetic peptides. *Proc Soc Exp Biol Med* 140:240–244, 1972.
10. Engel SL, Schaeffer TR, Waugh MH, et al: Effects of the nonapeptide SQ 20,881 on blood pressure of rats with experimental renovascular hypertension. *Proc Soc Exp Biol Med* 143:483–487, 1973.
11. Gavras H, Brunner HR, Laragh JH, et al: An angiotensin-converting enzyme inhibitor to identify and treat vasoconstrictor and volume factors in hypertensive patients. *N Engl J Med* 291:817–821, 1974.
12. Gavras H, Brunner HR, Laragh JH, et al: The use of angiotensin-converting enzyme inhibitor in the diagnosis and treatment of hypertension. *Clin Sci Mol Med* 48:57s–60s, 1975.
13. Johnson JG, Black WD, Vukovich RA: Treatment of patients with severe hypertension by inhibition of angiotensin-converting enzyme. *Clin Sci Mol Med* 48:53s–56s, 1975.
14. Case DB, Wallace JM, Keim HJ, et al: Possible role of renin in hypertension as suggested by renin–sodium profiling and inhibition of converting enzyme. *N Engl J Med* 296:641, 1977.
15. Gavras H, Brunner HR, Gavras I, et al: Hypotensive effect of angiotensin-converting enzyme inhibitor SQ 20,881. *Lancet* 2:353, 1974.
16. Margolius HS, Horwitz D, Pisano JJ, et al: Urinary kallikrein excretion in hypertensive man: Relationship to sodium intake and sodium retaining steroids. *Circ Res* 35:820–825, 1974.
17. Cushman DW, Pluščec J, Williams NJ, et al: Inhibition of angiotensin-converting enzyme by analogs of peptides from *Bothrops jararaca* venom. *Experientia* 29:1032–1035, 1973.
18. Cushman DW, Cheung HS: Spectrophotometric assay and properties of the angiotensin-converting enzyme of rabbit lung. *Biochem Pharmacol* 20:1637–1648, 1971.
19. Das M, Soffer RL: Pulmonary angiotensin-converting enzyme. Structural and catalytic properties. *J Biol Chem* 250:6762–6768, 1975.
20. Quiocho F, Lipscombe WN: Carboxypeptidase A: A protein and an enzyme. *Adv Protein Chem* 25:1–78, 1971.
21. Byers LD, Wolfenden P: Binding of the by-product analog benzylsuccinic acid by carboxypeptidase A.*Biochemistry* 12:2070–2078, 1973.

22. Ondetti MA, Rubin B, Cushman DW: Design of specific inhibitors of angiotensin-converting enzyme: New class of orally active antihypertensive agents. *Science* 196:441–444, 1977.
23. Cushman DW, Cheung HS, Sabo EF, et al: Design of potent inhibitors of angiotensin-converting enzyme. Carboxyalkanoyl and mercaptoalkanoyl amino acids. *Biochemistry* 16:5484, 1977.
24. Rubin B, Laffan RJ, Kotler DG, et al: SQ 14,225 (D-3-mercapto-2-methylpropanoyl-L-proline), a novel orally active inhibitor of angiotensin I-converting enzyme. *J Pharmacol Exp Ther* 204:271, 1978.
25. Laffan RJ, Goldberg ME, High JP, et al: Antihypertensive activity in rats of SQ 14,225, an orally active inhibitor of angiotensin I-converting enzyme. *J Pharmacol Exp Ther* 204:281, 1978.

Chapter 9

Captopril (Capoten®; SQ 14,225) (D-3-Mercapto-2-methylpropanoyl-L-proline)

A Novel Orally Active Inhibitor of Angiotensin-Converting Enzyme and Antihypertensive Agent

Bernard Rubin, Michael J. Antonaccio, and Zola P. Horovitz

Introduction

The enzymatic conversion of angiotensin I (AI) to angiotensin II (AII) and the inhibition of such conversion have been recently reviewed.[1-3] Angiotensin-converting enzyme (ACE) [E.C. 3.4.15.1] has also been designated as converting enzyme (CE), peptidyldipeptide carboxy hydrolase, kininase II, or "bradykininase." Hence, in vivo inhibition of ACE will reduce the pressor activity of AI, but not that of AII, and augment the vasodepressor activity of bradykinin (BK).

A successful attempt at designing orally active novel inhibitors of ACE based on a hypothetical model of the active site of this enzyme has recently been reported by our laboratories.[4] The most potent compound found to date is captopril (SQ 14,225; D-3-mercapto-2-methylpropanoyl-L-proline). The data presented here indicate that captopril is active both orally and parenterally and that captopril, on a weight basis, may be about 10 times as potent as the parenterally administered nonapeptide ACE inhibitor teprotide (SQ 20,881).[1,5-16] Furthermore, not only is captopril rapidly and markedly antihypertensive in several animal models of renal hypertension, but it is also antihypertensive in several types of genetically hypertensive animal models including spontaneously hypertensive rats.[16] Thus, there is a possibility that captopril may show an even wider spectrum of clinical effec-

BERNARD RUBIN, Ph.D., MICHAEL J. ANTONACCIO, Ph.D., and ZOLA P. HOROVITZ, Ph.D. · The Squibb Institute for Medical Research, Princeton, New Jersey 08540.

tiveness as an antihypertensive agent than previously considered for this class of agents.

In Vitro and in Vivo Inhibition of ACE by Captopril

In Vitro

We have previously described[13] the use of excised guinea pig ileum as an in vitro screening test for predicting inhibitor activity of ACE in vivo. Captopril, at concentrations of about 5 and 0.7 ng/ml, respectively, inhibited the contractile response of excised guinea pig ileum to AI (0.025 μg/ml) and augmented the contractile response to BK (0.01 μg/ml).[15] Captopril in vitro was 3–12 times as potent as teprotide in the guinea pig ileum preparation. The relative specificity of the inhibitory activity of captopril against ACE was indicated by its failure to alter the contractile response to autacoids such as acetylcholine (ACh) or to AII at concentrations about 20,000 times that needed to inhibit the contractile response to AI. Similar findings were obtained in several other types of excised smooth muscle contracted or relaxed with as many as nine other agonists, including dopamine, histamine, *dl*-isoproterenol, nicotine, *l*-norepinephrine, prostaglandin E_1, prostaglandin $F_{1\alpha}$, serotonin, and barium chloride.[15] The relative specificity of the inhibitory activity of captopril against ACE was further demonstrated[16,17] in that 230 to 70,000 times higher concentrations of captopril were needed to inhibit five other peptidases.

In Vivo

Monitoring of direct arterial blood pressures in unanesthetized Sprague–Dawley rats and mongrel dogs before and after intravenous or oral dosage with captopril was conducted by procedures similar or identical to those used previously with teprotide (SQ 20,881).[7,8,12,18,19] In normotensive rats, the changes in both the aortic pressor response to intravenous (iv) AI and AII and in the vasodepressor responses to iv BK and ACh were determined.[15] In related tests in normotensive dogs, the systemic pressor response to iv AI and AII were determined; in most of these tests with captopril, heart rate, transthoracic EKGs, and peripheral venous plasma renin activity (PRA) were monitored.[20]

Normotensive Rats. In fasted unanesthetized normotensive rats (NR), single oral doses of 0.1, 0.3, and 1.0 mg/kg of captopril produced, within the first 5–10 min, dose-related inhibition of the pressor response to AI; half-recovery times ($t_{1/2}$) ranged from about 75 to 145 min (Figure 1).

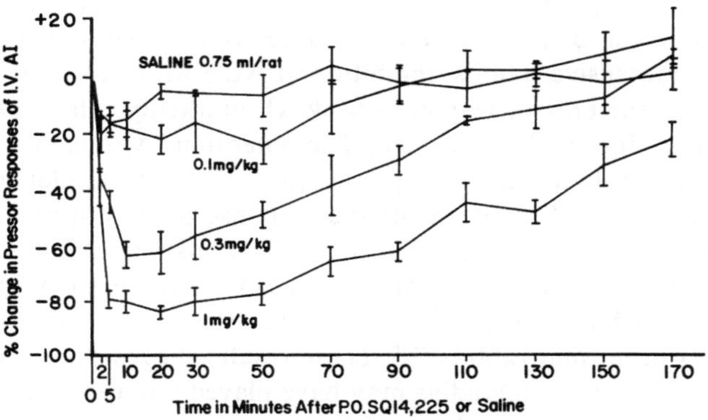

FIGURE 1. Graded inhibition of pressor responses to AI (310 ng/kg, iv) by single oral doses of SQ 14,225 (captopril) in 3 groups of 4 unanesthetized, overnight-fasted normotensive rats. A fourth group was dosed orally with saline. (Reproduced with permission.[15])

However, the pressor responses to AII or to *l*-norepinephrine, as well as resting mean blood pressure (MBP), were unaltered by these oral doses of captopril.[15]

Graded inhibition of pressor effects of AI was obtained in conscious NR receiving single iv doses of 0.01–1.0 mg/kg of captopril, although $t_{1/2}$s were much shorter than after oral dosage, ranging from about 8 to 55 min. Similarly, the pressor responses to AI as well as resting MBP were unchanged. Single oral doses of captopril were about one-eighth as effective as iv doses in terms of *maximum* inhibition, but the duration of inhibition of orally administered captopril was about 3–4 times longer than that achieved after iv captopril. The oral (po) and iv ID_{50}s of captopril were about 0.17 and 0.02 mg/kg, respectively, in the NR.[15] Little or no change in the reproducibility of captopril-induced inhibition of the pressor effect of AI occurred after short-term repeated iv or po doses of captopril in NR.[15]

In unanesthetized NR, single oral doses of 0.01, 0.1, and 1.0 mg/kg of captopril augmented and prolonged, by at least twofold, the transient vasodepressor effect of BK but not that of ACh, particularly after the two higher doses. Resting MBP showed little or no change after the two lower doses. After 1.0 mg/kg of captopril, MBP showed a gradual average decrease of about 10%–20%, possibly related to the interaction with residual BK still circulating after the relatively larger doses of BK.[15]

Normotensive Rabbits. Intravenous doses of captopril (0.031–1.0 mg/kg) inhibited the pressor response to AI but not to norepinephrine in conscious rabbits; the AII pressor response was somewhat enhanced by the higher doses of captopril. The vasodepressor responses in rabbits to iv isoproterenol, ACh, or prostaglandin E_2 were not affected by captopril.[21] In conscious normotensive rabbits, inhibition of ACE with captopril, as judged by inhibition of the pressor responses to iv AI, markedly enhanced the magnitude and duration of the BK-induced hypotension. Although in anephric rabbits the control hypotensive responses to iv BK were similar to those of normal rabbits, the enhancement of the response by captopril was significantly smaller than that observed in normal rabbits.[21,22] Indomethacin, 2.5 mg/kg iv, markedly attenuated the enhanced response to bradykinin in normal rabbits, while in anephric rabbits, the attenuation was smaller than that observed in normal rabbits.[21,22] These results suggest that after inhibition of ACE, renal prostaglandins may have played a major role in the BK-induced hypotension, while any contribution of extrarenal prostaglandins may have been small. Since indomethacin did not interfere with ACE inhibition induced by captopril or alter the pressor effect of AII and norepinephrine in these rabbits, the possibility of a mechanism other than inhibition of prostaglandin biosynthesis in explaining the observed effects appears to be unlikely.[22] Bilateral nephrectomy in rabbits did not interfere with the inhibitory effects of captopril on AI pressor responses.[22]

Normotensive Dogs. Unanesthetized normotensive dogs that had received single oral doses (0.03–3.0 mg/kg) of captopril showed graded inhibition in degree and/or duration of the iv AI pressor responses. About 85%–95% inhibition of the AI pressor response occurred within 15–30 min after 0.1–3.0 mg/kg po; $t_{1/2}$s were generally longer than those seen in the rat after comparable doses. All oral doses of captopril in unanesthetized dogs produced either little or no inhibition of the pressor response to AII.[20]

In anesthetized open-chest dogs, captopril caused a dose-dependent inhibition of the pressor as well as the renal vasoconstrictor effects of AI.[23] The renal vasoconstrictor effects of AI were more susceptible ($ID_{50} < 10$ $\mu g/kg$ iv) to inhibition by captopril than were the pressor effects ($ID_{50} = 37$ $\mu g/kg$ iv). Maximal inhibition of the pressor and vasoconstrictor effects of AI was seen after 100 $\mu g/kg$ iv of captopril. Pressor responses to AII were not affected by captopril, whereas the renal vasoconstrictor effects were enhanced.[23]

Normotensive Cats. In chloralose-anesthetized cats, captopril antagonized the pressor responses to iv AI in a dose-related manner (maximum inhibition at 310 $\mu g/kg$ iv) but did not alter the responses to AII. Intravenous captopril had no effect on pressor responses to centrally administered AI or AII, whereas centrally administered captopril produced dose-related decreases in centrally administered AI but not AII. Thus, captopril does not appear to cross the blood–brain barrier to any significant degree but can inhibit central ACE if administered directly into the brain.[24]

Normotensive Primates. In anesthetized rhesus monkeys, captopril had an ID_{50} of 6 μg/kg iv against AI pressor response.[15]

In normotensive conscious humans, captopril produced dose-dependent reductions of AI pressor responses after oral administration of 1–20 mg. Onset of action occurred within 15 min and declined to 40%–50% after 4 hr. The threshold inhibitory dose was about 1 mg, with a maximal effect occurring at 20 mg. Captopril had no effect on AII pressor responses.[25]

Effects of Captopril on Blood Pressure

Normotensive Animals

Groups of salt-replete male normotensive rats of the Wistar–Kyoto strain received captopril 3.0, 10, 30, or 100 mg/kg per day by gavage for 2 days.[18] One other group received only 0.9% saline, 5.0 ml/kg, po. The average predose initial mean blood pressure (MBP) per group ranged from 118 to 123 mm HG; the average initial predose heart rates per group ranged from 339 to 345 beats/min. The saline-treated controls showed a maximum decrease of about 7 mm Hg, equivalent to a 6% decrease in MBP. The maximum decrease in mean blood pressure on the first dose day ranged from 12 to 14 mm Hg, generally occurring within 1.5–3 hr after po doses of 3–100 mg/kg of captopril; these decreases in MBP represented about a 10% decrease in blood pressure, which was only about 4% greater than that obtained with saline alone (Figure 2). In contrast to renal hypertensive rats or spontaneously hypertensive rats, normotensive rats showed relatively little blood pressure lowering after dosage with captopril. In all of the NR groups, the slight, transient decreases in MBP occurred primarily within the first few hours after dosage. Also, in all the NR groups including the saline control groups, heart rates increased about 10%–20% after each oral dose, suggesting that no significant changes attributable to captopril alone were apparent.[18]

Other investigators[26] found that salt-replete NR (Sprague–Dawley rats) dosed orally with captopril for 7 days showed a decrease in MBP of about 11 mm Hg and a slight tachycardia (+15%), accompanied by increases of water intake, urine output, and urine sodium excretion. In sodium-depleted NR dosed with captopril, however, MBP decreased 22–24 mm Hg, and a slight tachycardia (+12%) was observed along with increased water intake, urine output, and urinary sodium excretion.[26]

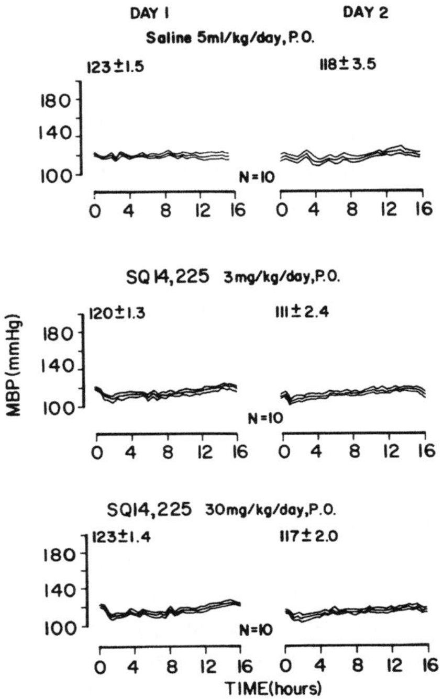

FIGURE 2. Effects on mean blood pressure (MBP) of single daily oral doses of SQ 14,225 (captopril) to 2 groups of 10 unanesthetized NR. A third group of 10 such rats received only saline (5 ml/kg per day) orally. The initial MBP ± SE (mm Hg) is shown for each daily plot. The 3 lines in each panel refer to the MBP ± SE. (Reproduced with permission.[18])

In conscious normotensive dogs, the highest oral doses of captopril produced about 20 mm Hg decreases in resting mean blood pressure within the first hour; recovery to or near predose levels occurred in most instances during the fourth to fifth hours.[20] After 0.03 or 0.1 mg/kg, captopril produced little or no effect on resting MBP in these dogs. Heart rate changes, if any, were slight to moderate and inconsistent after dosage with captopril. Orthostatic hypotension was not observed in these dogs following single po doses of captopril. No gross alterations of transthoracic EKG were observed.[20]

During long-term administration of captopril to Na^+-depleted normotensive dogs, arterial pressure, glomerular filtration rate, plasma aldosterone, and urinary kallikrein activity decreased, whereas plasma renin activity, urinary sodium excretion, renal blood flow, and blood and urinary kinin increased. It was concluded that the hypotensive and natriuretic effects of captopril were due to a combination of decreased circulating and renal levels of AII and increased circulating and renal levels of kinins.[27]

The mechanism of the hypotensive response produced by captopril was studied in other pentobarbital-anesthetized normotensive dogs. Captopril, 3.1 mg/kg iv, caused a rapid marked decrease in blood pressure of intact dogs. The hypotensive response was attenuated in a separate group of dogs that had been nephrectomized 16–18 hr previously. However, captopril persisted in significantly reducing blood pressure in these animals even though plasma renin activity was negligible. Captopril also lowered blood pressure in intact dogs following the blockade of angiotensin II receptors by infusing Sar^1,Ala^8-angiotensin II, 10 μg/kg per min. In addition, teprotide, at 10 mg/kg, iv, significantly lowered blood pressure in nephrectomized dogs. These findings led the authors to suggest that the angiotensin-covert-ing enzyme inhibitors, captopril and teprotide, may lower blood pressure of anesthetized normotensive dogs at relatively high intravenous doses via a mechanism unrelated to either the renin–angiotensin system or the renal kinin system.[28]

Renal Hypertension

Acute and Subacute Antihypertensive Effects. The antihypertensive effects of captopril were demonstrated in several animal models. An accelerated severe hypertension resembling a malignant type of renin-mediated renal hypertension[29] was induced in male Sprague–Dawley rats within several days after ligation of the aorta midway between the origin of the two renal arteries. Several such rats, anesthetized with urethane and atropinized 4–7 days after surgery, were given an iv infusion of between 0.3 and 1.0 mg/kg per min of captopril for 10 min. Moderate to marked decreases in mean blood pressure occurred within the first several minutes and persisted for at least the next 2 hr. The decreases in diastolic blood pressure (BP) were greater than those observed in systolic BP.[18]

In two-kidney Goldblatt renal hypertensive rats (RHR), a model that has been considered typical of renin–angiotensin-dependent hypertension in both the initial and established phases for at least the first several weeks,[30,31] captopril was administered the sixth week after unilateral clipping of one renal artery.[18] Direct mean blood pressure and heart rate were recorded from conscious rats for at least a 2-day dose period. Rats were dosed by gavage with each dose level of captopril once each day for at least 2 consecutive days. The average initial predose mean blood pressure per 10-rat group ranged from 187 to 201 mm Hg; the average predose heart rates ranged from 351 to 388 beats/min. Within 1–4 hr after po doses of 1.0–30 mg/kg of captopril, the maximum decreases in mean blood pressure on the first dose day ranged from about 10 to 65 mm Hg, which were equivalent to 10%–32% decreases in blood pressure (Figure 3). Half-recovery times ($t_{1/2}$s) were roughly 6–10 hr on the first and second days of dosage. It was also noted that at the time of the second daily dose, mean blood pressure had not completely returned to predose levels.

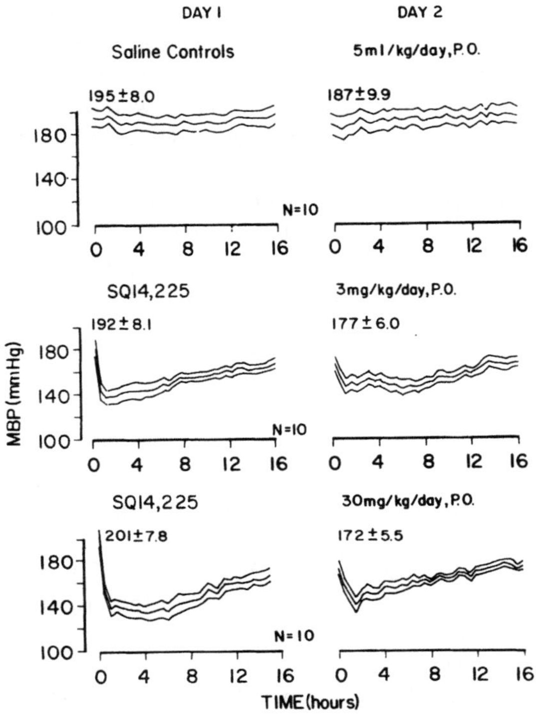

FIGURE 3. Antihypertensive effects of single daily oral doses of SQ 14,225 (captopril) to 2 groups of 10 unanesthetized two-kidney renal hypertensive rats (2-K-RHR). A third group of 10 such rats received only saline (5 ml/kg per day) orally. The initial MBP ± SE (mm Hg) is shown for each daily plot. The three lines in each panel refer to MBP ± SE. (Reproduced with permission.[18])

Other investigators also studied captopril in two-kidney renovascular hypertensive rats (Sprague–Dawley strain). In those rats with very high plasma renin activity, a precipitous fall in arterial pressure occurred after initiation of dosage with captopril; in those rats with normal plasma renin activity, a progressive but slow decrease in pressure was observed during 7 days of dosage. These decreases in pressure were accompanied by increased urinary volume and sodium excretion. Heart rates remained apparently unchanged or actually decreased.[24]

Studies have shown[26,32] (B. Rubin, unpublished results) that in one-kidney renal hypertensive rats, arterial blood pressure decreased about 25–50 mm Hg over a 4- or 7-day period of daily dosage with captopril.

Other investigators gave captopril orally to one-kidney dogs and rats for 1 day before and for several days after renal artery constriction, but this short term dosage failed to prevent the ultimate development of chronic renovascular hypertension in the dog[33] and rat.[34]

Chronic Antihypertensive Effects. Captopril (30 mg/kg) reduced systolic blood pressure of conscious two-kidney renal hypertensive rats (2-K-

RHR) previously clipped unilaterally for 6 wk.[35] In addition, captopril maintained its antihypertensive action after daily oral administration for over 6 mo. Only slight and inconsistent tolerance was noted in 2-K-RHR. In all studies, captopril consistently produced a rapid reduction in systolic blood pressure (SBP), usually within 4 hr after the first dose. In contrast, return of blood pressure to predrug levels after cessation of captopril dosage required from 5 to 7 days.[35] The reason for these differences in onset and duration of action of captopril are unknown at this time but may be related to differences between the immediate effects of angiotensin-converting enzyme inhibition and the chronic effects, such as bradykinin accumulation or inhibition of aldosterone secretion.

Although hydralazine caused an initially greater reduction in SBP of 2-K-RHR than did captopril, rapid and virtually complete tolerance developed to its antihypertensive effect within 4 wk of daily oral dosing.[35] Relative lack of tolerance to the effects of captopril may be related to lack of Na^+ retention,[26] which normally occurs with other antihypertensives.

Intermittent or chronic diuretic therapy had no effect on SBP of 2-K-RHR, results similar to those of other studies using either dietary Na^+ restriction or diuretics.[36-39] However, diuretic administered together with captopril, either intermittently or chronically, caused greater reductions in systolic blood pressure than either drug alone both in acute and chronic 2-K-RHR.[35]

Daily treatment of 2-K-RHR with captopril resulted in a significant reduction in relative heart weights in comparison with vehicle-treated RHR within 30 days of dosage, which was maintained throughout the 6- to 12-mo dosage period.[35,40] The survival of 2-K-RHR showed a dramatic increase in rats receiving captopril alone, and an even further increase when captopril was combined with the diuretic hydrochlorothiazide in comparison with either water-treated controls or rats receiving only diuretic.[35] The increased survival is probably related to the antihypertensive effect, since neither hydrochlorothiazide alone nor hydralazine chronically reduced systolic blood pressure or increased survival rate. Coadministration of guanethedine with captopril normalized blood pressure[40]; the above results demonstrated the long-term efficacy of captopril and suggest (1) a sympathetic component and (2) a volume-dependent mechanism in the maintenance of chronic two-kidney renal hypertension.[40]

Four weeks after surgery, in a group of 14 cellophane two-kidney perinephritic hypertensive trained unanesthetized dogs, 7 dogs were dosed orally each day for the next 9 wk with a capsule containing 31 mg/kg of captopril, and the other 7 dogs were dosed similarly with 31 mg/kg of lactose placebo. The indirect mean blood pressures of the captopril-treated group were about 25–50 mm Hg lower then those of the placebo-treated group (Figure 4). Blood pressures gradually returned to hypertensive levels

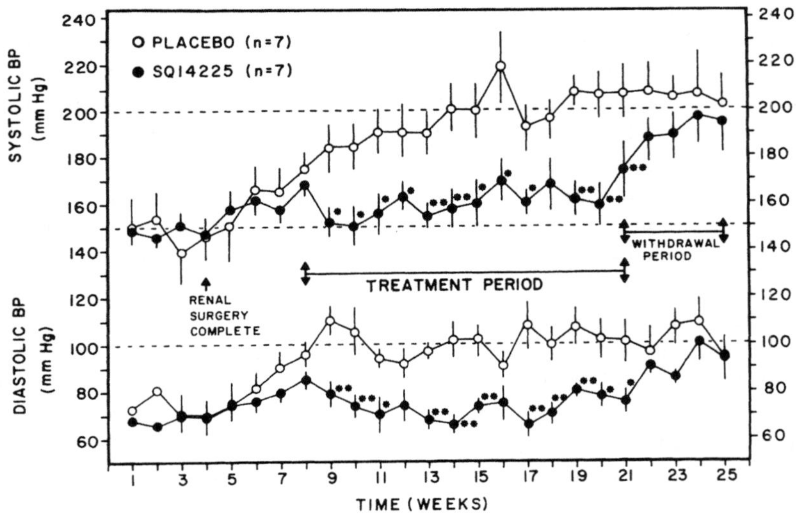

FIGURE 4. Two-kidney perinephritic hypertensive dogs. Treatment with SQ 14,225 (captopril), 31.0 mg/kg per day po, or lactose, 31.0 mg/kg per day po, was initiated at the beginning of week 8 and continued until the end of week 20. The pressure values shown during the treatment period were obtained immediately before each daily dose of SQ 14,255 was given, i.e., 24 hr after the previous dose. Asterisks indicate that pressure in the SQ 14,225 treated group is significantly less than in the placebo group ($p < 0.001$, Student's t test for unpaired comparisons). Vertical bars are ± SE.

similar to those of the placebo-treated group after the captopril dosage was stopped during the next 4 wk (R.R. Vollmer et al., unpublished results).

Genetic (Spontaneous) Hypertension

Acute and Subacute Antihypertensive Effects. Groups of male conscious spontaneously hypertensive rats (SHR) (Taconic Farms) of the Wistar–Kyoto strain, approximately 12 wk old, were used in these studies with captopril. Six groups of 10 rats each were used: one group each received one of the following oral doses by gavage once a day for at least 2 consecutive days: 0.9% saline control (5.0 ml/kg) or captopril 0.3, 1.0, 3.0, 10, 30, and 100 mg/kg per day. Aortic blood pressures and heart rates were monitored for at least 16 hr/day as described previously.[18,19] The average initial predose mean blood pressures and heart rates per group ranged from 163 to 180 mm Hg and from 341 to 374 beats/min, respectively. Captopril caused a dose-dependent fall in mean blood pressure.[18] The maximum decrease in mean blood pressure on the first dose day ranged from about 23 to 40 mm Hg, generally within 1–3 hr after these oral doses. These absolute changes in MBP represented 13%–22% decreases. The saline-treated controls showed a maximum decrease of about 3 mm Hg, equivalent to only a 2% decrease in mean blood pressure (Figure 5). Half-recovery times ($t_{1/2}$s) were about 8–14 hr on the first and second days of dosage with captopril. Heart rates in all groups of spontaneously hypertensive rats (SHR) treated with either captopril or with saline transiently increased during the first hour about 10%–25%. Thereafter, heart rates were increased only about 10% or less during the ensuing 14 hr; no major differences were observed in heart rates between control and drug-related groups.[18] Similar antihypertensive results were obtained with captopril by other investigators in the SHR.[41] Furthermore, no changes in body weight, diuresis, natriuresis–kaliuresis, and cardiac output were found as blood pressure was lowered; total peripheral vascular resistance was decreased in 1-yr-old conscious SHR.[41]

Other acute studies[42] have indicated that captopril (1) markedly decreased blood pressure in a conscious, stroke-prone high-renin substrain of SHR, (2) moderately decreased blood pressure in SHR, and (3) did not significantly affect blood pressure in normotensive rats.[42]

In another series of tests in 2 groups of spontaneously hypertensive rats, daily oral doses of captopril, 3 or 30 mg/kg per day, were repeated for 11 consecutive days. Initial average mean blood pressure per group ranged from 169 to 188 mm Hg. The moderate antihypertensive effects of captopril

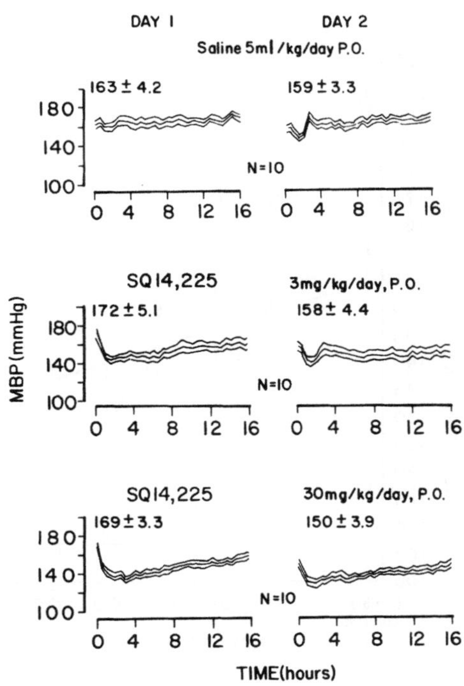

FIGURE 5. Effects on MBP of single oral daily doses of SQ 14,225 (captopril) to 2 groups of 10 unanesthetized Wistar–Kyoto spontaneous hypertensive rats (SHR). A third group of 10 such rats received only saline (5 ml/kg per day) orally. The inital MBP ± SE (mm Hg) is shown for each daily plot. The 3 lines in each panel refer to MBP ± SE. (Reproduced with permission.[18])

tended to remain generally similar during the 11-day period. The daily maximum decreases in mean blood pressure ranged from 15% to 20% after the 3 mg/kg dose and from 20% to 25% after the 30 mg/kg dose. A preliminary experiment was conducted with captopril in bilaterally nephrectomized spontaneous hypertensive rats about 18 hr after surgery; no significant decrease in mean blood pressure occurred after 3 mg/kg po in these animals.[18] Adrenalectomy, however, did not affect the antihypertensive effect of captopril in SHR.[43]

In the New Zealand strain of genetically hypertensive rats, captopril (30 mg/kg po) caused a reduction in mean arterial blood pressure of conscious rats of about 35 mm Hg (J. P. High, unpublished observations).

A comparison of the oral dose–response relationships occurring on the first test day for captopril in normotensive rats, spontaneously hypertensive rats, and two-kidney renal hypertensive rats[16] indicated (Figure 6) that there was (1) no linear regression in the normotensive rat model, (2) significant regression ($p < 0.01$) in the spontaneous hypertensive rat model, and (3) significant linear regression ($p < 0.001$) in the renal hypertensive rat model. Furthermore, the slope in the renal hypertensive rat was significantly steeper ($p < 0.01$) than that in the spontaneous hypertensive rat model.[18]

B. Rubin et al. (unpublished observations) and others[44,45] found that captopril was ineffective in lowering the blood pressure of DOCA–salt

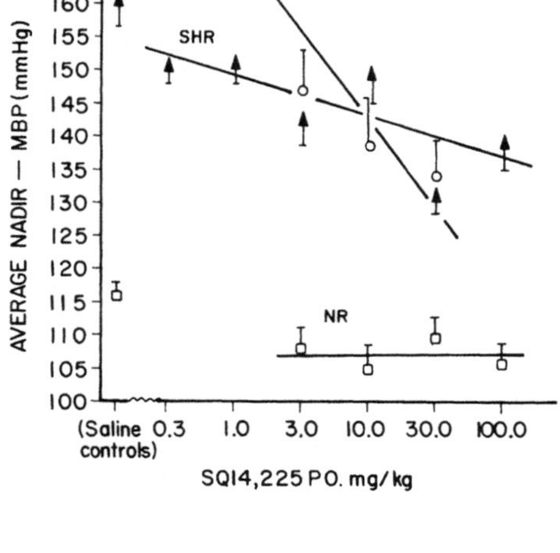

FIGURE 6. Comparison of maximum antihypertensive effects of single oral doses of SQ 14,225 (captopril) to unanesthetized 2-K RHR (○), Wistar–Kyoto SHR (▲), and Wistar–Kyoto normotensive rats (NR; □). The MBP ± SE is shown on each of the 3 lines. (Reproduced with permission.[18])

hypertensive rats after daily oral dosage for 4–21 days (10–1000 mg/kg). On the other hand, captopril was antihypertensive in an angiotensin II-salt hypertensive rat model.[46]

Chronic Antihypertensive Effects. The effects of hydralazine (3 mg/kg) and captopril (100 mg/kg) on mean arterial blood pressure, urinary Na^+, K^+. and aldosterone excretion were examined in Wistar–Kyoto spontaneously hypertensive rats after daily oral dosing for 2 wk or 3 or 6 mo. Captopril caused progressive, cumulative reductions in blood pressure resulting in normalization of pressure after 6 mo of dosing. No tolerance was observed. Hydralazine had less effect on blood pressure with no accumulation being noted. Reductions in heart size paralleled the changes in blood pressure, with normalization of cardiac hypertrophy occurring after captopril but not hydralazine.[47-49]

Dosage of weanling SHR with captopril for 4 mo prevented the development of hypertension; discontinuation of captopril treatment resulted in the usual development of hypertension.[50]

Hemodynamic Effects

In anesthetized normotensive dogs, captopril (0.31 mg/kg, iv) decreased systolic, diastolic, and mean blood pressures as well as total and renal vascular resistance. Heart rate was only transiently and slightly increased, whereas cardiac output, left ventricular dP/dt, mean pulmonary pressure, and pulmonary vascular resistance were unchanged.[23] Despite the decrease in blood pressure, renal blood flow increased significantly after captopril.[23]

Similarly, in conscious spontaneous hypertensive rats, captopril decreased total peripheral resistance with either no change[41] or an increase in cardiac output.[51] Captopril increased blood flow to all organs examined in spontaneous hypertensive rats, significantly so in heart and splanchnic organs.[52]

In human hypertensives treated with captopril for at least 3–7 days, mean arterial pressure decreased significantly; this reduction in pressure resulted from a reduction in total peripheral resistance without any significant change in cardiac index, heart rate, pulmonary wedge pressure, pulmonary artery pressure, or vascular resistance.[53,54] Plasma volume was slightly increased.[53]

Plasma Renin Activity (PRA), Aldosterone, and Na^+

In normotensive rats, mice, rabbits, and dogs as well as in renal hypertensive rats and dogs and spontaneously hypertensive rats[20,28,35,47,48]

(D.N. Harris et al., unpublished observations), and in hypertensive man, captopril causes 2- to 15-fold increases in PRA. These increases in plasma renin activity are thought to be mainly a result of inhibition of a negative feedback mechanism of AII on the juxtaglomerular apparatus. Reductions of circulating AII caused by angiotensin-converting enzyme inhibition with captopril should result in an increased renal secretion of renin in an attempt by the body to restore reduced AII levels. In hypertensive models, the reduction of blood pressure by captopril might also contribute to the elevated plasma renin activity through a compensatory reflex increase in sympathetic nerve activity to the kidney.

Captopril reduced aldosterone levels in hypertensive animals[56] and in hypertensive man,[57-59] presumably as a result of reductions in AII levels.

Captopril has been reported to either produce diuresis and natriuresis in animals or man[55-57,59] or to have little or no effect on water and sodium excretion.[26,49,55]

Miscellaneous Effects of Captopril

Captopril had no significant effect in rabbits on cardiovascular responses to serotonin, tyramine, norepinephrine, acetylcholine, vasopressin, isoproterenol, or PGE_2[21,22]; also, in dogs anesthetized with pentobarbital, captopril did not alter sympathetic funcction at the ganglionic, neuronal, or adrenergic receptor level at doses that were 10 and 100 times the level necessary to maximally inhibit the pressor activity of AI (R. R. Vollmer and J. A. Boccagno, unpublished results).

The augmentation by captopril of vasodepression produced by exogenous BK may be mediated by the release of renal prostaglandins in rabbits,[20] specifically prostacyclin.[60] This also appeared to be implicated in the (lack of) effects of captopril on heart rate. Captopril was reported to effect a decrease in baroreflex sensitivity.[61,62] Furthermore, the cyclooxygenase inhibitor indomethacin reversed the tachycardia but not the augumented hypotension produced by exogenous BK following captopril dosage in rabbits.[62] Thus, captopril, by possibly causing reflex vagal activation directly through BK or indirectly by release of prostaglandin, could have prevented or reduced reflex tachycardia. The effects of captopril on plasma BK levels in animals or man are thus far controversial; BK levels have been reported either as being largely unaltered[63,64] or as increased.[27,65]

Captopril was very effective in ameliorating low-output or[66,67] high-output failure in animal models of congestive heart failure[64,66] as well as in human congestive heart failure.[68,69]

Discussion

Inhibition of the pressor responses to AI without inhibition of the pressor responses to AII indicates that captopril is a potent inhibitor of angiotensin-converting enzyme after oral doses of 0.03–3 mg/kg in conscious animals. Furthermore, captopril thus far has shown no agonistic or antagonistic effect unrelated to angiotensin-converting enzyme inhibition after single or acute doses. It is about eight times more potent after iv doses than after oral doses in terms of maximum inhibitor effects in rats. The maximum inhibitory effects typically occur within 5–30 min after oral doses and persist about 3–4 times longer than after iv administration of the same dose in conscious rats. At present, we can speculate that the oral route maintains a longer and effective concentration of captopril or of unknown active metabolite(s) at the receptor sites of angiotensin-converting enzyme. A similar intensity and duration of AI inhibition in normal human subjects receiving single oral doses of 1–20 mg of captopril (equivalent to about 0.015–0.30 mg/kg) have been reported.[25] Similar types of studies in normal human subjects were conducted earlier with parenterally administered teprotide.[70,71]

Captopril has a relatively large margin of acute safety in the rat following oral administration. For example, the acute oral LD_{50} in rats is about 6000 mg/kg,[72] a dose that is (1) 25,000 times the oral ID_{50} against the pressor response to AI in conscious normotensive rats and (2) about 150–1500 times the oral antihypertensive dose range in the two-kidney Goldblatt-type renal hypertensive rats.

Captopril augments the vasodepressor effects of exogenously administered bradykinin in experimental animals. This action is intrinsic to the anticipated effects of an inhibitor of angiotensin-converting enzyme. As mentioned previously, captopril may slightly lower mean blood pressure even in unanesthetized normotensive rats, especially when accompanied by intermittent, high (10 μg/kg) iv doses of bradykinin.

In long-term studies with two-kidney renal hypertensive rats, daily doses with captopril alone produce prompt, moderate to marked antihypertensive effects, which do, however, tend to become more moderate after several months; little or no tachycardia has been observed. Addition of daily dosage with a thiazide diuretic augments both the antihypertensive effects and survival rate in two-kidney renal hypertensive rats.

It is possible that the antihypertensive responses to captopril result both from inhibition of AII formation and from accumulation of endogenous bradykinin which, in turn, could lead to increased release of prostaglandins,[73,74] especially in the renal vascular bed. Whether the latter effects are significant factors in the antihypertensive actions still remains uncertain.

Also uncertain at this time are the possible mechanism(s) of the more moderate antihypertensive effects of acute or subacute doses of captopril in the Wistar–Kyoto spontaneous hypertensive rats. The flatter dose response curves obtained with captopril in this model along with published controversial data concerning levels of plasma renin activity and concentration in the model and the failure of captopril to show its usual antihypertensive activity in bilaterally nephrectomized spontaneously hypertensive rats emphasize the need for further studies with captopril in this model of hypertension. Finally, prolonged daily dosage of spontaneously hypertensive rats with captopril reduces mean blood pressure to or near normotensive levels. Relative heart weights decrease in both spontaneous hypertensive rats and two-kidney renal hypertensive rats dosed chronically with captopril.

In the pharmacological studies conducted thus far, single or acute doses of captopril do not appear to significantly affect cardiovascular–autonomic function in normotensive animals. Furthermore, very little or no captopril crosses the blood–brain barrier in cats. Systemic administration of this compound in chloralose-anesthetized cats does not suppress the pressor effects of centrally injected AI or AII. Central administration of captopril, however, inhibits the pressor response to centrally injected AI (but not AII); but not the pressor responses to peripherally (iv) injected AI or AII.[24]

In studies conducted to date, captopril shares many of the properties of the previously described peptide, teprotide. The possible roles of the renin–angiotensin–aldosterone system and of the kallikrein–kinin–prostaglandin systems in various clinical disease states may be better understood after further studies with captopril have been conducted in models of animal or human hypertension and various renovascular disorders. Recently published clinical studies[55,57,59,75] have demonstrated the antihypertensive efficacy of captopril in malignant, renovascular, and essential hypertension as well as in hypertension of renal failure; the patients included subgroups with high, normal, and low renin levels.

Summary

Relatively potent and specific in vitro and in vivo (oral or intravenous) inhibition of angiotensin-converting enzyme by a nonpeptidic compound, captopril (SQ 14,255; D-3-mercapto-2-methylpropanoyl-L-proline), was demonstrated in excised guinea pig ileum and in rats, rabbits, cats, dogs, and monkeys. The design of captopril was based on a hypothetical model of the active site of the enzyme. Captopril, in vitro or in vivo, was about 10 times as potent as teprotide. Inhibition of angiotensin-converting enzyme was evaluated in vitro and in vivo by inhibition of contractile or vasopressor activity of angiotensin I or by augmentation of the contractile or vasodepressor activity of bradykinin. Acute or subacute dosage with captopril moderately to markedly lowered the blood pressure of the renin-dependent aortic-ligated and the conscious two-kidney Goldblatt hypertensive rat; in the latter, the effect was intensified by concomitant dosage with a thiazide diuretic. Furthermore, the life-prolonging effects of captopril in renal hypertensive rats were augmented by a thiazide diuretic. In the two-kidney Goldblatt rat, acute captopril (po) was about 10 times as potent as teprotide (sc) in lowering blood pressure. Acute or subacute oral doses of captopril moderately reduced the blood pressure of the spontaneously hypertensive Wistar-Kyoto rat; chronic dosage normalized blood pressure. Bilateral nephrectomy virtually abolished the hypotensive activity of captopril in the spontaneous hypertensive rat. The results suggest that captopril acts in large part by inhibiting the renin–angiotensin–aldosterone system to reduce elevated blood pressure, especially in renin-dependent models of hypertension; the roles of the kallikrein–kinin–prostaglandin systems and sodium balance remain to be elucidated. Captopril also lowers blood pressure in apparently nonrenin-dependent types of hypertension by mechanisms that are as yet undefined.

References

1. Erdös EG: Conversion of angiotensin I to angiotensin II. *Am J Med* 60:740, 1976.
2. Soffer, RL: Angiotensin-converting enzyme and the regulation of vasoactive peptides. *Annu Rev Biochem* 45:73, 1976.
3. Skeggs LT, Dorer FE, Kahn JR, et al: The biochemistry of renin–angiotensin system and its role in hypertension. *Am J Med* 60:737, 1976.
4. Ondetti MA, Rubin B, Cushman DW: Design of specific inhibitors of angiotensin-converting enzyme: A new class of orally active antihypertensive agents. *Science* 196:441, 1977.
5. Ondetti MA, Williams NJ, Sabo EF, et al: Angiotensin-converting enzyme inhibitors from the venom of *Bothrops jararaca*. Isolation, elucidation of structure and synthesis. *Biochemistry* 10:4033, 1971.
6. Cheung HS, Cushman DW: Inhibition of homogenous angiotensin-converting enzyme of rabbit lung by synthetic venom peptides of *Bothrops jararaca*. *Biochim Biophys Acta* 293:451, 1973.
7. Engel SL, Schaeffer TR, Gold BI, et al: Inhibition of pressor effects of angiotensin I and augmentation of depressor effects of bradykinin by synthetic peptides. *Proc Soc Exp Biol Med* 104:240, 1972.
8. Keim GR Jr, Kirpan J, Peterson AE, et al: Inhibition of angiotensin I-initiated hemodynamic changes in anesthetized dogs by a synthetic nonapeptide. *Proc Soc Exp Biol Med* 140:149, 1972.
9. Engel SL, Schaeffer TR, Waugh MH, et al: Effects of the nonapeptide SQ 20,881 on blood pressure of rats with experimental renovascular hypertension. *Proc Soc Exp Biol Med* 143:483, 1973.

10. Muirhead EE, Brooks B, Arora KK: Prevention of malignant hypertension by the synthetic peptide SQ 20,881. *Lab Invest* 30:129, 1974.
11. O'Keefe EH, Kotler DG, Waugh MH, et al: Inhibition and augmentation of peptide SQ 20,881 of contractile effects of angiotensin I (AI) and of bradykinin (B), respectively, on excised smooth muscle. *Fed Proc* 31:511, 1972.
12. Bianchi A, Evans DB, Cobb M, et al: Inhibition of SQ 20,881 of vasopressor responses to angiotensin I in conscious animals. *Eur J Pharmacol* 23:90, 1973.
13. Rubin B, O'Keefe EH, Kotler DG, et al: Use of excised guinea pig ileum as a predictive test for inhibitors in vivo of angiotensin-converting enzyme (ACE). *Fed Proc* 34:770, 1975.
14. Greene LJ, Camargo ACM, Krieger EM, et al: Inhibition of the conversion of angiotensin I to II and potentiation of bradykinin by small peptides present in *Bothrops jararaca* venom. *Circ Res* 31:II-62, 1972.
15. Rubin B, Laffan RJ, Kotler DG, et al: SQ 14,225 (D-3-mercapto-2-methylpropanoyl-L-proline), a novel orally active inhibitor of angiotensin I-converting enzyme. *J Pharmacol Exp Ther* 204:271, 1978.
16. Cushman DW, Cheung HS, Sabo EF, et al: Development of specific inhibitors of angiotensin I converting enzyme (kininase II). *Fed Proc* 38:2778, 1979.
17. Cushman DW, Cheung HS, Sabo EF, et al: Design of potent competitive inhibitors of angiotensin-converting enzyme. *Biochemistry* 16:5484, 1977.
18. Laffan RJ, Goldberg ME, High JP, et al: Antihypertensive activity in rats of SQ 14,225, an orally active inhibitor of angiotensin I-converting enzyme. *J Pharmacol Exp Ther* 204:281, 1978.
19. Laffan RJ, Peterson A, Hitch SW, et al: A technique for prolonged continuous recording of blood pressure of unrestrained rats. *Cardiovasc Res* 6:319, 1972.
20. Harris DN, Heran CL, Goldenberg HJ, et al: Effect of SQ 14,225 (D-3-mercapto-2-methylpropanoyl-L-proline) an orally active inhibitor of angiotensin converting enzyme on blood pressure, heart rate and plasma renin activity of conscious normotensive dogs. *Fed Proc* 37:718, 1978.
21. Murthy VS, Waldron TL, Goldberg ME, et al: Inhibition of angiotensin-converting enzyme by SQ 14,225 in conscious rabbits. *Eur J Pharmacol* 46:207, 1977.
22. Murthy VS, Waldron TL, Goldberg ME: The mechanism of bradykinin potentiation after inhibition of angiotensin converting enzyme (ACE) by SQ 14,225 in conscious rabbits. *Circ Res* 43(suppl I):40, 1978.
23. Murthy VS, Waldron TL, Goldberg ME: Inhibition of angiotensin converting enzyme by SQ 14,225 in anesthetized dogs: Hemodynamic and renal vascular effects. *Proc Soc Exp Biol Med* 157:121, 1978.
24. Vollmer RR, Boccagno JA: Central cardiovascular effects of SQ 14,225, an angiotensin-converting enzyme inhibitor in chloralose anesthetized cats. *Eur J Pharmacol* 45:117, 1977.
25. Ferguson RK, Brunner HR, Turini GA, et al: A specific orally active inhibitor of angiotensin-converting enzyme in man. *Lancet* 1:775, 1977.
26. Bengis RG, Coleman TG, Young DB, et al: Long-term blockade of angiotensin formation in various normotensive and hypertensive rat models using converting enzyme inhibitor (SQ 14,225). *Circ Res* 43(suppl I):45, 1978.
27. McCaa RE, Hall JE, McCaa CS: The effects of angiotensin I-converting enzyme inhibitors on arterial blood pressure and urinary sodium excretion. *Circ Res* 43(suppl I):32, 1978.
28. Vollmer RR, Boccagno JA, Harris DN, et al: Hypotension induced by inhibition of

angiotensin-converting enzyme in pentobarbital anesthetized dogs. *Eur J Pharmacol* 51:39, 1978.

29. Carretero OA, Kuk P, Piwonska S, et al: Role of the renin–angiotensin system in the pathogenesis of severe hypertension in rats. *Circ Res* 29:654, 1971.
30. Gavras H, Brunner HR, Thurston H, et al: Reciprocation of renin dependency with sodium volume dependency in renal hypertension. *Science* 188:1316, 1975.
31. Douglas JR Jr, Johnson EM Jr, Heist JF, et al: Is the peripheral sympathoadrenal nervous system necessary for renal hypertension? *J Pharmacol Exp Ther* 196:35, 1976.
32. Sen S, Smeby RR, Bumpus FM, et al: Role of renin–angiotensin system in chronic renal hypertensive rats. *Hypertension* 1:427, 1979.
33. Watkins BE, Davis JO, Freeman RH, et al: Continuous angiotensin II blockade throughout the acute phase of one-kidney hypertension in the dog. *Circ Res* 42:813, 1978.
34. Freeman RH, Davis JO, Watkins BE, et al: Effects of continuous converting enzyme blockade on renovascular hypertension in the rat. *Am J Physiol* 236:F21, 1979.
35. Rubin B, Antonaccio MJ, Goldberg ME, et al: Chronic antihypertensive effects of captopril (SQ 14,225), an orally active angiotensin I-converting enzyme inhibitor, in conscious 2–kidney renal hypertensive rats. *Eur J Pharmacol* 51:377, 1978.
36. Redleaf P, Tobian L: Sodium restriction and reserpine administration in experimental renal hypertension. A correlation of arterial blood pressure responses with the ionic composition of the arterial wall. *Circ Res* 6:343, 1958.
37. Brown TC, Davis JO, Olichney MJ, et al; Relation of plasma renin to sodium balance and arterial pressure in experimental renal hypertension. *Circ Res* 18:475, 1966.
38. Miksche LW, Miksche U, Gross F: Effect of sodium restriction on renal hypertension and on renin activity in the rat. *Circ Res* 27:973, 1970.
39. Gavras H, Oliver JA, Cannon PJ: Interrelations of renin, angiotensin II, and sodium in hypertension and renal failure, in Creger WP, Coggins CH, Hancock EW (eds): Annual Reviews of Medicine. Palo Alto, Annual Reviews, 1976, p 485.
40. Antonaccio MJ, Rubin B, Horovitz ZP, et al: Long-term efficacy of captopril (SQ 14,225) in 2–kidney renal hypertensive rats. *Clin Exp Hypertension* 1:505, 1979.
41. Muirhead ER, Prewitt RL Jr, Brooks B, et al: Antihypertensive action of the orally active converting enzyme inhibitor (SQ 14,225) in spontaneously hypertensive rats. *Circ Res* 43(suppl I):53, 1978.
42. Watanabe TX, Sokabe H: Acute vasodepressor effect of D-3-mercapto-2-methylpropanoyl-L-proline (SQ 14,225) in the stroke-prone substrain of spontaneously hypertensive rats (SHRSP). *Jpn J Pharmacol* 29:133, 1979.
43. Antonaccio MJ, High JP, Schaeffer T, et al: Renal, but not adrenal, contribution to the acute antihypertensive action of captopril (SQ 14,225) in spontaneously hypertensive rats (SHR). *Proc 6th Mtg International Soc Hypertension*, Goteborg, Sweden, June 11–13, 1979.
44. Douglas BH, Langford HG, McCaa RE: Failure of an angiotensin I converting inhibitor to alter desoxycorticosterone acetate–sodium chloride (DCA–NaCl) hypertension. *Clin Res* 26:510, 1978.
45. Dean HG, Ingham S: The effect of SQ 14,225 on fluid intake in DOCA/salt hypertensive rats. *Br J Pharmacol* 64:390P, 1978.
46. Muirhead EE, Brooks B, Brosius WL: Captopril in sodium–volume expanded hypertension. *Fed Proc* 38:1439, 1979.
47. Horovitz ZP, Rubin B, Antonaccio MJ, et al: Antihypertensive effects of SQ 14,225 (D-3-mercapto-2-methylpropanoyl-L-proline), an orally active angiotensin I-converting enzyme inhibitor, in spontaneously hypertensive rats (SHR) during chronic therapy. *Fed Proc* 37:718, 1978.

48. Antonaccio MJ, Rubin B, High J, et al: Chronic effects of SQ 14,225, an orally active angiotensin I-converting enzyme inhibitor in renal (RHR) and spontaneously hypertensive (SHR) rats. *Proceedings of the Seventh International Congress of Pharmacology, IUPHAR*, Paris, France, July 16–21, p 662, 1978.
49. Antonaccio MJ, Rubin B, Horovitz ZP, et al: Effects of chronic treatment with captopril (SQ 14,225), an orally active inhibitor of angiotensin I-converting enzyme, in spontaneously hypertensive rats. *Jpn J Pharmacol* 29:275, 1979.
50. Ferrone RA, Antonaccio MJ: Prevention of the development of spontaneous hypertension in rats by captopril (SQ 14,225). *Eur J Pharmacol* 60:131, 1979.
51. Ferrone RA, Kardon MB, Walsh GM: Systemic hemodynamic effects of converting enzyme inhibitor (CEI, SQ 14,225) during acute renovascular hypertension. *Fed Proc* 37:718, 1978.
52. Ferrone RA, Heran CL: Hemodynamic effects of SQ 14,225 and guanethidine in spontaneously hypertensive rats. *Circulation* 57–58(suppl II):II-44, 1978.
53. Cody RJ Jr., Tarazi RC, Bravo EL, et al: Hemodynamics of orally-active converting enzyme inhibitor (SQ 14,225) in hypertensive patients. *Clin Sci Mol Med* 55:453, 1978.
54. Sullivan JM, Ginsburg BA, Ratts TE, et al: Hemodynamic and antihypertensive effects of captopril, an orally active angiotensin converting enzyme inhibitor. *Am J Cardiol* 43:417, 1979.
55. Case DB, Atlas SA, Laragh JH, et al: Clinical experience with blockade of the renin–angiotensin–aldosterone system by an oral converting-enzyme inhibitor (SQ 14,225, captopril) in hypertensive patients. *Prog Cardiovasc Dis* 21:195, 1978.
56. McCaa RE, McCaa CS, Bengis RG, et al: Role of aldosterone in experimental hypertension. *J Endocrinol* 81:69P, 1979.
57. Atlas SA, Case DB, Sealey JE, et al: Interruption of the renin–angiotensin system in hypertensive patients by captopril induces sustained reduction in aldosterone secretion, potassium retention and natriuresis. *Hypertension* 1:274, 1979.
58. Bravo EL, Tarazi RC: Converting enzyme inhibition with an orally active compound in hypertensive man. *Hypertension* 1:39, 1979.
59. Brunner HR, Gavras H, Waeber B, et al: Oral angiotensin-converting enzyme inhibitor in long-term treatment of hypertensive patients. *Ann Intern Med* 90:19, 1979.
60. Moncada S, Mullane KM, Vane JR: Prostacyclin release by bradykinin in vivo. *Br J Pharmacol* 66:96P, 1979.
61. Heavey DJ, Reid JL: The effect of SQ 14,225 on baroreceptor reflex sensitivity in conscious normotensive rabbits. *Br J Pharmacol* 64:389P, 1978.
62. Murthy VS, Waldron TL: Modification of chronotropic effects on bradykinin (BK) by captopril (C) and indomethacin (I) in conscious rabbits. *Fed Proc* 38:738, 1979.
63. Matthews G, McGrath B, Johnston C: Hormonal changes with long-term converting enzyme inhibition by captopril in essential hypertension. *Proc 6th Sci Mtg Int Soc Hypertension*, Goteborg, Sweden June 11–13, 1979.
64. Millar JA, Johnston CI: The effect of captopril (SQ 14,225) on circulating levels and clearance of angiotensin I and bradykinin in man, dog, and rabbit. *Proc 6th Sci Mtg Int Soc Hypertension*, Goteborg, Sweden, June 11–13, 1979.
65. McKinstry DN, Singhvi SM, Kripalani KJ, et al: Disposition and cardiovascular–endocrine effects of an orally active angiotensin-converting enzyme inhibitor, SQ 14,225, in normal subjects. *Clin Pharmacol Ther* 23:121, 1978.
66. Freeman RH, Davis JO, Williams GM, et al: Effects of the oral converting enzyme inhibitor, SQ 14,225, in a model of low cardiac output in dogs. *Circ Res* 45:540, 1979.
67. Williams GM, Davis JO, Freeman RH, et al: Effects of the oral converting enzyme inhibitor, SQ 14,225, in experimental high output failure. *Am J Physiol* 236:F541, 1979.

68. Davis R, Ribner HS, LeJemtel TH, et al: Treatment of chronic congestive heart failure with captopril, an oral inhibitor of angiotensin-converting enzyme. *N Engl J Med* 301:117, 1979.
69. Levine TB, Cohn JN, Carlyle PF, et al: Hemodynamic response to captopril, an oral angiotensin converting enzyme inhibitor, in congestive heart failure. *Clin Res* 27:439A, 1979.
70. Collier JG, Robinson BF, Vane JR: Reduction of pressor effects of angiotensin I in man by synthetic nonapeptide (B.P.P. 9a or SQ 20,881) which inhibits converting enzyme. *Lancet* 1:72, 1973.
71. Vukovich RA, Willard DA, Brannick LJ: Endocrine and cardiovascular consequences of angiotensin converting inhibition. *J Int Med Res* 5:1, 1977.
72. Sibley PL, Keim GR, Keysser CH, et al: SQ 14,225, an orally active inhibitor of angiotensin converting enzyme: Acute and subacute toxicity in animals. *Toxicol Appl Pharmacol* 45:315, 1978.
73. McGiff JC, Itskovitz HD, Terragno A, et al: Modulation and mediation of the action of the renal kallikrein–kinin system of prostaglandins. *Fed Proc* 35:175, 1976.
74. McGiff JC, Nasjletti A: Kinins, renal function and blood pressure regulation. *Fed Proc* 35:172, 1976.
75. Gavras H, Brunner HR, Turini CA, et al: Antihypertensive effect of the oral angiotensin converting-enzyme inhibitor SQ 14,225 in man. *N Engl J Med* 298:991, 1978.

Chapter 10

Toxicologic and Drug Metabolic Studies of SQ 14,225 in Animals

G. R. Keim

Introduction

The historical development of SQ 14,225 as a potential therapeutic agent for the treatment of hypertension has been described by Cushman et al. and Rubin et al. in other chapters in this volume. This chapter will delineate the results of a number of studies that characterized the acute and subacute toxicities of SQ 14,225 in laboratory animals. Some metabolic data from preliminary studies in rats and dogs are also included.

Methods

Acute Toxicities in Mice and Rats

Median lethal doses (LD_{50}) of SQ 14,225, in aqueous solution, were determined by intravenous administration to mice and by oral administration to mice and rats. Single doses were given to groups of 10 or 15 animals. A series of graded doses was used such that the lowest dose caused no deaths, the highest dose caused 85 to 100% deaths, and at least one intermediate dose caused lethality between the two extremes. The LD_{50} and LD_2 (the dose expected to cause death in 2% of the animals) were estimated from a graphic plot of percentage death versus dose.

In order to determine the effect of reduced liver or kidney function on the acute oral toxicity of SQ 14,225, similar studies were also conducted in mice with chemically induced hepatic damage (5.6 ml of CCl_4/kg orally) or renal damage [9.0 mg of $UO_2(NO_3)_2 \cdot 6H_2O$/kg intravenously].

Acute Oral Toxicities in Dogs and Monkeys

Single doses of SQ 14,225 in aqueous solution, ranging from 200 to 600 mg/kg, were given by gavage to two young adult male purebred beagles

G. R. KEIM, D.V.M. · The Squibb Institute for Medical Research, New Brunswick, New Jersey 08903.

with at least 48 hr between treatments. Both dogs had unilateral carotid cannulae surgically implanted 1 week prior to the first administration of SQ 14,225. For each test, a dog was placed in a cage, and carotid pressure, ECG, and heart rate were recorded by cabling to a polygraph. A continuous record was taken from 1 hr prior to 4 hr after dosing.

In addition, doses of 250, 500, and 1000 mg of SQ 14,225/kg were given by gavage, each dose to a different male rhesus monkey, and 375, 675, and 1500 mg/kg were given by gavage, each dose to a different female rhesus monkey. Physical examinations that included opthalmoscopy and electrocardiography were conducted before and at intervals up to 48 hr after dosing.

Cardiovascular and Renal Safety in Dogs

SQ 14,225 was injected intravenously (over 2 min), into two male beagles anesthetized with sodium pentobarbital, at doses of 10, 30, and 100 mg of SQ 14,225/kg given 60 min apart. Left renal blood flow and right femoral blood flow were monitored by means of electromagnetic flow probes placed around the arteries. Carotid pressure, Lead II ECG, and heart and respiratory rates were also recorded continuously. Creatinine was added to a buffered mannitol intravenous infusate that provided adequate urine flow, and urine was collected from ureteral cannulae for successive 20-min periods during the 4-hr studies. Creatinine clearance was determined and used as a measure of glomerular filtration rate. Arterial blood samples were taken midway during each urine collection period for determinations of hematocrit and serum osmolality, total protein, creatinine, sodium, and potassium.

Epinephrine interaction studies were conducted in unanesthetized dogs. Two beagles, standing partially restrained in a sling, were prepared for recording the ECG and heart rate. Three control responses to an intravenous dose of 2 μg of epinephrine/kg were obtained prior to giving 20 mg of SQ 14,225/kg intravenously. The epinephrine injection was repeated 15, 45, and 75 min after dosing with SQ 14,225.

One-Month Oral Toxicologic Studies in Rats, Dogs, and Monkeys

Groups of six male and six female Charles River rats, 5 weeks old, were given daily doses of 0, 50, 150, and 450 mg of SQ 14,225/kg, divided b.i.d., by gavage, 7 days a week for 1 month. Another group was given daily doses that began at 50 mg/kg and were gradually increased to 3000 mg/kg, divided b.i.d., for the last week of the study. Hematologic and serum chemical tests that included urea nitrogen (BUN), creatinine, glucose, cholesterol, total protein, glutamate pyruvate transaminase, alkaline phosphatase, and creatine phosphokinase were conducted during the last week of the study. Ophthalmoscopic examinations by a veterinary ophthalmologist and urinalyses were also conducted during the last week of the study. At the end of the study, 21-hr urine samples from the 450 mg/kg and control groups were analyzed for their calcium, magnesium, copper, and zinc contents, and the concentrations of these metals were determined in heart samples and, along with iron, in liver samples taken from the same groups at necropsy. Gross and histopathological examinations were done on all rats.

Groups of male and female young adult purebred beagles were given 0, 25, 75, and 225 mg of SQ 14,225/kg daily, divided b.i.d., by gavage, 7 days a week for 1 month. Hematologic and serum chemical tests as described for rats were conducted before dosing began and during the second and fourth weeks; serum bilirubin was determined during the fourth week; and plasma renin activity was measured before dosing began and on one day during each week of the study. All dogs were tested for intravenous glucose tolerance 1 hr after a morning dose during the fourth week, and serum retention of intravenously administered bromsulfalein, as a measure of liver function, was determined before dosing began and during the fourth week. An electrocadiographic profile was obtained before dosing began and during the first, second, and fourth weeks. Ophthalmoscopic examinations by a veterinary ophthalmologist were made during the third week. Urinalyses were conducted on all dogs before dosing began and again during the second and fourth weeks of the study. Other urine samples, collected for 48 hr before dosing began and again during the fourth week, were analyzed for calcium, magnesium, copper, zinc, and iron. At necropsy, heart and liver samples were taken from dogs in the high-dose and control groups and analyzed for calcium, magnesium, copper, and zinc, and liver samples were also tested for iron. Gross and histopathological examinations were done on all dogs.

Groups of male and female adolescent rhesus monkeys were given 0, 25, 75, and 225 mg of SQ 14,225/kg daily, divided b.i.d., by gavage, 7 days a week for 1 month. In addition to the usual hematological and serum chemical tests done before dosing began and during the first, second, and fourth weeks of the study, plasma renin activity was measured at these same times. Serum retention of intravenously administered bromsulfalein, as a measure of liver function, was determined before dosing began and during the last week of the study. An electrocardiographic profile was obtained before dosing began and during each week of the study. Ophthalmoscopic examinations were made during the last week, and urinalyses were done before dosing began and during the second and fourth weeks. At necropsy, heart and liver samples were taken from monkeys in the high-dose and control groups and analysed for calcium, magnesium, copper, and zinc. Gross and histopathological examinations were done on all monkeys.

Acute Oral Toxicity Interaction in Mice

Because SQ 14,225 may be used in man along with other medications, some knowledge of acute toxicity interactions of such combinations might be helpful. Five compounds have been tested in mice for their effects on the SQ 14,225 oral LD_{50}. The compounds were hydralazine, hydrochlorothiazide, methyldopa, nadolol (a new β-blocking agent), and spironolactone. Each compound was given orally to groups of 10 to 20 mice at its LD_2 or lower. The SQ 14,225 oral LD_{50} was determined in mice for each combination in a manner similar to that described for mouse acute toxicity (LD_{50}) studies. By appropriate graphic treatment of the LD_{50} data for mice dosed with SQ 14,225 alone and in combination with another drug, the results were interpreted as simple additive toxicity or as potentiation (when the SQ 14,255 LD_{50} in combination with another compound was much lower than would be expected, based on the lethal dose of each compound alone).

Absorption and Excretion in Rats

Single doses of 50 mg of SQ 14,255-^{35}S/kg were given orally and intravenously to groups of four rats, and the excretion of radioactivity in the urine and feces was followed for 4 days.

Pharmacokinetics in the Dog

In a preliminary study, 25 mg of SQ 14,225-^{35}S/kg was given orally and intravenously on two different occasions to the same unanesthetized beagle with a biliary fistula. Bile was collected for 8 hr after dosing, and urine and feces were collected for 4 days. Venous blood samples, taken at various times after dosing for 4 days, were used to determine plasma half-life and percentage plasma protein binding.

Results

Acute Toxicities in Mice and Rats

The results of the acute toxicity studies in rodents are summarized in Table 1. SQ 14,225 has a very low order of acute toxicity as evidenced by the high LD_{50} values. The intravenous LD_{50} in mice was about 1000 mg/kg,

TABLE 1. Acute Toxicity of SQ 14,225 in Rodents

Species	Conditions	Route	LD_{50} (mg/kg)	LD_2 (mg/kg)
Mouse	Normal	iv	1040	830
		po	6000	3850
	Hepatic damage	po	3650	1600
	Renal damage	po	3900	1900
Rat	Normal	po	5800	3900

and the oral LD_{50}s in mice and rats were approximately 6000 mg/kg. In mice with hepatic or renal damage, SQ 14,225 was only slightly more toxic than in normal mice.

Acute Oral Toxicities in Dogs and Monkeys

The results of the oral single-dose toxicity studies in dogs and monkeys are summarized in Table 2. Emesis occurred in dogs at 300 mg/kg and above and in monkeys (along with loose feces) at 500 mg/kg and above. In dogs, there were dose-related decreases in arterial pressure of 10 to 25%. No ECG changes or overt toxicity were observed in either species. Higher doses were not given to dogs and monkeys because emesis caused a significant loss of the administered dose. These results, like those from rodents, indicate that SQ 14,225 has a very low single-dose toxicity.

Cardiovascular and Renal Safety in Dogs

The results of these studies are summarized in Table 3. In anesthetized dogs, renal blood flow increased after each injection; the greatest change

TABLE 2. Acute Oral Toxicity of SQ 14,225 in Dogs and Monkeys

Animal	Single doses	Results
Beagle	200, 300, 400, and 600 mg/kg	Emesis at 300 and above Blood pressure decreases (10–25%) No ECG changes No overt toxicity
Rhesus monkey	250, 375, 500, 675, 1000, and 1500 mg/kg	Emesis and loose feces at 500 and above No ECG changes No overt toxicity

TABLE 3. Intravenous Cardiovascular and Renal Safety Studies of SQ 14,225 in Dogs

Study	Dose (mg/kg)	Results
CV and renal safety tests in two anesthetized dogs	10, 30, and 100	Renal blood flow increase Femoral blood flow decrease Arterial pressure decrease Myocardial contractility increase Glomerular filtration unchanged
Epinephrine interaction in two unanesthetized dogs	20	No sensitization of myocardium to epinephrine-induced arrhythmias

occurred after the 10-mg/kg dose. In contrast, the femoral blood flow generally decreased, but to a lesser degree than the increase in renal blood flow. Slight decreases (approximately 9%) in arterial pressure, primarily diastolic, occurred in both dogs after the 10-mg/kg dose. There were no other changes in blood pressure except for a transient period of mild hypotension after the 100-mg/kg dose in each dog. A significant shortening of the preejection period after the 10-mg/kg dose in both dogs may indicate that SQ 14,225 increased myocardial contractility. The glomerular filtration rate remained unchanged.

In the epinephrine interaction study, the electrocardiograms disclosed no evidence of enhanced cardiac automaticity after the administration of SQ 14,225 in either dog.

Thus, there were no adverse cardiovascular or renal effects after treatment with SQ 14,225 in either the cardiovascular and renal safety study or the epinephrine interaction study. Rather, some of the compound-induced changes, viz., increased renal blood flow and myocardial contractility, have definite therapeutic potential.

One-Month Oral Toxicologic Studies in Rats, Dogs, and Monkeys

The results of the rat study are summarized in Table 4. Dose-related retardations of growth and increases in mean serum urea nitrogen were found for the three higher-dose groups. Some rats given 3000 mg/kg during the last week showed slight decreases in hemoglobin, hematocrit, and erythrocyte counts, and slight increases in leukocyte counts. All treated groups had a slightly increased mean water intake. No drug-related pathological lesion was seen in any rat. Analyses of urine, heart, and liver samples from the 450-mg/kg and control groups for certain metals disclosed no significant differences in the mean values for the two groups.

TABLE 4. One-Month Oral Toxicologic Study of SQ 14,225 in Rats

Group number	Number of animals	Total daily dose (mg/kg)	Results[a, b]
I	12 (6M; 6F)	3000[c]	Retardation of growth (M:20%; F:8%) Slight decrease in RBC parameters Slight increase in WBCs Moderate increase in BUN
II	12	450	Retardation of growth (M:15%) Slight increase in BUN No effect on tissue or urinary metals
III	12	150	Retardation of growth (M:10%) Slight increase in BUN
IV	12	50	—
V	12	0	—

[a] Slight increase in water intake in all treatment groups.
[b] No drug-induced gross or histological lesions.
[c] Dose progressively increased during study; 3000 mg/kg for final week.

The results of the dog study are summarized in Table 5. Slight decreases in erythrocytic parameters were found for all four high- and two of four intermediate-dose dogs. There were slight increases in mean urinary calcium excretion in the high- and intermediate-dose groups. There were no significant changes in the urinary excretion of magnesium, sodium, or potassium, nor did the serum concentrations of the latter two cations or calcium change significantly. Water consumption and urine output were

TABLE 5. One-Month Oral Toxicologic Study of SQ 14,225 in Dogs

Group number	Number of animals	Total daily dose (mg/kg)	Results[a, b]
I	4 (2M; 2F)	225	Slight decrease in RBC parameters (4/4) Increase in urinary calcium excretion No effect on tissue metals
II	4	75	Slight decrease in RBC parameters (2/4) Increase in urinary calcium excretion
III	4	25	—
IV	4	0	—

[a] Plasma renin activity increase in all treatment groups.
[b] No drug-induced gross or histological lesions.

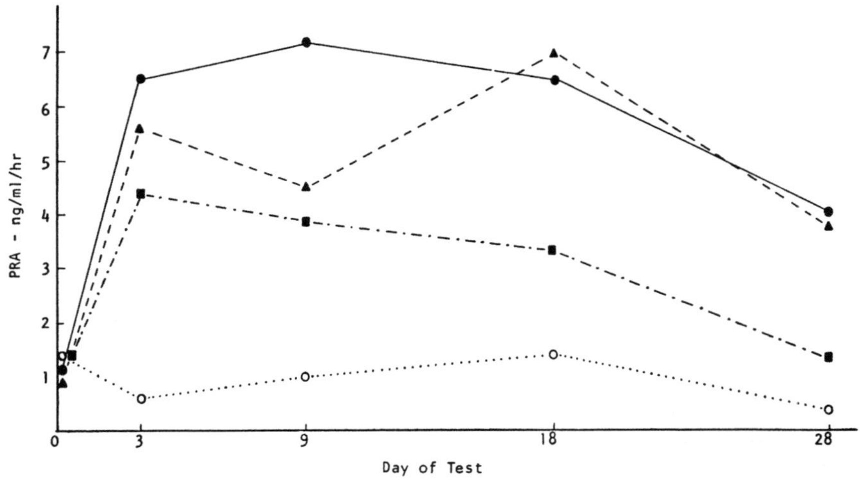

FIGURE 1. Plasma renin activity during a 1-month study of SQ 14,225 in beagles with daily oral doses of 0 (○), 25 (■), 75 (▲), and 225 (●) mg/kg. Each point is the mean for four dogs.

similar for treated and control dogs. No significant differences in the mean metal contents of livers and hearts were found between the high-dose and control groups. No drug-related pathological lesion was seen in any dog. Results of the analyses for plasma renin activity are shown in Figure 1. Mean plasma renin activity, measured 2 hr after dosing, showed a dose-related increase by the third day of the test, showed little change through the eighteenth day of dosing, and appeared to be returning toward control levels at the end of 4 weeks.

The results of the monkey study are summarized in Table 6. There were no significant differences in the metal contents of heart and liver tissues from the high-dose and control groups, no indications of toxicity, and no drug-related pathological lesions. Results of the analyses for plasma

TABLE 6. One-Month Oral Toxicologic Study of SQ 14,225 in Monkeys

Group number	Number of animals	Total daily dose (mg/kg)	Results
I	3	225	Plasma renin activity increases
II	3	75	No effect on tissue metals
III	3	25	No toxicity or drug-induced pathological lesions
IV	3	0	

renin activity are shown in Figure 2. Plasma renin activity was slightly elevated in all treated groups by the third day and was markedly elevated by the ninth day. The means on the ninth day were greater than 150 ng of angiotensin I generated/ml per hr. These are at least 35 times the values obtained prior to the first dose and are in marked contrast to mean values obtained in the dog studies which were always less than 10 ng/ml per hr. At the end of 4 weeks of dosing, the means for all treated groups had decreased to 40 ng/ml per hr or less.

Acute Oral Toxicity Interaction in Mice

There was no potentiation of SQ 14,225 acute oral toxicity in mice that had also been dosed with hydrochlorothiazide, nadolol, or spironolactone. There was, however, potentiation of SQ 14,225 toxicity in mice that had been given hydralazine or methyldopa.

Absorption and Excretion in Rats

The results of this study are summarized in Table 7, which lists group mean values. Based on the ratio of the percentage of an oral dose of SQ 14,225 excreted in urine to the percentage of an intravenous dose excreted by the same route, SQ 14,225 was well absorbed after oral administration to rats. Oral absorption ranged from 69 to 87% of the dose for four rats, with

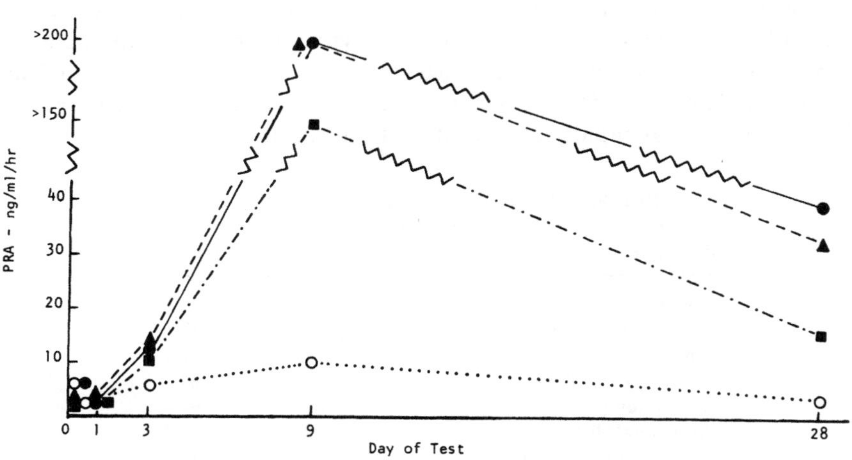

FIGURE 2. Plasma renin activity during a 1-month study of SQ 14,225 in rhesus monkeys with daily oral doses of 0 (○), 25 (■), 75 (▲), and 225 (●) mg/kg. Each point is the mean for three monkeys.

TABLE 7. Absorption and Excretion of SQ 14,225-^{35}S in Rats

Number of animals	Route	Excretion (%) Urine 7 hr	Urine 96 hr	Feces 96 hr	Absorption (%)
4 (2M; 2F)	iv	71	82	15	100
4 (2M; 2F)	po	56	63	23	77 (69–87)

[a] 50 mg/kg administered.

a mean of 77%. The results also show that the primary route of excretion was via the urine.

Pharmacokinetics in the Dog

The results of a preliminary study in the dog are summarized in Table 8. As was seen with rats, the major portion of the administered dose of SQ 14,225 was excreted in the urine. The extent of oral absorption in this dog was 60% of the administered dose; however, since only about 80% of the dose had been recovered in urine and feces within 4 days, the estimate of oral absorption may be low. Plasma half-life was approximately 2.5 hr, and 31 to 35% of the radioactivity in plasma was bound to plasma proteins. Radioactivity in the urine of rats and dogs was predominately as the disulfide with one or two minor metabolites. In vitro biotransformation studies in plasma, liver and intestinal homogenates, and simulated gastric and intestinal fluids of rats, dogs, monkeys, and man (where applicable) revealed that SQ 14,225 was rapidly converted to the disulfide.

TABLE 8. Pharmacokinetics of SQ 14,225-^{35}S in a Dog[a]

Parameter	iv Dose	po Dose
Excretion		
urine (% in 4 days)	99	59
bile (% in 8 hr)	5.5	1.2
feces (% in 4 days)	0.4	20
Absorption (%)	100	60
Plasma half-life (hr)	2.6	2.3
Plasma protein binding (%)	35	31

[a] 25 mg/kg administered.

Summary

The results of these preclinical studies have disclosed no toxic signs that would preclude initial clinical testing of SQ 14,225. The compound has a very low order of acute toxicity and produced only minor adverse effects at the higher doses in repeat-dose studies. Increases in plasma renin activity were not associated with any detrimental effects. Finally, the absence of significant changes in fluid and electrolyte parameters indicates that SQ 14,225's potential inhibition of aldosterone has little effect in normal animals.

Chapter 11

Captopril

An Oral Angiotensin-Converting Enzyme Inhibitor Active in Man

Hans R. Brunner, Haralambos Gavras, B. Waeber, G. A. Turini, and J. P. Wauters

Introduction

Two types of inhibitors of the renin–angiotensin system have been available for clinical research.[1,2] They both have the severe shortcoming that they must be administered parenterally, which makes chronic blockade of the system practically impossible. Furthermore, saralasin, a competitive inhibitor of the active hormone angiotensin II, has the disadvantage of inherent agonistic properties.[3,4] On the other hand, because angiotensin-converting enzyme is identical with kininase II, its inhibitor teprotide (SQ 20,881) not only blocks angiotensin II generation but simultaneously may increase bradykinin,[5] a potentially vasodilating hormone.

These two compounds have made it possible to investigate the participation of the renin–angiotensin system in the maintenance of abnormally high blood pressure in different types of hypertension. In renovascular hypertension, saralasin provided a useful tool to identify individuals whose hypertension is dependent on angiotensin II.[3,6] The bulk of the data obtained with saralasin seemed to suggest that angiotensin II plays an active role only when its levels are increased.[3,6] However, the physiological significance of these results has been questioned because of the inherent agonistic properties of the drug.[3,4,7] In contrast, teprotide has induced significant blood pressure reduction even in patients with "normal" renin essential hypertension.[8,9] Based on the findings of these studies, it was postulated that

HANS R. BRUNNER, M.D., B. WAEBER, M.D., G. A. TURINI, M.D., and J. P. WAUTERS, M.D. · Department of Medicine, Université de Lausanne, and Department of Medicine, Hôpital Cantonal Universitaire, CH-1011 Lausanne, Switzerland. HARALAMBOS GAVRAS, M.D. · Department of Medicine, Boston University School of Medicine, and Hypertension Section, Boston City Hospital, Boston, Massachusetts 02118.

renin and sodium acting together are the main determinants of blood pressure. Indeed, sodium has been recognized as participating actively in the development and maintenance of essential hypertension.[4]

In patients with impaired renal function, the renin levels have most frequently been found "normal" or low, and it seems likely that the sodium factor plays a key role in the pathogenesis of their hypertension.[10-12] However, several investigators have pointed out that these renin levels, though seemingly "normal," may be inappropriately high in relation to the corresponding total body sodium.[13,14] When patients with renal failure need treatment by hemodialysis, about 80% are hypertensive.[15] Blood pressure is then usually normalized by reducing total body sodium by ultrafiltration of extracellular fluid.[15] However, a minority of patients exhibits so-called "dialysis-resistant" hypertension, and these tend to have high renin levels.[16] To control their blood pressure, bilateral nephrectomy has been used.[17,18] Based on the hypothesis that the blood pressure of these patients may be sustained by an excess of plasma renin activity, saralasin has been infused, and this has often resulted in acute blood pressure reduction.[19]

The renin–angiotensin system has also been shown to participate in the control of afterload in normotensive patients with congestive heart failure. Blockade of the renin system by intravenous administration of saralasin has been used to acutely decrease systemic resistance, and this has resulted in improved cardiac function.[20,21]

An orally active inhibitor of the angiotensin-converting enzyme, captopril (SQ 14,225), has recently been developed. In normal man, it is a powerful inhibitor of the pressor effect of exogenous angiotensin I.[22] The present chapter summarizes some short- and long-term effects obtained with this drug in patients with different types of hypertension, the effects of captopril on renal function of patients with essential hypertension, and the acute hemodynamic responses to captopril administration in normotensive patients with severe congestive heart failure.

Methods

Patients

Fourteen healthy male volunteers aged 21 to 32 and weighing between 63 and 73 kg were studied to evaluate the efficacy of captopril in inhibiting pressor responses to exogenous angiotensin I. The subjects were maintained on their regular salt intake and were admitted to hospital for 24 hr. on the morning of the study.

Thirty-nine hypertensive patients, 28 men and 11 women aged 10 to 65, were then included in a second study. Nine patients had renovascular hypertension; thirteen, essential hypertension; and two, primary hyperaldosteronism. Seven patients had chronic renal failure with plasma creatinine levels > 1.5 mg/dl. Eight additional patients were on chronic hemodialysis treatment for 6 mo to 7 yr; all of them had hypertension refractory to ultrafiltration and to conventional antihypertensive therapy.

The effect of captopril on renal hemodynamics and function was assessed in an additional eight untreated patients with essential hypertension maintained on an unrestricted sodium intake.

In still another study, six nonhypertensive men with refractory congestive heart failure (four with idiopathic congestive cardiomyopathy, one with ischemic cardiomyopathy, and one with myotonic dystrophy) were included. Two patients were bedridden and unable to walk without shortness of breath for 3 and 6 mo despite treatment with salt restriction, digitalis, and diuretics. The other four were symptomatic on minimal exertion. Serum creatinine was elevated in two patients at 2.7 and 1.7 mg/dl.

Procedures

In each normotensive volunteer, a dose–response relation for angiotensin I was first determined using Ileu^5-angiotensin I (Schwartz–Mann). A single dose of captopril was then given by mouth, and 15 min later the intravenous dose of angiotensin I that had previously caused the maximum pressure rise was reinjected. If this was ineffective because of the blocking action of the inhibitor, larger doses (3- to 8-fold) of angiotensin I were administered subsequently. Increasing doses of captopril (1, 2.5, 5, 10, and 20 mg) were tested similarly.[22]

The protocol used to initiate captopril treatment in hypertensive patients has been described.[23] In short, antihypertensive medication was discontinued whenever possible 3 wk prior to the study. The patients were hospitalized and maintained on a constant sodium and potassium intake of 100 mEq and 60 to 80 mEq per day, respectively. Then captopril was started following a placebo period of 3 days. Blood samples, for the measurement of plasma renin and angiotensin-converting enzyme activities and of plasma aldosterone and catecholamine levels, were drawn on the last day of placebo and on days 4 to 6 after starting captopril, 1 hr following the morning dose.

The protocol for the patients on maintenance hemodialysis differed in that all determinations were always done before and after hemodialysis. In some patients treatment by captopril had to be complemented with salt subtraction, i.e., following conventional dialysis, 1–2 liters of ultrafiltrate were replaced by equal volumes of 5% glucose.[24]

After discharge from the hospital, all patients continued treatment with captopril, 50–200 mg twice daily. Diuretics were added in seven patients with essential hypertension and in five patients with nonterminal chronic renal failure. An ambulatory blood pressure profile was obtained in 17 patients using a portable recorder (Remler Corp., San Francisco) 13 ± 2 wk after starting captopril.

Renal plasma flow and glomerular filtration rate were estimated by a constant infusion technique employing as reference substance [^{131}I]-*o*-iodohippurate and [^{125}I]sodium iothalamate (Amersham Radiochemical Pharmaceuticals). Following determination of two 20-min control clearances, 50 mg of captopril were given po. Renal clearances were determined during 4 periods of 20 min each between the 20th and the 100th minute after captopril administration. Sodium and potassium were determined in each urine collection. The two control renal clearances were averaged (control value) as were the two determinations obtained between the 20th and the 60th minute (E_1) and between the 60th and the 100th minute (E_2) after captopril administration.[25]

The patients with congestive heart failure underwent cardiac catheterization in the supine position. After a resting period of 30 min, baseline hemodynamic measurements were obtained at 15-min intervals. Thereafter, 25 mg of captopril were administered orally. Hemodynamic measurements were repeated every 30 min for the following 2 hr and hourly thereafter until values had returned to baseline.[26]

Analytical Methods

Plasma renin activity, plasma aldosterone levels, and 24-hr urinary excretion of aldosterone were measured by radioimmunoassay.[23] The patient's renin activity was classified as "low," "normal," or "high" according to a method described earlier.[27] Plasma angiotensin-converting enzyme activity was determined by a radioenzymatic method using a radiolabeled acylated tripeptide as substrate (Ventrex Corp., Portland, Maine).[23] Plasma catecholamines also were quantitated by a radioenzymatic method.[28] Clearances were proportioned by conversion to 1.73 m^2 body surface area. Filtration fraction (FF) was expressed as GFR/ERPF. Renal resistance was calculated as the ratio of the mean arterial blood pressure (MAP) to renal blood flow [ERPF/(1 − hematocrit)].

Results

The time course of the changes in pressor responsiveness to exogenous angiotensin I after oral captopril is shown in Figure 1. The pressor response to angiotensin I is expressed as a percentage of the control response

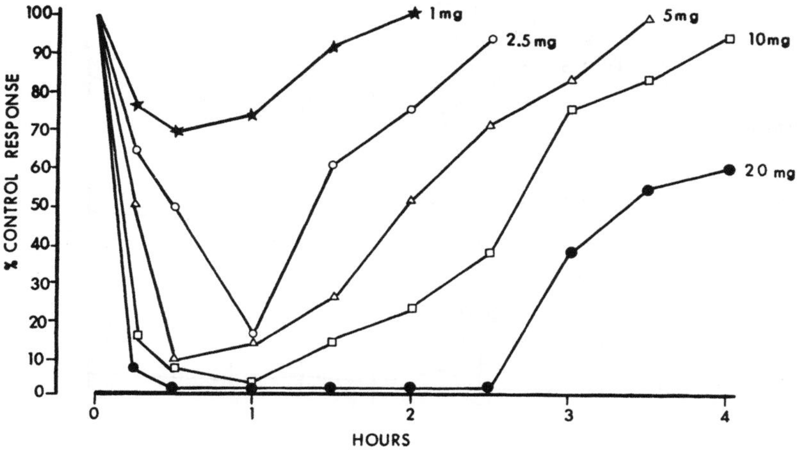

FIGURE 1. Inhibition of systolic pressor responses to angiotensin I in 14 healthy men after incremental doses of oral captopril. Mean responses of 3 subjects are shown for each dose of captopril except for 20 mg where data are derived from 2. (From Ferguson et al.[22])

determined before drug administration (time zero). Time–response curves for each dose of captorpil were averaged. The magnitude and duration of inhibition were dose-related. Captopril, 1 mg produced only slight (30%) inhibition and thus appeared to come close to a threshold dose. At this dose, near-complete recovery of responsiveness had occurred by 1.5 hr. Increasing doses of captopril produced progressively greater inhibition as well as measured duration of effect. Onset of inhibition was rapid and varied with the dosage. For example, the 20-mg dose produced nearly complete inhibition at 15 min which lasted for over 2 hr; at 4 hr, the average systolic response was still inhibited by 40%.

Figure 2 illustrates the time course of the blood-pressure-lowering effect of three different doses of captopril observed in six hypertensive patients on three consecutive days. With 25 mg, mean blood pressure decreased from a control of 130 ± 8 to 125 ± 11 mm Hg ($p < 0.05$) at 15 min and to 111 ± 7 mm Hg ($p < 0.001$) at 60 min after administration of captopril. It returned to baseline levels of 127 ± 8 mm Hg at 360 min. Blood pressure reduction induced by 100 mg showed a similar pattern, whereas 200 mg clearly had a prolonged antihypertensive effect, since after 6 hr, blood pressure was still reduced by 9 ± 4%. Thus, larger doses did not produce a greater blood pressure fall but prolonged its duration.

The blood-pressure-lowering effect according to clinical diagnosis during the first 4–6 days of hospitalization is shown in Figure 3. Blood pressure in patients with essential hypertension was reduced from 169/111 ± 5/3 to

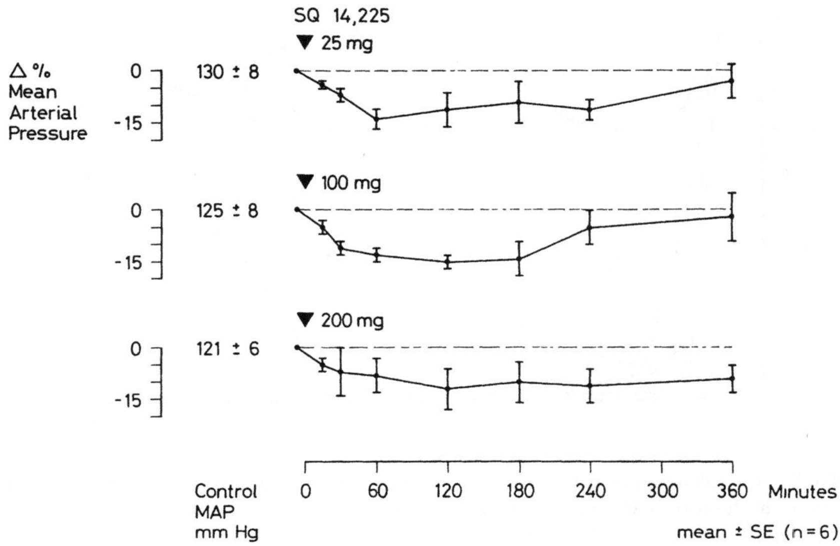

FIGURE 2. Magnitude and duration of antihypertensive effect obtained with three different doses of captopril (SQ 14,225) administered on 3 successive days. Note that starting mean blood pressure (MAP) is different each time. (From Brunner et al.[23])

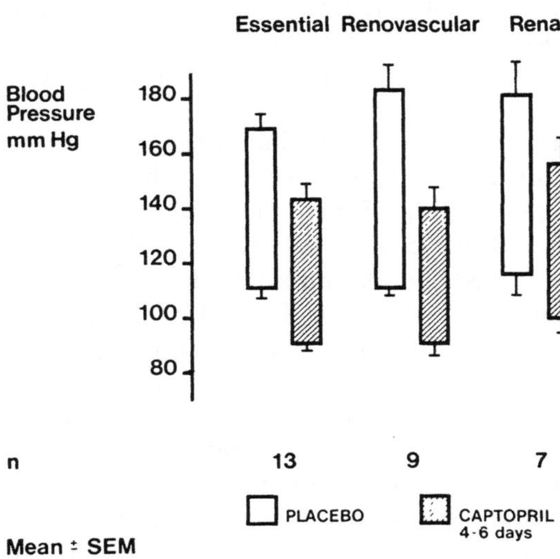

FIGURE 3. Changes in blood pressure achieved with captopril in subgroups of patients classified according to cause of hypertension.

143/91 ± 5/2 mmHg ($p < 0.001$), in those with renovascular hypertension from 183/111 ± 9.2 to 140/91 ± 7/4 mm Hg ($p < 0.001$), and in those with chronic renal failure from 181/116 ± 12/7 to 156/100 ± 9/5 mm Hg ($p < 0.05$).

In Figure 4 the diastolic blood pressure changes are depicted which were obtained in 39 hypertensive patients 1 hr after the first dose of cap-

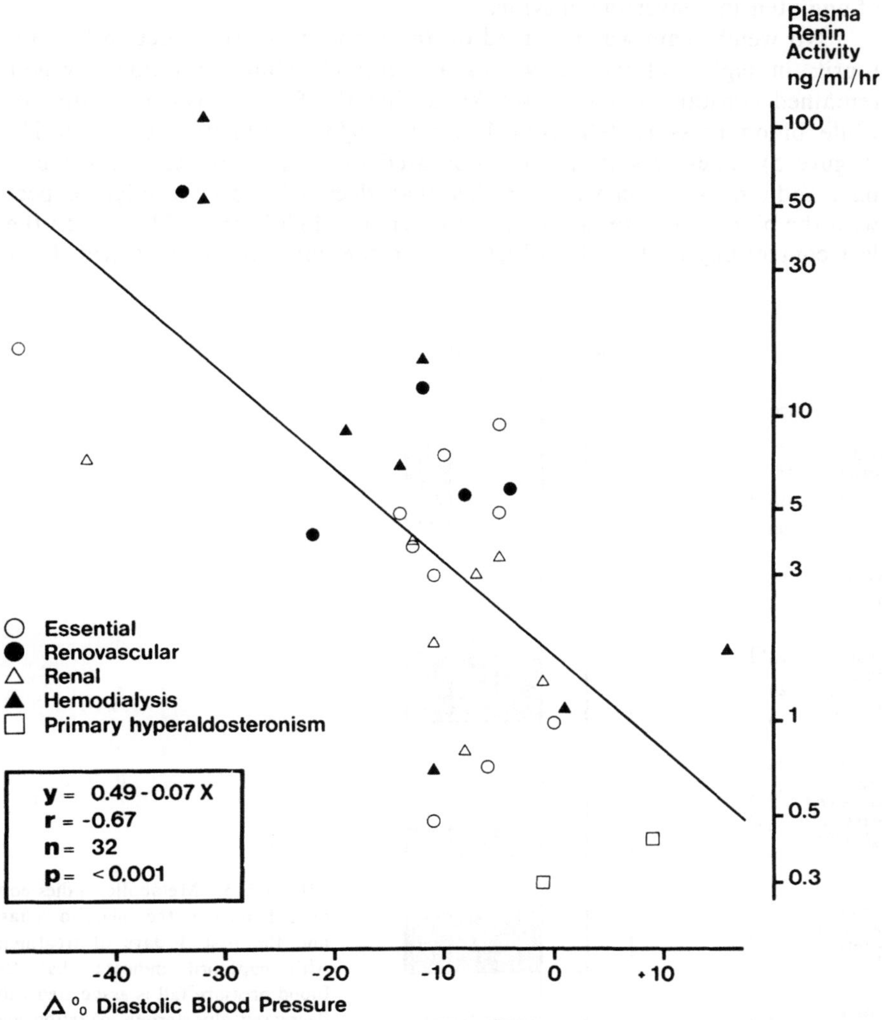

FIGURE 4. Correlation between control plasma renin activity and induced diastolic blood pressure reduction 1 hr following the first dose of captopril in 32 patients with different types of hypertension.

topril. There was a significant correlation between pretreatment plasma renin activity and the fall in diastolic blood pressure ($r = -0.67, p < 0.001$). Patients with high plasma renin activity showed the greatest blood pressure fall, but in those with normal and even low renin levels blood pressure was also reduced. In the two patients with primary hyperaldosteronism and the lowest renin levels, the blood pressure did not decrease following inhibition of angiotensin-converting enzyme.

No weight gain was observed during blood pressure reduction by captopril; in eight patients in whom a metabolic study was done, weight remained constant at 63.5 ± 4.5 kg during the first 3 days of treatment, while blood pressure fell from 172/110 ± 9/5 to 144/96 ± 6/4 mm Hg (Figure 5). These results are corroborated by measurements of 24-hr urinary sodium excretion which, rather than decreasing as one might expect with the blood pressure fall, tended to increase slightly from 74 ± 15 on the last control day to 97 ± 18 mEq/24 hr on the third day of treatment. Dur-

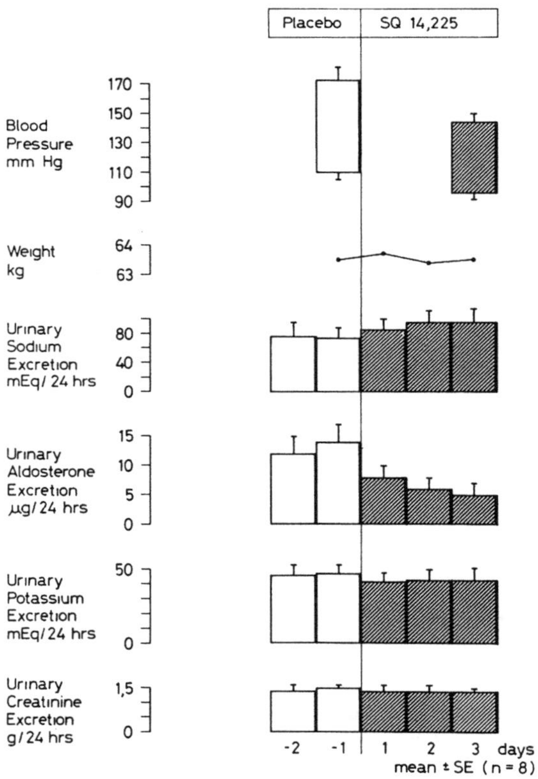

FIGURE 5. Metabolic studies conducted during the placebo phase and the first 3 days of treatment with captopril indicate that the blood pressure fall is associated with decreased aldosterone excretion and a slight increase in sodium excretion. Weight and renal function do not change. (From Brunner et al.[23])

ing the same period, 24–hr urinary excretion of aldosterone fell sharply from 13.6 ± 3 to 5.3 ± 2 μg/24 hr ($p < 0.01$). Twenty-four-hour excretion of potassium and creatinine remained practically unchanged.

The effects of captopril on the arterial pressure and renal hemodynamics of eight patients with essential hypertension are summarized in Table 1. At the end of period E_2, arterial pressure was reduced by 8.8 ± 1.8% (range 1–17.3). A significant increase in renal plasma flow of 11.8 ± 4% (range 6–33) ($p < 0.01$) occurred after captopril, while calculated renal resistance decreased by 16.4 ± 4.1% ($p < 0.01$). Glomerular filtration rate and urinary sodium excretion were not altered by captopril.

In seven patients with essential hypertension and in five patients with chronic renal failure, captopril alone did not normalize blood pressure, and diuretics had to be added before or after discharge from the hospital in order to control the patients' blood pressure. On previous therapy consisting of β-blockers and diuretics and, in some, of an additional vasodilating drug, the blood pressure remained high at 178/115 ± 6/2 mm Hg (Figure 6). In the hospital, with all antihypertensive therapy withdrawn, it was slightly higher at 182/118 ± 6/4 mm Hg. Captopril alone during the initial 4 to 6 days reduced blood pressure to 150/96 ± 6/4 mm Hg ($p < 0.001$). With the addition of diuretics, the blood pressure decreased further to 132/88 ± 5/3 mm Hg ($p < 0.05$). Administration of captopril increased plasma renin activity form 5.1 ± 1.4 to 17.5 ± 6.5 ng/ml per hr ($p < 0.05$), while plasma aldosterone fell from 22.6 ± 5.8 to 10.6 ± 1.8 ng/100 ml, and plasma angiotensin-converting enzyme activity decreased form 79 ± 6 to 17 ± 4 nmol/ml per hr ($p < 0.001$). The addition of diuretics increased renin further, whereas plasma aldosterone levels and plasma converting enzyme activity hardly changed.

Figure 7 shows the typical example of a 29-year-old male with insulin-dependent diabetes, hypertension, and chronic renal failure (plasma creatinine level at 1.7 mg/dl). Previous therapy consisting of propranolol 160 mg/day, spironolactone 100 mg/day, chlorthalidone 100 mg/day, and dihydralazine 100 mg/day did not control his blood pressure which averaged, over a period of 60 days, 195/118 ± 6/3 mm Hg. Three weeks following discontinuation of this conventional therapy, blood pressure in the hospital was little changed. On the third day of captopril, blood pressure still averaged 201/122 ± 3/1 mm Hg. Beginning on the 4th day of captopril therapy, furosemide 120 mg/day orally was added, and this contributed to a cumulative weight loss of 4 kg up to the 7th day of therapy, when the patient was discharged with a blood pressure of 166/94 ± 7/6 mm Hg.

After discharge, blood pressure continued to fall and reached a low of 90/70 mm Hg on the 14th day, when the patient complained of dizziness. Furosemide was interrupted during 2 days and readministered at only 40

TABLE 1. Effect of Captopril on Mean Arterial Pressure (MAP) and Renal Function in Eight Patients with Essential Hypertension on Unrestricted Sodium Intake[a,b]

	MAP (mm Hg)	GFR (ml·min^{-1})	ERPF (ml·min^{-1})	FF	$U_{Na}V$ (μmol·min^{-1})	$U_K V$ (μmol·min^{-1})
Control	119 ± 9	130 ± 4	518 ± 34	0.26 ± 0.02	183 ± 39	70 ± 11
Period E_1	111 ± 8**	122 ± 5 NS	556 ± 43**	0.23 ± 0.02**	181 ± 42 NS	49 ± 11**
% change	−6.8 ± 1.2	−6 ± 3.7	+9.8 ± 1	−13.4 ± 3.3	−1.2 ± 10	−32 ± 9
Period E_2	109 ± 8**	129 ± 7 NS	582 ± 47**	0.23 ± 0.02**	160 ± 30 NS	40 ± 6**
% change	−8.8 ± 1.8	−1.4 ± 2.9	+11.8 ± 4	−11.3 ± 2.6	−3 ± 13	−38 ± 8

[a] GFR and ERPF are proportioned by conversion to 1.73 m^2 body surface area.
[b] NS, not significant; *, $p < 0.05$; **, $p < 0.01$ (paired Student's *t*-test).

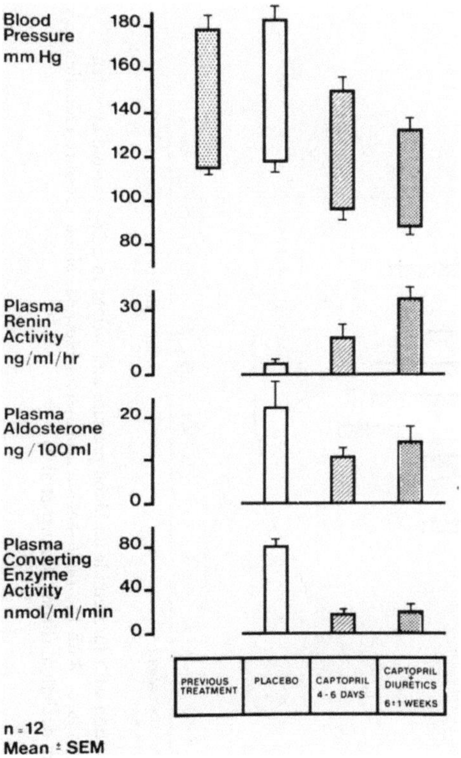

FIGURE 6. Effect of captopril alone and in combination with diuretics on blood pressure, plasma renin activity, plasma aldosterone, and angiotensin-converting enzyme activity. Blood pressure on previous therapy is depicted as a basis for the evaluation of the efficacy of captopril and diuretics.

mg/day thereafter. Weight increased again (0.8 kg) together with blood pressure which stabilized at 120/85 mm Hg.

Following blockade of the renin–angiotensin system, blood pressure becomes closely dependent on total body sodium. This is illustrated in Figure 8 which depicts the results of a 23-year-old severely hypertensive patient with chronic renal failure (plasma creatinine of 3 mg/dl). On captopril treatment, there exists a close correlation ($r = 0.86$, $p < 0.001$) between this patient's diastolic blood pressure and his body weight which, over a period of 8 months, varied considerably because of variations in sodium intake and changing doses of furosemide.

A similar observation in a patient with primary aldosteronism resulting from an adenoma of the zona glomerulosa is illustrated in Figure 9. Initially, without any other therapy, captopril had no effect on blood pressure which averaged 163/125 mm Hg. Four weeks of treatment with spironoloctone 600 mg/day decreased weight form 74.7 to 71.5 kg and blood pressure to 119/98 mm Hg, while plasma renin activity increased

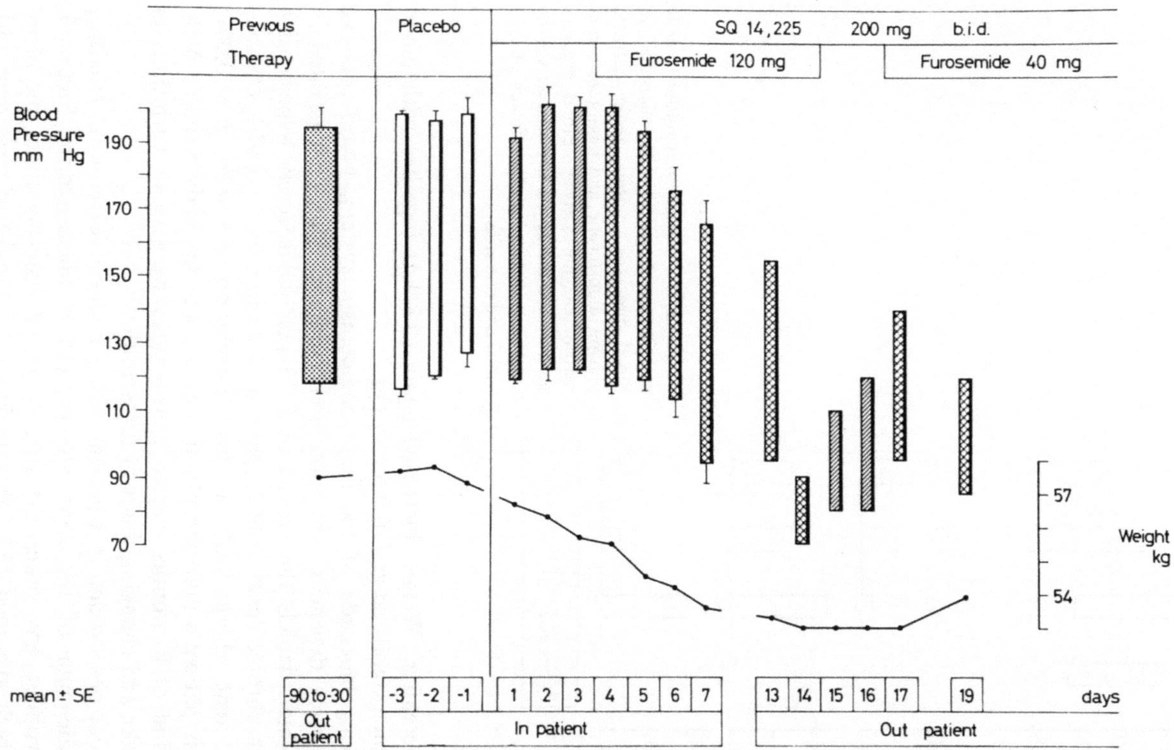

FIGURE 7. Effect of captopril alone and in combination with furosemide on blood pressure and weight in a 28-year-old hypertensive patient with diabetes mellitus and chronic renal failure. With the renin–angiotensin system blocked, blood pressure reduction paralleled the weight loss, reflecting progressive sodium depletion. (From Brunner et al.[31])

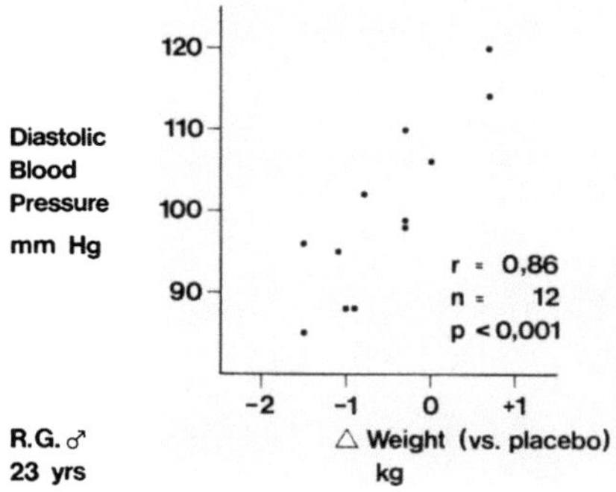

FIGURE 8. Relationship between furosemide-induced weight changes and diastolic blood pressure in a patient treated with captopril. Weight changes were based on the weight measured during the placebo period. (From Brunner et al.[36])

from 0.3 to 0.83 ng/ml per hr. Readministration of one dose of captopril now normalized blood pressure at 100/83 mm Hg.

In the eight patients on chronic hemodialysis with "uncontrollable" hypertension, blood pressure on previous therapy averaged 179/105 ± 6/3 mm Hg (Figure 10). After 4 to 6 days of captopril, blood pressure was lower at 164/90 ± 10/4 mm Hg but not normalized in all patients: four responded well, and their blood pressures remained under control for up to 9 months of treatment with captopril alone. Those four patients had the

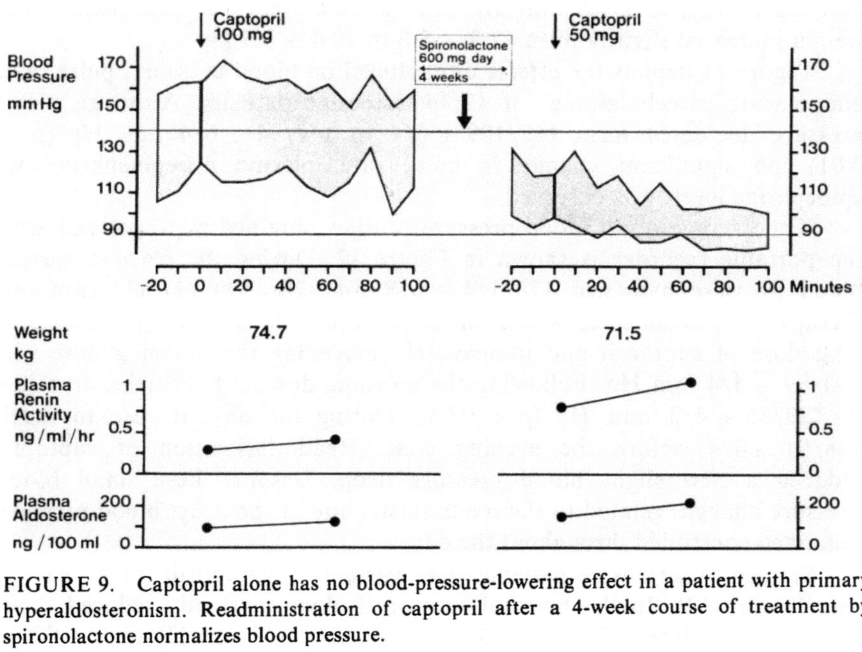

FIGURE 9. Captopril alone has no blood-pressure-lowering effect in a patient with primary hyperaldosteronism. Readministration of captopril after a 4-week course of treatment by spironolactone normalizes blood pressure.

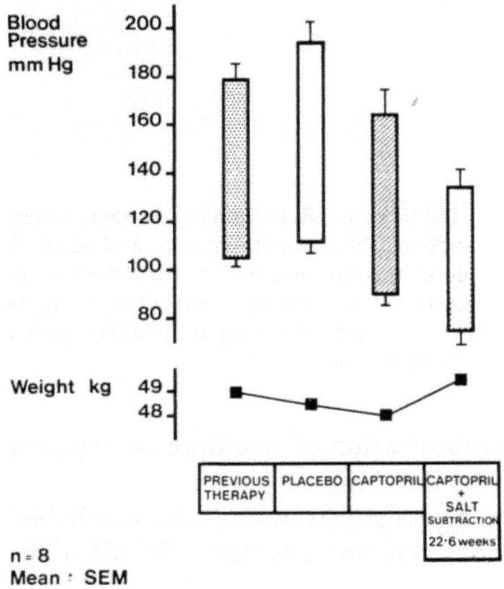

FIGURE 10. Effect of captopril alone or combined with salt subtraction on blood pressure and weight in chronic hemodialysis patients with hypertension resistant to ultrafiltration and conventional therapy.

highest renin values (8.9–97 ng/ml per hr). In the four other patients with the lowest renin values (0.71–6.9 ng/ml per hr), additional salt subtraction was necessary. This made it possible to control blood pressure in all eight patients at 134/76 ± 7.5 mm Hg after 22 ± 6 weeks of treatment, while weight increased slightly form 47.9 ± 5.8 to 49.4 ± 5.9 kg.

Figure 11 depicts the effects of captopril on blood pressure, pulse rate, and plasma catecholamines of 12 hypertensive patients. Although blood pressure decreased form 167/109 ± 6/4 to 144/94 ± 6/4 mm Hg ($p < 0.01$), no significant change in pulse rate, plasma norepinephrine, or epinephrine levels was observed.

The average of all blood pressure profiles obtained in 17 patients with the portable recorder is shown in Figure 12. During the placebo period, blood pressure averaged 178/114 ± 6/3 mm Hg. On chronic captopril therapy for a mean of 13 weeks, blood presure 14 hr after the previous evening dose of captopril and immediately preceding the morning dose was 140/89 ± 4/4 mm Hg. Following the morning dose, it fell further to a low of 129/85 ± 4/3 mm Hg ($p < 0.05$). During the day, it rose to reach 138/91 ± 4/4 before the evening dose. Readministration of captopril induced a new slight blood pressure drop. Despite these small blood pressure changes related to the readministration of the drug, blood pressure remained controlled throughout the day.

Sixteen hypertensive patients were treated by captoprill for at least 1 year (Figure 13). In the hospital, captopril alone markedly reduced their blood pressure from 176/113 ± 6/4 to 144/90 ± 6/2 mm Hg ($p < 0.001$).

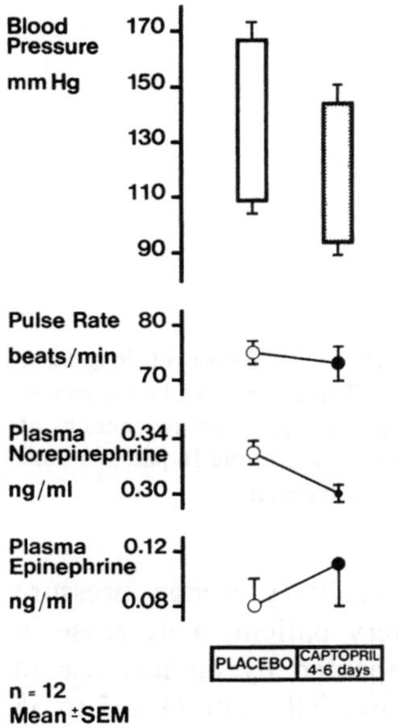

FIGURE 11. Effect of captopril on heart rate and catecholamines. Captopril does not seem to change the activity of the sympathetic nervous system.

In eight of them, a diuretic was added after discharge from the hospital in order to control their blood pressure. Following 6 and 12 months of continued treatment, blood pressure remained low at 133/90 ± 5/2 and 129/88 ± 4/3 mm Hg respectively.

Figure 14 summarizes some results obtained in patients with congestive heart failure without hypertension and depicts the relationship for each

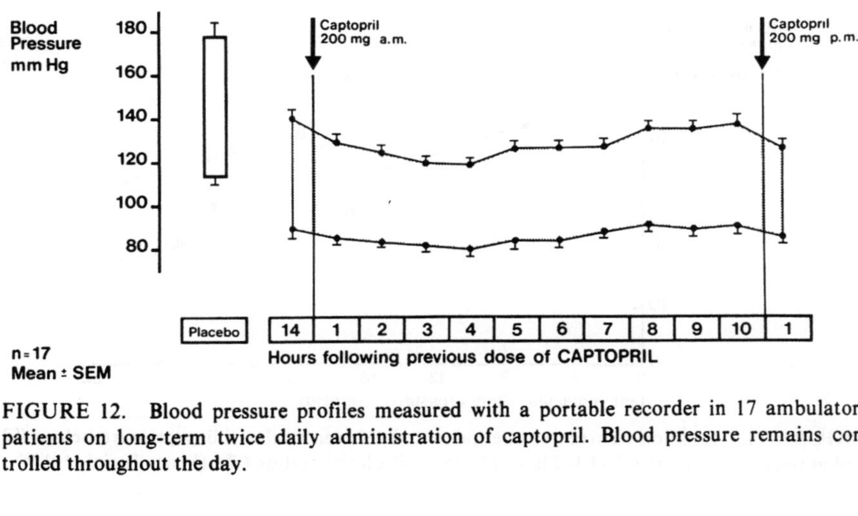

FIGURE 12. Blood pressure profiles measured with a portable recorder in 17 ambulatory patients on long-term twice daily administration of captopril. Blood pressure remains controlled throughout the day.

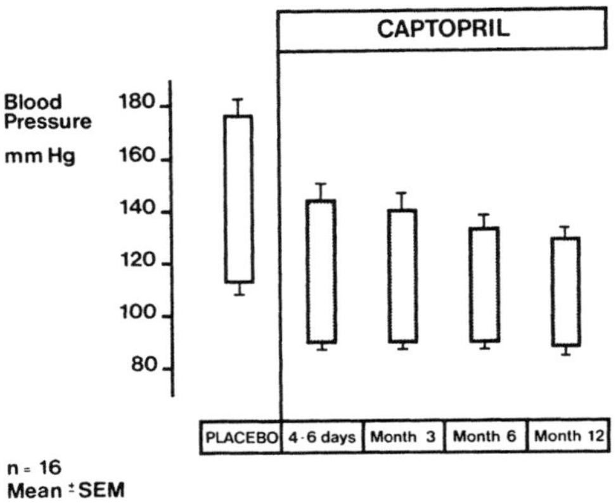

FIGURE 13. Effect of long-term therapy. There seems to be no escape from the antihypertensive action of captopril. Eight of the 16 patients took additional diuretics.

patient between stroke index and pulmonary capillary wedge pressure before and after captopril administration. In every patient, a decrease in pulmonary capillary wedge pressure was accompanied by an increase in stroke index. Simultaneously, mean arterial pressure fell from 73 ± 5 to 55 ± 7 mm Hg.

Some hormonal responses of these patients to captopril are illustrated in Figure 15. Plasma renin activity was high in five of the patients. It increased in all six from 21 ± 9.4 to 46 ± 17.4 ng/ml per hr ($p < 0.05$) at the time of maximal hemodynamic response to captopril. Plasma norepinephrine levels were high in all patients, the two with the most severe functional limitations exhibiting the highest values of 1.52 and 2.92 ng/ml

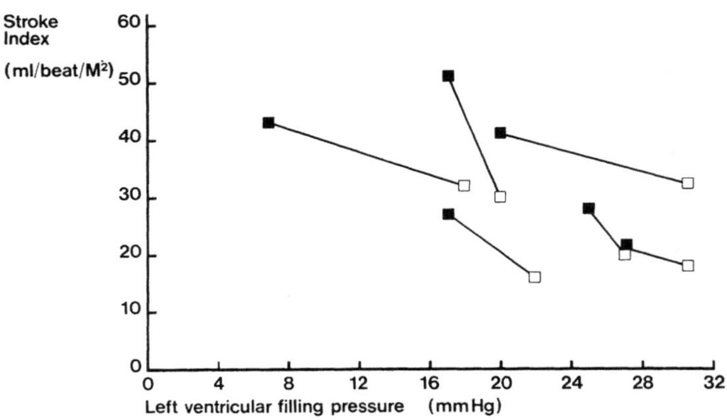

FIGURE 14. Relation between stroke index and left ventricular filling pressure before (□) and at time of maximum effect 1–3 hr after captopril administration (■). (From Turini et al.[26])

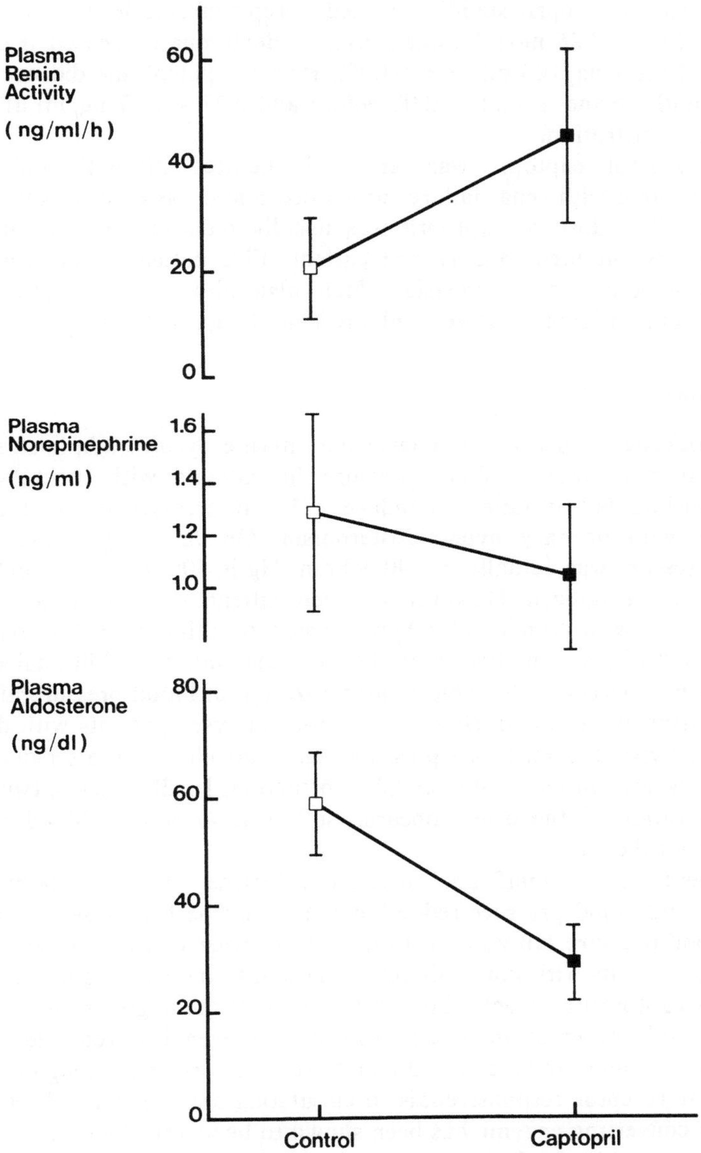

FIGURE 15. Effect of captopril on plasma renin activity, plasma norepinephrine, and plasma aldosterone levels in 6 patients with congestive heart failure. Placebo phase (□) and maximum hemodynamic effect of captopril (■) are shown.

respectively. Captopril slightly reduced norepinephrine levels from 1.29 ± 0.37 to 1.04 ± 0.26 ng/ml while plasma aldosterone decreased from 60 ± 10.3 to 30 ± 7 ng/100 ml ($p < 0.005$). Plasma epinephrine did not change significantly, being at 0.26 ± 0.08 before and 0.27 ± 0.07 ng/ml after captopril administration.

In general, captopril was very well tolerated. Notwithstanding, five patients (three with renal failure) developed a skin rash which was of short duration. The dose of captopril was usually reduced, and the drug was actually discontinued in only one patient. Five patients (four with renal failure) experienced hypogeusia which also disappeared spontaneously. None of our patients has developed any sign of nephrotoxicity.

Discussion

Blockade of angiotensin-converting enzyme by oral administration of captopril has lowered blood pressure in patients with most types of hypertension, but it failed to induce a blood pressure drop in the two patients with primary hyperaldosteronism. On captopril therapy alone, blood pressure was actually < 140/90 mm Hg in 30% of our patients while they were hospitalized. However, in seven patients with essential hypertension, in one with renovascular hypertension resulting from bilateral renal artery stenosis, and in five with chronic renal failure, additional diuretic therapy was necessary to achieve normalization of blood pressure after discharge from the hospital. Similarly, in four dialysed patients with dialysis-resistant hypertension, blood pressure was controlled only after decreasing total body sodium by additional salt subtraction. In all patients, twice daily administration of the drug appeared sufficient to control blood pressure throughout the day.

There was a significant correlation between baseline plasma renin activity and blood pressure reduction 1 hr after the first dose of captopril. The blood pressure fall was most marked in patients with high renin levels, but even patients with low renin levels showed some pressure drop. Assuming that captopril acts only through blockade of the angiotensin-converting enzyme, this observation would suggest that even low renin levels may contribute to maintining elevated blood pressure, possibly through increased arteriolar receptor responsiveness to circulating angiotensin II.[29] However, because converting enzyme has been shown to be identical with kininase II,[5] blockade may also lead to accumulation of bradykinin. Thus, the possibility that blood pressure reduction observed in our patients with low renin levels may be partly the result of a bradykinin effect cannot be ruled out.[23]

Blood pressure reduction was rapid, and maximal antihypertensive effect could generally be achieved within the first 2 hr of treatment. At the doses used, the amplitude of the blood pressure fall was not dose-dependent. Indeed, 25 mg of captopril was sufficient to induce on an antihypertensive effect comparable to the one obtained subsequently with higher doses. This is in total agreement with the findings in normal volunteers who exhibited a complete blockade of angiotensin conversion for more than 2 hr after ingestion of 20 mg of captopril.[22] Increasing the dose prolonged the blocking effect, which was still apparent for more than 6 hr after administration of 200 mg of captopril.

The blood pressure-lowering effect of angiotensin-converting enzyme inhibition may be so substantial because reduction of angiotensin II levels not only reverses arteriolar constriction but also decreases secretion of aldosterone.[30] Unlike most antihypertensive drugs which almost invariably induce sodium retention, captopril had no such effect. The lack of sodium retention can be explained by this reduced aldosterone secretion. Moreover, antagonizing intrarenal effects of the renin system may also counteract sodium retention. Thus, in patients with essential hypertension maintained on unrestricted sodium intake, acute administration of captopril was associated with an increase in renal plasma flow, the magnitude of which was positively correlated with plasma renin activity (not shown in Table 1). In addition, since glomerular filtration rate was not altered, filtration fraction fell in all patients. These results strongly suggest that angiotensin II participates actively in the regulation of renal vascular tone, and more precisely at the level of the efferent arterioles of the glomeruli.[25] Because sodium depletion has a potentiating effect on blood pressure reduction induced by converting enzyme blockade,[8] the lack of sodium retention can be expected to enhance therapeutic efficacy of captopril.

Sodium depletion and diuretics have long been used to treat essential hypertension and hypertension associated with chronic renal failure. If these measures alone often fail to normalize blood pressure, it may be because of the well-known compensatory rise in renin induced by sodium depletion. It now appears that this renin response, rather than being appropriate, is excessive, since specific blockade of angiotensin II generation leads to normalization of blood pressure in paractically all patients.[23,31] Thus, blockade of the pressor effect of the compensatory rise in renin induced by diuretics makes it possible to "titrate" the amount of sodium that has to be removed to normalize blood pressure. Figures 6, 7, and 8 illustrate the blood pressure behavior when captopril and diuretics are used together. The decrease in total body sodium induced by furosemide shifts the blood pressure from a renin-independent state to a situation of exquisite renin dependency. Accordingly, following blockage of the renin–angiotensin system, blood pressure is adjusted only by changing the dose of diuretics. Moreover, if hypertension occurs, the dose of captopril should not be reduced, since even very small doses still inhibit angiotensin conversion.[22,31,32] Blood pressure recovers after a short withdrawal of the diuretic.

Captopril was also effective in lowering blood pressure of chronic hemodialysis patients with previously "uncontrollable" hypertension. In these patients, whenever plasma renin activity was high, captopril was effective alone. However, when renin values were not clearly elevated, additional salt subtraction was necessary to control blood pressure.[24]

β-Blocking agents have been thought to lower blood pressure, at least in part, by lowering renin secretion.[33] Nevertheless, the patient data presented in Figure 6 strongly suggest that, in combination with diuretics, specific angiotentin-converting enzyme inhibition by captopril is more effective in lowering blood pressure than is β-blockade, since in all of them β-blocking agents were the mainstay of the previous therapy that did not control their blood pressure. Furthermore, the dose of diuretics that was needed to normalize blood pressure together with captopril therapy was, in each patient, equal to or smaller than the dose taken before in addition to the β-blockers.

The data obtained with captopril in patients with chronic congestive heart failure suggest that blockade of the renin system improves their cardiac function. The marked decrease in systemic vascular resistance (not shown in the figure) resulted, in these patients, in increases in stroke index and cardiac output. In addition to afterload, right atrial pressure and preload were also reduced, and this further decreased left ventricular filling pressure and, possibly, myocardial oxygen consumption. Whether these beneficial effects of inhibition of the renin–angiotensin system on cardiac function persist when captopril is administered chronically remains to be established. If so, captopril might be a useful new vasodilator agent for treating congestive heart failure. Notwithstanding, these date are in complete agreement with earlier observations suggesting that the renin system plays an important role in determining pre- and afterload of normotensive patients with congestive heart failure.[20,21,26,34,35]

In summary, captopril is a powerful and well tolerated drug effective in lowering blood pressure of hypertensive patients and in enhancing cardiac function of patients with congestive heart failure. When given together with diuretics or other means of salt subtraction, practically any hypertension can be reduced.

References

1. Pals DT, Masucci FD, Sipos F, Denning GS Jr: A specific competitive antagonist of the vascular action of angiotensin II. *Circ Res* 29:664–672, 1971.
2. Ondetti MA, Williams NJ, Sabo EF, Plusec J, Weaver ER, Kocy O: Angiotensin-

converting enzyme inhibitors from the venom of *Bothrops fararaca:* Isolation, elucidation of structure and synthesis. *Biochemistry* 10:4033–4039, 1971.
3. Streeten DHP, Anderson GH, Freiberg JM, Dalakos TG: Use of angiotensin II antagonist (saralasin) in the recognition of "angiotensinogenic" hypertension. *N Engl J Med* 292:657–662, 1975.
4. Gavras H, Ribeiro A, Brunner HR, Gavras I: Reciprocal relationship between renin dependency and sodium dependency in essential hypertension. *N Engl J Med* 295: 1278–1283, 1976.
5. Erdös EG: Angiotensin I converting enzyme. *Circ Res* 36:247–255, 1975.
6. Brunner HR, Gavras H, Laragh JH, Keenan R: Hypertension in man. Exposure of the renin and sodium components using angiotensin II blockade. *Circ Res* (suppl)1:35–45, 1974.
7. Vaughan ED, Peach MJ Jr: Saralasin. *Kidney Int* 15(Suppl 9), 1979.
8. Gavras J, Brunner HR, Laragh JH, Sealey JE, Gavras I, Vukovich RA: The use of an angiotensin converting enzyme inhibitor to identify and treat vasoconstrictor and volume factors in hypertensive patients. *N Engl J Med* 291:817–821, 1974.
9. Case DB, Wallace JM, Keim HJ, Weber MA, Drayer JIM, White RP, Sealey JE, Laragh JH: Estimating renin participation in hypertension: Superiority of converting enzyme inhibitor over saralasin. *Am J Med* 61:790–796, 1976.
10. Nielsen I, Clausen E, Jensen G: Plasma renin activity in chronic nephropathy. *Acta Med Scand* 188:351–354, 1970.
11. Brown JJ, Düsterdieck G, Fraser R, Lever AF, Robertson JIS, Iree M, Weir RJ: Hypertension and chronic renal failure. *Br Med Bull* 27:128–135, 1971.
12. Weidmann P, Maxwell MH, Lupn AN, Lewin AJ, Massry SG: Plasma renin activity and blood pressure in terminal renal failure. *N Engl J Med* 285:757–762, 1971.
13. Schalekamp MA, Beevers DG, Briggs JD, Brown JJ, Davies DL, Fraser R, Lebel M, Lever AF, Medina A, Morton JJ, Robertson JIS, Tree M: Hypertension in chronic renal failure. An abnormal relation between sodium and the renin–agiotensin system. *Am J Med* 55:379–390, 1973.
14. Weidmann P, Beretta-Piccoli C, Steffen F, Blumberg A, Reubi FC: Hypertension in terminal renal failure. *Kidney Int* 9:294–301, 1976.
15. Weidmann P, Maxwell MH: Hypertension, in: Massry SG and Sellers AL (eds), Clinical aspects of Uremia and Dialysis. Springfield, Charles C Thomas, pp 100–145, 1976.
16. Vertes V, Cangiano JL, Berman LB, Gould A: Hypertension in end-stage renal disease. *N Engl J Med* 280:978–981, 1969.
17. Lazarus JM, Hampers CL, Bennett AH, Vandam LD, Merrill JP: Urgent bilateral nephrectomy for severe hypertension. *Ann Intern Med* 76:733–739, 1972.
18. Onesti G, Swartz C, Ramirez O, Brest AN: Bilateral nephrectomy for control of hypertension in uremia. *Trans Am Soc Artif Intern Organs* 14:361–366, 1968.
19. Mimran A, Shaldon D, Barjon P, Mion C: The effect of an angiotensin antagonist (saralasin) on arterial pressure and plasma aldosterone in hemodialysis-resistant hypertensive patients. *Clin Nephrol* 9:63–67, 1978.
20. Turini GA, Brunner HR, Ferguson RK, Rivier JL, Gavras H: Improvement of cardiac function by angiotensin II blockade. *Clin Res* 25:258A, 1977.
21. Turini GA, Brunner HR, Ferguson RK, Rivier JL, Gavras H: Congestive heart failure in normotensive man. Haemodynamics, renin, and angiotensin II blockade. *Br Heart J* 40:1134–1142, 1978.
22. Ferguson RK, Turini GA, Brunner HR, Gavras H, McKinstry D: A specific orally active inhibitor of angiotensin-converting enzyme in man. *Lancet* 1:775–778, 1977.
23. Brunner HR, Gavras H, Waeber B, Kershaw GR, Turini GA, Vukovich RA, McKinstry

DN, Gavras I: Oral angiotensin-converting enzyme inhibitor in long-term treatment of hypertensive patients. *Ann Intern Med* 90:19–23, 1979.

24. Wauters JP, Waeber B, Brunner HR, Guignard JP, Turini GA, Gavras H: Blockade of the renin system by captorpil in patients with "uncontrollable" hypertension on hemodialysis. *Kidney Int* 15:588, 1979.
25. Mimran A, Brunner HR, Turini GA, Waeber B, Brunner D: Effect of captopril on renal vascular tone in patients with essential hypertension. *Clin Sci* 57:421s–423s, 1979.
26. Turini GA, Brunner HR, Gribic M, Waeber B, Gavras H: Improvement of chronic congestive heart-failure by oral captopril. *Lancet* 1:1213–1216, 1979.
27. Brunner HR, Laragh JH, Baer L, Newton MA, Goodwin FT, Krakoff LR, Bard RH, Bühler RT: Essential hypertention: Renin and aldosterone, heart attack and stroke. *N Engl J Med* 286:441–449, 1972.
28. Peuler JD, Johnson G: Simultaneous single isotope radioenzymatic assay of plasma norepinephrine, epinephrine and dopamine. *Life Sci* 21:625, 1977.
29. Brunner HR, Chang P, Wallach R, Sealey JE, Laragh JH: Angiotensin II vascular receptors: Their avidity in relationship to sodium balance, the autonomic nervous system and hypertension. *J Clin Invest* 51:58–67, 1972.
30. Gavras H, Brunner HR, Turini GA, Kershaw GR, Tifft CP, Cuttelod S, Gavras I, Vukovich RA, McKinstry DN: Antihypertensive effect of the oral angiotensin converting-enzyme inhibitor SQ 14,225 in man. *N Engl J Med* 298:991–995, 1978.
31. Brunner HR, Waeber B, Wauters JP, Turini GA, McKinstry DN, Gavras H: Inappropriate renin secretion unmasked by captopril (SQ 14,225) in hypertension of chronic renal failure. *Lancet* 2:704–707, 1978.
32. Brunner HR, Waeber B, Gavras H: Rational use of captopril. *Lancet* 1:832, 1979.
33. Bühler FR, Laragh JH, Baer L, Vaughan ED, Brunner HR: Propranolol inhibition of renin secretion. A specific approach to diagnosis and treatment of renin-dependent hypertensive diseases. *N Engl J Med* 287:1209–1214, 1972.
34. Gavras H, Faxon DP, Berkoben J, Brunner HR, Ryan TJ: Angiotensin converting enzyme inhibition in patients with congestive heart failure. *Circulation* 58:770–776, 1978.
35. Curtiss C, Cohn JN, Vrobel T, Franciosa JA: Role of the renin–angiotensin system in the systemic vasoconstriction of chronic congestive heart failure. *Circulation* 58:763–770, 1978.
36. Brunner HR, Wauters, JP, Waeber, B, Gavras, H: The renin–angiotensin system in hypertensive patients with chronic renal failure. *Mitt Klin Nephrologi* 8:4–14, 1979.

Part III · Clinical Use of Converting Enzyme Inhibitors

Chapter 12

The Renin System in High Blood Pressure, from Disbelief to Reality

Converting Enzyme Blockade for Analysis and Treatment

John H. Laragh

Introduction

Captopril is the newly developed orally active inhibitor of the enzyme that controls formation of the pressor hormone, angiotensin II, from its inactive precursor, angiotensin I. Based on previous experience with an intravenously given nonapeptide inhibitor, the compound was developed as a potential antihypertensive agent, and, as described in this volume, it has proven to be extremely potent. This treatment focuses once more on the renin–angiotensin system as a vital participant in sustaining the blood pressure of hypertensive patients.

In this chapter on oral converting enzyme blockade, I will review the renin–angiotensin–aldosterone control system, how it was discovered in hypertensive patients, how we have learned to analyze its behavior in terms of its normal relationship to the sodium ion that it controls via aldosterone, and how, using a series of semispecific but differently acting pharmacological probes as antihypertensive agents, we have learned more and more of its participation in the spectrum of human hypertension and also about its status as a unique biological control system that regulates normotension and electrolyte balance.

Prior to the development of captopril, three different types of pharmacological probes had been used to evaluate the renin system. These

Reprinted from *Progress in Cardiovascular Diseases* 21(3):159–166, 1978, by permission of the author and the publisher, Grune & Stratton.

JOHN H. LARAGH, M.D. · Cardiovascular Center and Division of Cardiology, New York Hospital–Cornell Medical Center, New York, New York 10021.

agents block the system at the point of renin release (β-adrenergic blocking drugs), at the formation point of angiotensin II (converting enzyme blockade), or at the vascular receptor site of action of the hormone angiotensin II (saralasin). With these agents, growing and reinforcing evidence has been put forth for the active participation of the renin system in most patients with essential hypertension. This sequence of events had led to the development and use of the first orally active inhibitor of angiotensin-converting enzyme, captopril—the subject of this volume.

Discovery of the Renal–Adrenal Interaction

That a renal substance could produce hypertension is an idea that has been waiting for its time to come since 1898 when Tigerstedt and Bergmann[1] injected a saline extract of minced rabbit kidneys (they called it renin) into another rabbit and produced a pressor response. The idea lost credence when other investigators failed to duplicate the experiment, was revived in 1934 when Goldblatt clamped the renal artery of the dog and produced hypertension indistinguishable from the human form,[2] and then again fell into disrepute because of the difficulties of assaying renin and because no investigator was able to find increases consistently associated with any form of hypertension.

For an equally long time, an association between salt balance and hypertension was known or suspected, and research in this area was aimed at defining renal and extrarenal mechanisms of electrolyte regulation as a first step to the understanding of pathogenesis. This was the research pathway that led our group back to renin some 20 yr ago. We had been studying the control of fluid volume by aldosterone, the sodium-retaining and kaliuretic adrenocortical hormone, using a laborious but precise double isotope dilution method to measure it. We expected and found very excessive aldosterone secretion rates in primary aldosteronism, a rare and mild hypertensive disorder cured by removing an autonomous adrenal tumor. We did not expect, however, and were startled to discover, extraordinarily high aldosterone levels in patients with malignant hypertension.[3] This was the first identification of a humoral pathophysiological abnormality in a common hypertensive disease.

We asked why this should be so. Was malignant hypertension analogous to primary aldosteronism? This analogy disintegrated when we removed the adrenals of some of the patients only to find no effect on the inexorable course of the disease. Moreover, these adrenal glands were tumor-free and revealed instead bilateral hyperplasia. This meant that they were reacting to an abnormal stimulus. The question was, what? It seemed reasonable to us to suspect that the source was the kidney, since that organ exhibits the greatest pathologic change in malignant hypertension.

This supposition returned us to the puzzlie posed 60 yr earlier by Tigerstedt and Bergmann, and even to a version of their experiment. We were not about to inject minced human kidneys into human volunteers, nor had we access to renin. However, it was now known that renin's interaction with a plasma protein substrate produced angiotensin II, a powerful vasoconstrictor octapeptide. Moreover, angiotensin II had recently been synthesized and was available for clinical trial.

Consequently, we infused angiotensin II into volunteers and induced striking increases in their adrenocortical secretion of aldosterone.[4] No other pressor substance produced this response—neither epinephrine, norepinephrine, vasopressin, nor a series of synthetic analogues. The specificity of the response revealed the biological interaction[5] among three hormones that have come to be called the renin–angiotensin–aldosterone system.

Thus, in 1960 the renin system was exposed[4,5] as a circle of biochemical events capable of causing high blood pressure in two ways: both because of the vasoconstrictive effect of angiotensin and the volume-retaining effects of aldosterone. At that time, we suggested[5] that the new system worked as a closed feedback loop for normal regulation of blood pressure and electrolyte balance. The signal for renin release is lowered blood pressure at kidney, and the signal for its shutoff is the raised pressure at the kidney produced by the system itself. We felt that this could be a central regulating mechanism for all blood pressure phenomena, and our subsequent research has substantiated this feeling.

The Renin–Aldosterone System: Its Involvement in Malignant Hypertension

The behavior of the renin system can be understood by considering the hypothesis proposed to explain malignant hypertension[4,5] (Figure 1). When established hypertension produces a critical degree of renal damage, the renin-producing cells mistake the identity of a local phenomenon of reduced pressure beyond obstructed arterioles, and they react by releasing more and more renin into the bloodstream. Renin then reacts with a plasma globulin to produce angiotensin I, an inactive decapeptide which, in passage through the lungs, encounters the enzyme that converts it into the active octapeptide hormone, angiotensin II—the most potent endogenous pressor agent known. The resulting excessive vasoconstriction raises blood pressure. What is more, this angiotensin II concurrently summons a volume effect by stimulating the adrenal cortex to release aldosterone, which causes excessive

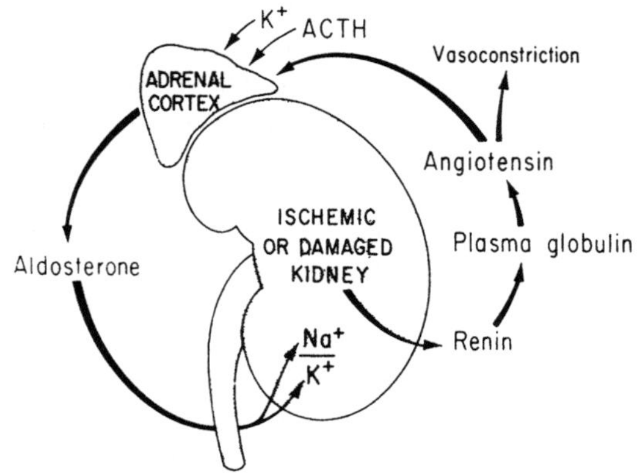

FIGURE 1. The renal-adrenal axis–a hormonal cascade involving renin, angiotensin, and aldosterone for regulation of sodium and potassium balance and blood pressure. The interaction is depicted as it was first discovered in the studies of patients with malignant hypertension in whom, because of defective feedback, it is involved in causation. Accordingly, there is a massive excess of both renin and aldosterone that cannot turn itself off. (Reproduced by permission.[5])

sodium retention, with concurrent fluid retention, and kaliuresis. This response would, under normal circumstances, restore blood pressure and renal flow and shut off the signal for renin release, but the damaged kidney cannot respond properly since the higher pressure and flow do not reach the sensor cells, and so the kidneys continue to release renin inappropriately, raising blood pressure further. The resulting vicious cycle—kidney damage, renin release, aldosterone production, sodium retention, heightened blood pressure, more kidney damage, more renin release, and finally more and more angiotensin II and aldosterone—becomes irreversible. Widespread systemic vascular damage and renal arteriolar necrosis and rupture are ultimately fatal (Figure 1).

A number of observations now support this hypothesis.[6] When renin and aldosterone are injected separately in animals, normal compensatory mechanisms tend to maintain blood pressure at viable levels; hypertension and vascular damage may ensue only after some time. However, if renin and aldosterone are injected simultaneously, the animals will die of vasculitis in a day or two. More significant is recent experience from dialysis wards that provides proof of the hypothesis: When the kidneys of a patient with malignant hypertension are removed, the blood pressure often drops to normal, and biopsies show healing of the arteriolar necrosis.

The Normal Operation of the Renin System

From this and other research,[6,7] it has been our view that the renin axis is designed to maintain arterial blood pressure and sodium balance simultaneously (Figure 2). Renin responds to factors that reduce arterial blood pressure and renal perfusion, such as shock, hemorrhage, or heart failure, or that reduce flow in the distal renal tubule, as in sodium depletion.

Angiotensin II, in turn, raises blood pressure quickly by constricting the arterioles. Aldosterone acts over the next several hours to cause renal sodium retention and potassium excretion. The retained sodium leads secondarily to water retention, expanding the extracellular fluid volume, and by restoring flow, giving further indirect support to the blood pressure. As the system is compensated by restoring systematic blood flow and renal perfusion, renin release is shut off by signals involving baroreceptor mechanisms in the afferent renal arterioles largely under α-adrenergic control[8] and by receptors in the macula densa portion of the renal tubules sensitive to changes in sodium supply.

Clinical Evaluation of the Renin System

Renin and aldosterone secretion normally fluctuate widely but predictably according to the state of sodium balance. Since this can vary quite considerably from day to day, we developed procedures called *renin–sodium profiling* and *aldosterone–sodium profiling* to evaluate the normality of the system.[7,9] The hormone measurements are referenced

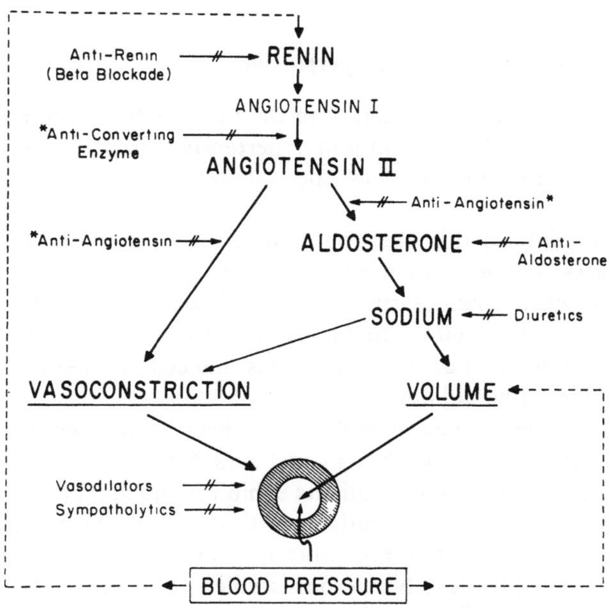

FIGURE 2. Site of intervention of various orally active antihypertensive drugs and of the two peptide inhibitors of angiotensin II formation or action. ---, Negative feedback; *, intravenous agents. (Reproduced by permission.[24])

against the concurrent 24-hr rate of urinary sodium excretion, which is used as an index of intake and balance,[7] and the values from patients are compared to curves obtained from studies of normal subjects. Blood for renin assay is collected in ambulatory patients so that the test includes the postural stimulus to renin secretion, which, for the most part, is neurogenically mediated.[8] A reliable assay for plasma renin activity that is sensitive enough to explore fully and discriminate the subnormal range is required.[7,9]

Even before the renin system was recognized, it had been known since 1955 that the excess aldosterone secretion of primary aldosteronism can cause a rare form of hypertension. Then, as already discussed, we showed that malignant hypertension was caused by an excess of both renin and aldosterone.[5] Curable unilateral renovascular hypertension is also probably caused by excess renin secretion,[10] and oral contraceptive hypertension[11] is associated with an excess renin substrate. Thus, abnormalities in the renin system play a causal role in three, and perhaps four, relatively uncommon hypertensive states. However, the lack of awareness of the role of the renin system in these particular hypertensive disorders can be appreciated when one realizes that in the recently reported National Cooperative Study of renovascular hypertension, renin measurements were not even used in the analysis.

The Renin System in Essential Hypertension

Even if a specific derangement in the renin–aldosterone axis causes at least three particular but uncommon hypertensive diseases, the question has remained whether or not, and how, the system might be involved in essential hypertension.

Our first clue on this question came from a study showing that very small increases in renin might cause hypertension. Ames and associates[12] showed that when angiotensin II was infused into normal volunteers, diminishingly small amounts could sustain an elevated pressure as sodium retention (via aldosterone stimulation) was induced. This effect was specific in that norepinephrine did not act similarly.[2]

Then, using renin–sodium profiling, we became convinced that essential hypertension is not all alike but in fact is a biochemically heterogeneous group of conditions with some patients exhibiting no and others excess renin involvement.[13] We found that patients with essential hypertension fall into three major subgroups exhibiting either low (about 30%), normal (55%), or high (15%) renin profiles. Numerous studies throughout the world have described generally similar distributions.

While this meant that only some 15% had truly high renin levels, we also observed that low renin patients appeared to suffer fewer heart attacks and strokes than either normal or high renin patients.[13] In fact, the "normal" renin group seemed almost at as much at risk as high renin patients. The validity of this observation has been questioned, but most such reports have not tested the proposal critically.[14] Actually, the stubborn fact remains that low renin patients are often more hypertensive than the normal renin group and are significantly older by at least 9 yr.[15] In the face of this more severe disease, the most likely explanation for the low renin group's greater longevity is that they enjoy a measure of protection from the cardiovascular damage associated with renin activity and its attendant vasoconstriction and that renin may be inappropriate even in so-called "normal renin" patients.

Altogether, the heterogeneity of the renin–sodium profiles led us to suspect that the varying levels of renin in essential hypertension reflect a reciprocation of vasoconstriction with volume factors supporting the hypertension. In this view, high renin patients would be the most vasoconstricted and hypovolemic, whereas, conversely, low renin patients would have the least vasoconstriction, and their hypertension would be largely due instead to overfilling of the circulation by an unknown mechanism causing sodium–volume excess with resultant suppression of renin secretion. This vasoconstriction–volume hypothesis[16] is supported by the established fact that most patients with low renin levels respond best to diuretic therapy, suggesting that their basic lesion does involve sodium and water retention.

Evolution of the Pharmacological Proof of Renin System Participation in Essential Hypertension

What was lacking in this hypothesis was direct evidence that plasma renin measurements in fact reflect the degree of its vasoconstriction. In the absence of this evidence, it is perhaps easy to understand how one might accept the alternative and more popular interpretation of the wide range of renin levels in essential hypertension, i.e., that they merely indicate that the renin system plays no pathophysiological role and is not involved in blood pressure support or control. This older view also gained apparent support from the fact that many patients exhibit ostensibly normal renin levels. Thus, a related question was: Are these values truly normal or are they in fact inappropriately high in the face of a maintained high blood pressure?

The first direct evidence for participation of renin in a majority of hypertensive patients emerged in 1972 when Bühler and associates[8] showed that the degree to which the β-adrenergic blocking drug, propranolol, lowered blood pressure was directly related to the height of the pretreatment plasma renin level and also to the degree that the drug reduced renin. In fact, propranolol alone was partially or completely effective in more than half of an unselected group of patients with essential hypertension—those with high renin and many with normal renin levels. Thus, this suggested that what had been considered a normal renin might be abnormal. In fact, recognizing that high pressure normally suppresses renin release, the normal response to hypertension ought to be a lowered renin secretion (Figure 2). More support for this concept came from the reciprocal observation that propranolol was without effect in the low renin subgroup.

While there have been many arguments put forth against the idea that renin participates in the blood pressure support of large fractions of hypertensive patients, this concept has been confirmed and extended in studies using drugs that block the action of angiotensin II (saralasin)[17,18] or its formation (converting enzyme inhibitor).[19,20] Experience with the later agent in particular, which unlike saralasin has no intrinsic pressor action, completely parallels and extends earlier observations with propranolol, indicating that a renin factor contributes to the hypertension in up to 70% of all patients with essential hypertension.[20,21]

Moreover, these studies establish that the renin level per se is a valid indicator of the extent of its active vasoconstriction in an individual patient, while the 24-hr urinary sodium measurement indicates the appropriateness of this vasoconstriction for the patient's sodium intake.[20]

Numerous reports now verify the differing response patterns of hypertensive patients both to β-blockade and to diuretic therapy (Table 1). Reciprocal effects reinforce these relationships; not only is propranolol usually ineffective in low renin patients, but like saralasin, it can be overtly *pressor* in them. Diuretics, uniquely effective in low renin patients, can be pressor in the high renin patients who are presumably already vasoconstricted and hypovolemic and react to more dehydration with an excessive renin response. The renin–volume interplay appears as a see-saw. Some patients given diuretics respond with vigorous hyperreninemia, explaining the failure of their blood pressure to fall.[19] Conversely, patients given antirenin agents may not respond because of reactive sodium retention.

Altogether, these results, based on many different approaches to the same question, all support the view that renin measurements reveal the degree to which blood pressure is supported by angiotensin-induced vasoconstriction and can be used to predict the antihypertensive response of individual patients to different types of therapy.

Long-Term Converting Enzyme Blockade: A New Era of More Specific and Potent Antirenin System Therapy

In this setting, the orally active converting-enzyme inhibitor, captopril, was developed. Its discovery was based, on the one hand, on fundamental

TABLE 1. The Selective Effectiveness of Antihypertensive Drugs

Beta-blockers are preferentially effective in high- and normal-renin patients	Diuretics are preferentially effective in low-renin patients
Bühler et al., *N Engl J Med* 287:1209, 1972	Crane et al., *Am J Med Sci* 260:311, 1970
Bühler et al., *Am J. Cardiol* 32:511, 1973	Spark et al., *Ann Intern Med* 75:831, 1971
Bühler et al., *Am J Cardiol* 36:652, 1975	Crane et al., *Am J Med* 52:457, 1972
Castenfors et al., *Acta Med Scand* 193:189, 1973	Carey et al., *Arch Intern Med* 130:849, 1972
Pettinger et al., *N Engl J Med* 292:1214, 1975	Adlin et al., *Arch Intern Med* 130:855, 1972
Karlberg et al., *Am J Cardiol* 27:642, 1976	Vaughan et al., *Am J Cardiol* 32:523, 1973
Hollifield et al., *N Engl J Med* 295:68, 1976	Castenfors et al., *Acta Med Scand* 193:189, 1973
Weidman et al., *Klin Wochenschr* 54:765, 1976	Distler et al., *Dtsch Med Wochenschr* 99:864, 1974
Menard et al., *Am J Med* 60:886, 1976	Douglas et al., *JAMA* 227:518, 1974
Stumpe et al., *Am J Med* 60:853, 1976	Karlberg et al., *Am J Cardiol* 37:642, 1976
MacGregor et al., *Clin Sci Mol Med* 50:18p, 1976	MacGregor et al., *Clin Sci Mol Med* 50:18p, 1976
Boerth, *Pediatr Res* 10:328, 1976	
Moore et al., *Lancet* 2:67, 1976	
Bahr et al., *Clin Pharmacol Ther* 20:130, 1976	
Zech et al., *Postgrad Med J* 53(*Suppl* 3):134, 1977	
Philipp et al., *Dtsch Med Wochenschr* 102:569, 1977	
Beta-blockers can actually raise pressure in low-renin patients	**Diuretics can actually raise pressure in high-renin patients**
Drayer et al., *Am J Med* 60:897, 1976	Baer et al., *Ann Intern Med* 86:257, 1977

studies of the nature and properties of the angiotensin-converting enzyme and, on the other hand, on clinical studies of the effect of the blockade of the enzyme with the intravenous nonapeptide described previously.

From a fundamental standpoint, this research process perhaps began with the landmark studies of Leonard Skeggs and his group,[22] who discovered converting enzyme and described its properties and the existence of two forms of angiotensin. Following this, work by Soffer and his associates and by Cushman and his group and by others cited by them in two chapters of this volume, greatly increased our knowledge of the biochemistry of the converting enzyme. The discovery of the nonapeptide inhibitor of converting enzyme by Ferreira and Greene[23] led to the clinical research by Case and associates[20,21] of our group, described above, which implicated a renin factor in maintaining part or all of the hypertension in some 70% of patients with essential hypertension. Indeed, these studies with the nonapeptide were presented before publication at the Squibb Institute in January 1975 and perhaps acted as a catalyst to the masterful and ingenious studies of Cushman, Cheung, Sato, and Ondetti, summarized herein, that led to the development of the orally active compound, captopril.

Clinical findings to date suggest that the effects of captopril are basically a direct extension over a longer time course of those described for the intravenous nonapeptide converting enzyme inhibitor.[19,20] There does, however, appear to be a greater reduction in blood pressure with continued administration, which begins sometime after the third day. This is very likely a result of the suppression of aldosterone secretion with resultant changes in sodium and potassium balance—a bonus that takes several days or more for full expression.

Several lines of evidence presented in this volume by Case et al. strongly suggest that the main effect of captopril in lowering blood pressure in patients is mediated by inhibition of the generation of the two effector hormones of the renin system, angiotensin II and aldosterone. Indeed, in view of these impressive correlations, there now seems little need to assign any considerable role to bradykinin generation or to other possible factors in the blood pressure lowering, even though this issue must remain open until all the critical direct evidence is in hand.

The clinical results with captopril also support our previous suggestions that normal renin levels are in fact inappropriately high for patients with an elevated arterial pressure, and in this way too, these results complement findings using the nonapeptide or saralasin or β-blocking drugs. All four types of experience thus become reinforcing in pointing to a significant participation of the renin system in patients with either high renin or normal renin essential hypertension.

Oral converting-enzyme blockade could be a real breakthrough for both the acute and the long-term treatment of many patients with high blood pressure. Given alone, this modality appears more powerful and more effective in larger fractions of patients than any other known agent. Moreover, side effects seem even less of a problem than with other approaches. Because β-blocking drugs also inhibit renin activity, albeit less completely, and since they are also very well tolerated, this class of drugs appears to be the most likely clinical alternative to captopril. More work is necessary before valid comparisons can be made. Meanwhile, it is already clear that, in some instances, converting enzyme blockade will be effective when β-blockade fails.

In the excitement of the clinical promise of this new therapeutic mode, the conceptual value of the new information should not be underestimated, since it seems to be bringing us closer to a final solution of hypertension. In so doing, it points us again towards a central role for the kidneys in determining the blood pressure level, doing so via changes in renin–aldosterone system activity, which presides over both vasoconstriction and volume, the two final determinants of blood pressure and of blood flow to tissues. Understanding this control system is therefore the underpinning for new therapeutic strategies. However, one must as always be alerted to the exceptions to the working hypothesis that are so often clues for revealing other mechanisms. This growing awareness of the role of the renin–aldosterone system may not be quite what Tigerstedt and Bergmann or Harry Goldblatt had predicted, but it is certainly close enough to please them.

References

1. Tigerstedt R, Bergman PG: Niere und Kreislauf. *Scand Arch Physiol* 8:223–271, 1898.
2. Goldblatt HJ, Lynch RF, Hanzal RF, et al: Studies on experimental hypertension. Production of persistent elevation of systolic blood pressure by means of renal ischemia. *J Exp Med* 59:347–378, 1934.
3. Laragh JH, Ulick S, Januszewicz W, et al: Aldosterone secretion and primary and malignant hypertension. *J Clin Invest* 39:1091, 1960.
4. Laragh JH, Angers M, Kelly WG, et al: Hypotensive agents and pressor substances. The effect of epinephrine, norepinephrine, angiotensin II and others on the secretory rate of aldosterone in man. *JAMA* 174:234, 1960.
5. Laragh JH: The role of aldosterone in man: Evidence for regulation of electrolyte balance and arterial pressure by renal–adrenal system which may be involved in malignant hypertension. *JAMA* 174:293, 1960.
6. Laragh JH, Baer L, Brunner HR, et al: Renin, angiotensin and aldosterone system in pathogenesis and management of hypertensive vascular disease. *Am J Med* 52:633–652, 1972.
7. Laragh JH, Sealey JE: Renin sodium profiling: Why, how and when in clinical practice. *Cardiovasc Med* 2:1053–1075, 1977.
8. Bühler FR, Laragh JH, Baer L, et al: Propranolol inhibition of renin secretion. A specific approach to diagnosis and treatment of renin-dependent hypertensive disease. *N Engl J Med* 287:1209–1214, 1972.
9. Sealey JE, Laragh JH: How to do a plasma renin assay. *Cardiovasc Med* 2:1076–1092, 1977.

10. Vaughan ED Jr, Bühler FR, Laragh JH, et al: Renovascular hypertension: Renin measurements to indicate hypersecretion and contralateral suppression, estimate renal plasma flow and score for surgical curability. *Am J Med* 55:402–414, 1973.
11. Laragh JH, Sealey JE, Ledingham JG, et al: Oral contraceptives. Renin, aldosterone, and high blood pressure. *JAMA* 201:981–922, 1967.
12. Ames RP, Borkowski AJ, Sicinski AM, et al: Prolonged infusions of angiotensin II and norepinephrine and blood pressure, electrolyte balance, aldosterone and cortisol secretion in normal man and in cirrhosis with ascites. *J Clin Invest* 44:1171–1186, 1965.
13. Brunner HR, Laragh JH, Baer L: Essential hypertension: Renin and aldosterone, Heart attack and stroke. *N Engl J Med* 286:441–449, 1972.
14. Kirkendall WN, Hammond JJ, Overturf ML: Renin as a predictor of hypertensive complications. *Ann NY Acad Sci* 304:147–160, 1978.
15. Laragh JH: Renin as a predictor of hypertensive complications: Discussion. *Ann NY Acad Sci* 304:165–177, 1978.
16. Laragh JH: Vasoconstriction–volume analysis for understanding and treating hypertension: The use of renin and aldosterone profiles. *Am J Med* 55:261–274, 1973.
17. Brunner HR, Gavras H, Laragh JH: Angiotensin II blockade in man by Sar^1-ala^8-angiotensin II for understanding and treatment of high blood pressure. *Lancet* 2:1045–1048, 1973.
18. Brunner HR, Gavras H, Laragh JH: Hypertension in man. Exposure of the renin and sodium components using angiotensin II blockade. *Circ Res* 34–35 (Suppl I):I-35–I-45, 1974.
19. Gavras H, Brunner HR, Laragh JH, et al: An angiotensin converting enzyme inhibitor to identify and treat vasoconstrictor and volume factors in hypertensive patients. *N Engl J Med* 291:817–821, 1974.
20. Case D, Wallace JM, Keim HJ, et al: Possible role of renin in hypertension as suggested by renin-sodium profiling and inhibition of converting enzyme. *N Engl J Med* 296:641–646, 1977.
21. Case DB, Wallace JM, Keim HJ, et al: Estimating renin participation in hypertension. Superiority of converting enzyme inhibitor over saralasin. *Am J Med* 61:790–769, 1976.
22. Skeggs LT Jr, Dorer EF, Kahn JR, et al: The biochemistry of the renin–angiotensin system and its role in hypertension. *Am J Med* 60:737–748, 1976.
23. Ferreira SH, Greene LJ, Alabaster VA, et al: Activity of various fractions of bradykinin potentiating factor against angiotensin I converting enzyme. *Nature* 255:379, 1970.
24. Laragh JH: Modern system for treating high blood pressure based on renin-profiling and vasoconstriction–volume analysis: A primary role for beta-blocking drugs such as propranolol. *Am J Med* 61:797–809, 1976.

Chapter 13

Experiences with Blockade of the Renin System in Human Hypertension Using Converting Enzyme Inhibitor SQ 20,881 and Saralasin

David B. Case, Hans J. Keim, John M. Wallace, and John H. Laragh

Introduction

The development of agents which are capable of producing in vivo angiotensin II blockade has provided to investigators and clinicians alike the opportunity to determine and to quantify the extent to which the renin–angiotensin system participates in the maintenance of hypertensive states. High levels of plasma renin activity relative to the state of sodium balance have been documented in patients with malignant, surgically remediable renovascular hypertension and also in some patients with essential hypertension.[1] The recent development of the angiotensin II analogue sar^1-ala^8-angiotensin II (saralasin) provided evidence to support the concept that these elevated renin levels are in fact participating in the hypertensive state.[2-5] However, saralasin is not a pure competitive antagonist of angiotensin II, but is rather a partial agonist,[5,6] and it seems likely that responses to this drug might underestimate the true renin factor.[5]

Early studies using the nonapeptide converting enzyme inhibitor of angiotensin II formation suggested that the renin–angiotensin system may have a greater degree of involvement in the blood pressure of hypertensive patients, since pressure reductions were measured in 5 of 8 normal-renin patients studied in the supine position as well as in high-renin patients.[7] Our

DAVID B. CASE, M.D., and JOHN H. LARAGH, M.D. · Cardiovascular Center and Division of Cardiology, New York Hospital–Cornell Medical Center, New York, New York 10021. HANS J. KEIM, M.D. · Johannes Gutenberg-Universität, I. Medizinische Klinik und Poliklinik, 6500 Mainz, Germany. JOHN M. WALLACE, M.D. · Department of Medicine, University of Texas Medical College, Galveston, Texas 77550.

studies were designed to systematically evaluate responses in blood pressure and plasma renin activity of hypertensive patients who had been previously categorized by an established renin-sodium profile.[8] In addition, all of the studies were done in untreated patients in the seated position receiving either a normal or a low sodium diet.[9] A second important part of the study was to compare the converting enzyme inhibitor, SQ 20,881, to the competitive inhibitor, saralasin, in 39 matched studies.[10] A third and final component of the study involved the application of SQ 20,881 and saralasin in anephric patients.[10]

Methods

Patients

After complete clinical examination, 66 hypertensive patients were selected for study. All of these patients had been withdrawn from all antihypertensive medications for a period of a least 21 days before study or had never received treatment. Classification according to the renin–sodium profile was based on concurrent measurements of plasma renin activity (PRA) and 24-hr urinary sodium excretion obtained just prior to the time of study according to the methods previously described.[8] Distribution of the patients who received SQ 20,881 alone is shown in Table 1.

Thirty-nine hypertensive patients were selected to receive both saralasin acetate (Sar^1-ala^8-angiotensin II, P113) and the nonapeptide converting enzyme inhibitor. These patients also had different forms of hypertension and were subgrouped according to their renin–sodium profiles. Of the 6 patients with low-renin profiles, 2 had primary aldosteronism, 1 bilateral renal artery stenosis, and 3 essential hypertension. Of the 23 patients with normal-renin profiles, all had essential hypertension, except for 1 who had unilateral renal artery stenosis but symmetrical renal vein renin values. Four of the 10 patients with high-renin profiles had renal artery stenosis (1 bilateral), 2 had malignant hypertension, and 4 had essential hypertension.

In the third part of this study, we administered saralasin and SQ 20,881 to 6 patients who were in a chronic hemodialysis program and had undergone bilateral nephrectomy.

Study Procedure

All of the following studies were carried out with patients seated comfortably in a study room where a quiet, nondistracting atmosphere was maintained. Blood pressure was measured at 2-minute intervals by Arteriosonde® or continuously by direct arterial recordings. A diet of 100 mEq sodium/day or an unrestricted diet was used to represented a normal sodium intake. Sodium depletion was accomplished by using a 10-mEq

TABLE 1. Clinical Diagnosis and Sodium Intakes of Subjects[a]

	Number of patients	
	Normal-sodium intake	Low-sodium intake
High-renin (19)		
Renal artery stenosis	5	4
Malignant	1	2
Renal disease	3	0
Pheochromocytoma	1	0
Essential	3	0
Normal-renin (35)		
Borderline	10	8
Renal artery stenosis	1	0
Essential	11	4
Malignant	0	1
Low-renin (12)		
Renal artery stenosis	1	1
Renal disease	1	0
Primary aldosterosis	1	3
Essential	3	2

[a] Low sodium intake entailed a period of at least 5 days of sodium intake of 10 mEq/day with a urinary sodium excretion rate of less than 50 mEq on the day of study. Normal sodium intakes were achieved by a constant diet of 105 mEq sodium per day or an unrestricted diet. (Adapted from Case et al.[10] with permission of the editor of *The New England Journal of Medicine*.)

sodium diet for 5 days prior to the study. Diuretic pretreatment was not used in any patient. SQ 20,881 was given as a single 1-mg/kg intravenous bolus after the seated blood pressure had remained stable for at least 20 min. Blood samples for the determination of plasma renin activity were drawn through a previously positioned indwelling venous catheter prior to and 30 min after drug administration. The same procedure was followed for the comparative studies with saralasin except this latter agent was given by constant infusion at the rate of 10 μg/kg per min for 30 min. The comparative studies of saralasin and SQ 20,881 were done within the same 24-hr period but separated in time by no less than 1 hr during which blood pressure and plasma renin activity returned to pretreatment levels. Plasma renin activity was measured according to the method of Sealey and Laragh.[11]

Analytical Methods

The control blood pressure for each patient was the average blood pressure over 20 min prior to blood sampling. Unless otherwise stated, the maximal change in diastolic pressure, expressed as a percentage of the control pressure, was used for analysis. These maximal deflections were obtained as averages over 4–6 min periods only at 10, 20, or 30 min intervals after the initiation of drug administration.

As appropriate in small samples, often without a normal distribution, nonparametric statistical methods were used to detect differences between two groups (Wilcoxon's 2-sample test) and to calculate correlation coefficients between variables (Spearman's correlation coefficient). All results are expressed as means ± standard error of the mean (SEM).

Results

Blood Pressure Responses of Renin Subgroups to Converting Enzyme Inhibitor, SQ 20,881

Analysis of the blood pressure responses of all patients grouped according to their renin–sodium profiles revealed significant differences (Figure 1).

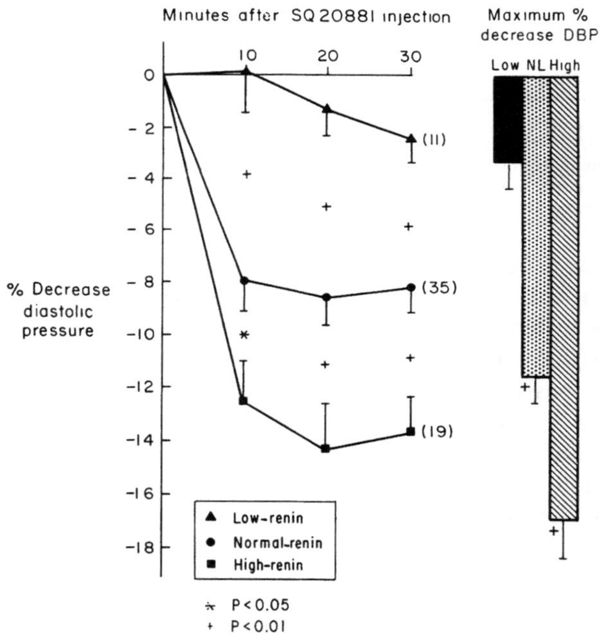

FIGURE 1. Diastolic blood pressure responses to converting enzyme inhibitor SQ 20,881 (1 mg/kg) in 65 hypertensive patients profiled as high-, normal- (NL), and low-renin. Values are mean ± SEM. The left panel represents the time course of the depressor responses, comparing the values of the low-renin (▲), and high-renin (■) patients. The right panel compares the maximal percent decreases in diastolic blood pressure of the three subgroups. Figures in parentheses denote number of patients. (Reproduced from Case et al.[9] with permission of the editor of *The New England Journal of Medicine*.)

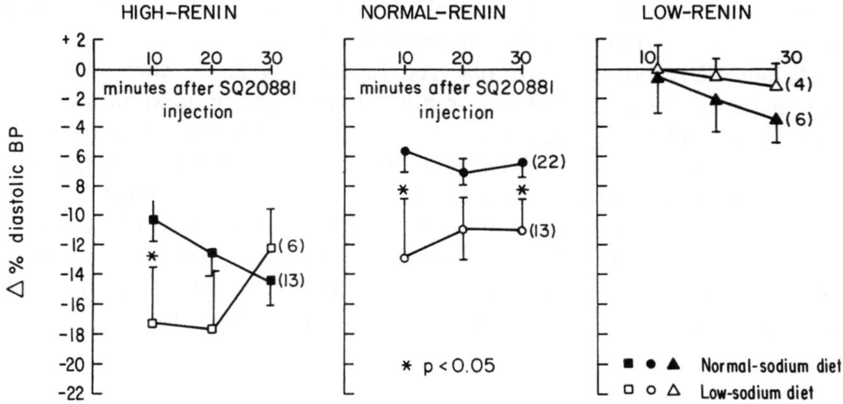

FIGURE 2. Effect of sodium intake on the response of mean diastolic blood pressure to converting enzyme inhibitor in the three renin subgroups. Symbols as in Figure 1. In each renin subgroup, patients on normal sodium intake are represented by closed symbols and those with moderate dietary sodium depletion by open symbols. (Reproduced from Case et al.[9] with permission of the editor of *The New England Journal of Medicine.*)

The high-renin patients had the greatest declines in blood pressure during all periods of observation; these, at the time of maximum decrease, averaged $-16.8 \pm 1.6\%$ of control diastolic pressure. These changes were greater than those observed in normal renin patients (maximum $-11.5 \pm 1.0\%$, $p < 0.01$). Both normal- and high-renin subgroups had greater falls at any time and at the time of maximal blood pressure decrease than did low-renin patients ($p < 0.01$ and 0.001, respectively). The average maximal decrease in diastolic pressure usually occurred by the 20-min observation period.

As shown in Figure 2, both before and after moderate dietary sodium depletion, diastolic pressures were reduced in all high-renin (maximum by -17.3 and -19.8% respectively) and in nearly all normal-renin patients (maximum -9.1 and -17.7%, respectively). This method of sodium depletion, however, did not produce significantly higher control renin levels in either the high- or the low-renin subgroups of patients, but it did in the normal-renin subgroup ($p < 0.01$).

Low-renin patients who were on either normal or low sodium intake failed to exhibit significant depressor responses (defined as a 5% or greater fall in diastolic pressure) to the nonapeptide converting enzyme inhibitor. Only 4 of 12 low-renin patients had slight decreases in diastolic pressure.

Sodium-depleted high-renin patients had maximal depressor responses within 10 min, more promptly than did a comparable group studied on normal sodium intake. However, comparable degrees of blood pressure reduction occurred in both high-renin groups. The group of sodium-depleted normal-renin subjects was indistinguishable from both groups of high-renin patients with respect to their control plasma renin values and their blood pressure responses to converting enzyme inhibitor.

When all responses were analyzed together, a direct correlation was found between the control plasma renin activity and the maximum percent decline in diastolic pressure (Figure 3, $r = 0.67$, $p < 0.001$). The regression line formed by this analysis intercepts the ordinate at a plasma renin value of approximately 2 ng angiotensin I(AI)/ml per hr. Of the 11 patients who had minimal changes in blood pressure (± 5% of control diastolic pressure) only 1 had a pretreatment plasma renin value greater than 2 ng/ml per hr (2.4 ng AI/ml per hr). Of all patients with blood pressure falls greater than 5%, only 2 had control renin levels of 2 ng AI/ml per hr or less.

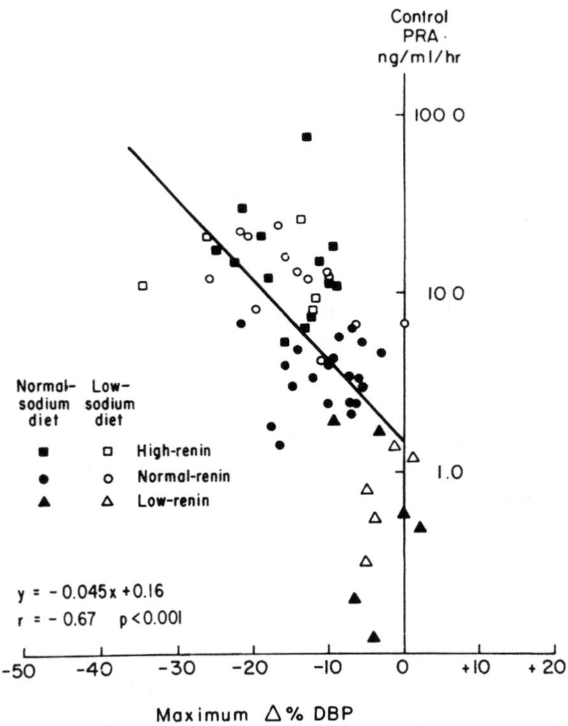

FIGURE 3. Relation between control plasma renin activity and the maximum percentage induced change in diastolic blood pressure in 62 hypertensive patients. Symbols as in Figure 1. A significant correlation if found irrespective of sodium diet ($p < 0.001$). The line of correlation intersects the vertical axis at a point corresponding to a plasma renin activity of about 2 ng angiotensin I/ml per hr, a theoretical level above which depressor responses would be predicted. (Reproduced from Case et al.[9] with permission of the editor of *The New England Journal of Medicine*.)

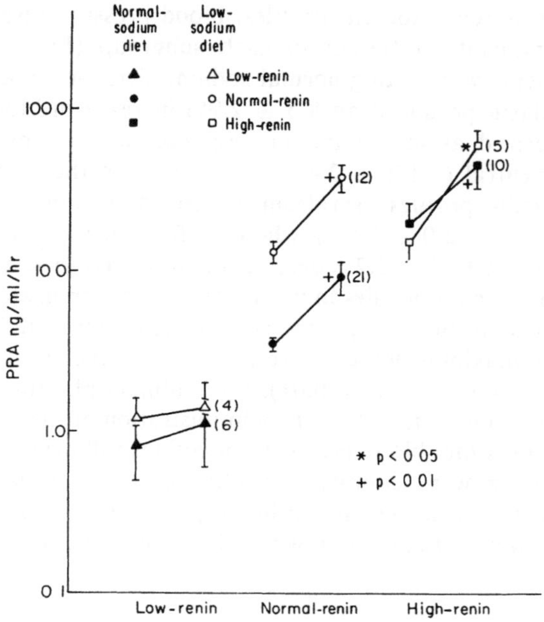

FIGURE 4. Effect of converting enzyme inhibitor SQ 20,881 on plasma renin activity in renin subgroups. The left symbol of each pair represents the pretreatment value, and the right one represents the value 30 min after injection of the inhibitor. The greatest changes were seen in sodium-depleted normal-renin patients and in both groups of high-renin patients, in all of whom comparable depressor responses to SQ 20,881 were induced. (Reproduced from Case et al.[9] with permission of the editor of *The New England Journal of Medicine*.)

In contrast to the relationship between renin and induced blood pressure changes, there was no correlation between the urinary sodium excretion and the change in blood pressure within each renin subgroup nor with all patients analyzed together.

SQ 20,881 produced significant increases in plasma renin activity (PRA) in all normal- and high-renin patients whether on normal or on a low sodium intake (Figure 4). In contrast, no significant rises in PRA were observed in low renin patients. The level to which PRA rose was clearly related to the control level of PRA ($r = 0.92$, $p < 0.001$). Moreover, a correlation ($r = 0.70$, $p < 0.001$) between the maximum decrease in diastolic pressure and the induced increment in PRA was demonstrated.

Comparison of Converting Enzyme Inhibitor and Saralasin

When the patients who were given both saralasin and converting enzyme inhibitor under matched conditions were divided into groups according to their renin–sodium profiles, blood pressure responses to each drug were significantly different in each subgroup (Figure 5). In these studies, all patients were eating normal sodium diets. Whereas the administration of saralasin produced an 8.5 ± 2.9% increase in blood pressure in patients categorized as low-renin, the response to the converting enzyme inhibitor was neutral (−1.2 ± 2.4%, $p < 0.05$). In the group of patients with normal-renin profiles, saralasin produced a minimal response in diastoloic pressure (+2.0 ± 1.5%), whereas after injection of the converting enzyme inhibitor, a 10.2 ± 1.2% decline was observed ($p < 0.001$). Even in patients with high-renin profiles in whom depressor responses occurred after the administration of both drugs, the converting enzyme inhibitor produced slightly greater maximal depressor responses than the saralasin (−18.7 ± 1.9% versus −13.6 ± 2.0%, $p < 0.01$). Pretreatment plasma renin levels did not differ in each subgroup before the administration of the blocking agents.

When the maximal blood pressure deflections following the administration of each drug were compared relative to the pretreatment level of plasma renin activity, decrements in blood pressure for any level of plasma renin activity were greater following the administration of converting

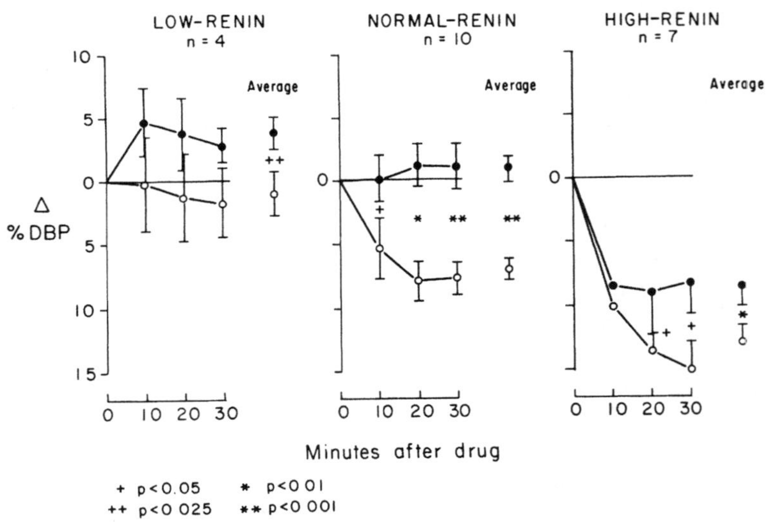

FIGURE 5. Comparison of the blood pressure responses to both saralasin (●) and SQ 20,881 (O) administration in 21 hypertensive patients previously profiled as low-, normal-, or high-renin. Changes in blood pressure are estimated as percent change in diastolic blood pressure. The average change for each 30-min period is shown at the right of each panel. Results are expressed as the mean ± SEM. (Reproduced from Laragh et al.[12] with permission of the editor of *The American Journal of Medicine*.)

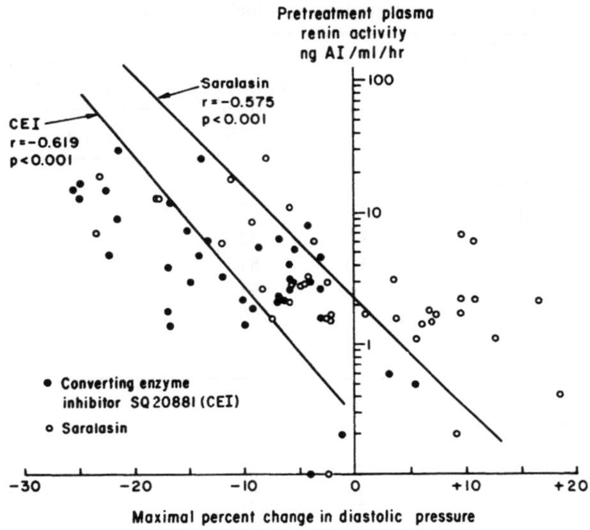

FIGURE 6. Comparison of the relationships between the pretreatment level of plasma renin activity and the maximum induced changes in diastolic pressure in patients treated with converting enzyme inhibitor (CEI) SQ 20,881 (●) or with saralasin (○). Both responses correlated well ($p < 0.001$) with pretreatment renin. However, at a given renin level, CEI lowered blood pressure more than did saralasin.

enzyme inhibitor than those following the administration of saralasin. However, the maximal depressor responses correlated well ($p < 0.001$ for both) with the pretreatment renin levels (Figure 6).

Effect of Converting Enzyme Inhibitor in Anephric Patients

In order to determine the effects of converting enzyme inhibitor in patients in whom there was no circulating renin, the drug was given to 6 anephric patients (see Table 2). The converting enzyme inhibitor produced no discernible trend in diastolic pressures, the mean change being +2.3 ± 2.0% after 10 min and +1.3 ± 2.3% after 20 min. In contrast, saralasin, in doses of 1 or 10 μg/kg per min, was uniformly pressor in 4 additional studies (11.5 ± 1.5% increase in diastolic pressure). Blood pressure in these studies, measured by Arteriosonde,® was unstable as is typical in anephric patients.

Discussion

Our experience with intravenous administration of the nonapeptide converting enzyme inhibitor SQ 20,881 and saralasin in seated hypertensive

TABLE 2. Effect of Angiotensin Blockade in Anephric Patients

		Control diastolic pressure (mm Hg)	Change in diastolic pressure (mm Hg) after:	
			10 min	20 min
Converting enzyme inhibitor SQ 20,881 (1 mg/kg)	A	72	−2	−6
	B	77	+11	+7
	C	82	−1	+3
	D	87	−1	−4
	E	91	+4	+8
	F	100	+3	0
Mean ± SE			+2.3 ± 2.0	+1.3 ± 2.3[a]
			15 min	
Saralasin (1 or 10 μg/kg per min)	G	62	+16	
	H	72	+10	
	F	89	+10	
	E	93	+10	
Mean ± SE			+11.5 ± 1.5	

[a] $p < 0.05$ when compared to diastolic pressure change in patients receiving saralasin. (Reproduced from Case et al.[10] with permission of the editor of *The American Journal of Medicine*.)

patients reveals that blood pressure responses to both agents are closely correlated with the pretreatment levels of PRA. However, it is from the side-by-side comparison of these two agents that the intrinsic agonism of saralasin becomes apparent. Thus, in low-renin and anephric patients where renin levels are very low or absent, saralasin is overtly pressor, while in the same patients the converting enzyme inhibitor produced neither pressor no depressor responses. Even when renin levels are high and both agents lower blood pressure, the converting enzyme inhibitor produced slightly greater responses. Accordingly, saralasin has distinct limitations in assessing renin-dependent blood pressure.[5]

In contrast to the saralasin experience, testing with converting enzyme inhibitor exposed degrees of renin-dependent blood pressure in all high- and in more than 90% of all normal-renin hypertensive patients. In contrast, low-renin patients exhibited no response even after moderate dietary sodium deprivation. These observations define a prevalent yet circumscribed pattern of response to converting enzyme inhibitor which corresponds closely to the biochemical measurement of the activity of the renin system. Despite this close correlation, mechanisms other than blockade of angiotensin II may be operative in the drug's antihypertensive action. It is therefore appropriate to review the evidence which bears on the mechanism of action of the converting enzyme inhibitor.

Mechanism of Action of Converting Enzyme Inhibitor

Although the findings are consistent with the interpretation that the major effect of the agent is to lower circulating angiotension II levels, this same enzyme (kininase II) also degrades the potent vasodilator bradykinin[13] in both animal and human tissue.[14-16] This latter reaction is also blocked by the converting enzyme inhibitor. In addition, there have been reports to indicate that plasma renin and angiotensin II levels move in parallel with bradykinin in response to alterations in sodium balance and in posture in normal human subjects.[17] Thus, it is conceivable that the depressor responses result both from angiotensin II inhibition and from brakykinin accumulation.

There are several lines of evidence which do not support the interpretation that bradykinin accumulation is a significant factor in producing the blood pressure changes after converting enzyme inhibitor. In previous studies, no increases in bradykinin levels were found after administation of SQ 20,881 in dogs with renovascular hypertension[18] or in nomotensive subjects, even when depressor responses were induced.[19] In our studies, low-renin patients as a group had no changes induced in blood pressure by SQ 20,881. This latter point is weakened by the finding that endogenous brakykinin and angiotensin II levels parallel each other. However, another line of evidence against bradykinin participation in this response comes from those studies in which both hypertensive and normotensive anephric subjects in whom renin levels were unmeasurably low and in whom converting enzyme inhibitor failed to lower the blood pressure. Another line of evidence against participation of bradykinin comes from the finding that there are at least four other peptide hydrolases, also located within the pulmonary capillary endothelium, which are capable of degrading bradykinin and which are unaffected by the converting enzyme inhibitor.[15,20,21]

On the other hand, there is considerable positive evidence that the induced depressor responses were largely related to blockade of angiotensin II formation. Neither depressor responses nor induced rises in renin activity occurred until pretreatment levels of PRA were 2 ng AI/ml per hr or greater. In addition, there were close correlations between pretreatment levels of renin activity and the induced increments in renin activity, as well as the levels to which renin activity rose. Most important were the significant correlations between the height of the pretreatment renin level and the magnitude of the induced fall in blood pressure. We have also shown a close parallel between the acute blood pressure response to converting enzyme inhibitor and that to another angiotensin-blocking drug, saralasin.

Haber and his colleagues, using depressor respones to converting enzyme inhibitor to assess the role of renin in blood pressure regulation in both dogs and humans[18,19] found that, despite large induced increases in PRA, there were no corresponding rises in plasma aldosterone, a finding indicating effective blockade of angiotensin II generation. Using the same interpretation applied by these authors[18,19] and others,[22] our present findings support the view that the blood-presure-lowering effect results from inhibition of angiotensin II formation. However, more extensive studies are required to exclude positively any role for bradykinin in the blood pressure response to converting enzyme inhibitor.

Another key consideration in the interpretation of our data relates to the incompleteness of the converting enzyme blockade, which at times might enable compensatory response of the renin–angiotensin system to overcome the pharmacological blockade. Animal studies indicate that doses of 1–2 mg/kg produce about at 80–90% blockade of convering enzyme,[15,23] and in the present study large reactive rises in PRA were observed. With an incomplete blockade, compensatory hypersecretion of renin could work to restore effective angiotensin II and blood pressure levels. In view of this possibility, only the early maximal response observed within the first 20 min was used in evaluating the blockade. Whatever the case in individual studies, it is clear that an incomplete converting enzyme blockade would only work to underestimate the true renin factor.

Responses to Converting Enzyme Inhibitor Provide Physiological Meaning to Renin Profiling

The close correlation between renin levels and the responses to converting enzyme inhibitor endows the measured PRA with physiological meaning, since the value reflects the extent of participation of renin activity in sustaining the blood pressure level. Thus, the physiological or pathological relevance of PRA can be estimated both by biochemical measurement and by functional testing using a converting enzyme inhibitor. Either method of renin estimation, however, relies on a concurrent measurement of the state of sodium balance, as reflected in the rate of urinary sodium excretion. In this way, it is possible to decide whether the renin activity is normal, high, or low for the physiological state of sodium balance.[8]

Accordingly, patients in each of the three renin-level subgroups exhibited characteristic responses to the nonapeptide, with changes in sodium intake which paralleled induced changes in control renin levels. Thus, moderate sodium depletion raised renin levels and enhanced the amplitude of depressor responses in normal-renin patients, whereas in low-renin patients with a minimal or absent renin response to dietary sodium depletion, there was no depressor response. Moreover, normal-renin patients can be separated from high-renin patients by their comparatively smaller depressor responses while on normal sodium intake. As might be predicted, mild dietary sodium depletion enables a more precise separation of low from normal renin patients when testing with a renin-blocking agent or by measurements of PRA.

Is Normal-Renin Hypertension "Normal"?

Since nearly all of our "normal-renin" hypertensive patients exhibited some degree of angiotenisn dependence of blood pressure, one may question the appropriateness of "normal" levels of this pressor hormone in the presence of elevated blood pressure resulting from sodium–volume excess. Niarchos and colleagues[24] have shown that SQ 20,881 lowers blood pressure in normotensive subjects and that this response can be exaggerated after prior dietary sodium depletion. However, one would expect that the baroreceptor stimulus from elevated blood pressure would work to suppress renin secretion. Viewed in this way, perhaps the kidneys of the low-renin group respond appropriately to increased arterial pressure, while the kidneys of normal- and high-renin patients secrete a relative or absolute excess of renin. For this reason it may be more appropriate to apply the term "*medium*" instead of "*normal*" to renin levels. Altogether, the nonapeptide converting enzyme inhibitor SQ 20,881 and saralasin lowered blood pressure in large fractions of patients with normal- and high-renin forms of hypertension. Of the two agents, SQ 20,881 reduced blood pressure to a greater extent and in more patients because it does not possess the weak angiotenisn II-like activity of saralasin. From these studies, it would seem desirable to develop orally active converting enzyme inhibitors as both diagnostic and therapeutic tools in hypertensive disease.

Summary

Converting enzyme inhibitor lowers blood pressure in hypertensive patients in direct relationship to the height of the pretreatment level of PRA. Thus, the response to SQ 20,881 can be used to predict or estimate the level of endogenous PRA. Therefore, knowing the state of sodium balance from the 24-hr urinary sodium excretion rate, one can profile hypertensive patients into normal-, low-, and high-renin subgroups by the magnitude of their blood pressure response to converting enzyme blockade.

Since depressor responses were observed in most normal-renin patients and all high-renin patients, the renin–angiotensin system may be responsible for sustaining some part of the hypertension in the majority of hypertenisve patients (except the low-renin group). Blood pressure responses to converting enzyme inhibitor and saralasin were parallel, but saralasin exhibited intrinsic agonist activity and therefore tested less sensitively for angiotensin dependency of blood pressure when judged by depressor responses.

It remains for further studies to determine whether this renin participation is primary and, if not, why this pressor system fails to shut off with elevated blood pressure. We also need to learn whether this renin participation is greater or less than its involvement in normal homeostasis.

References

1. Laragh JH, Sealey JE: The renin–angiotensin–aldosterone hormonal system and regulation of sodium, potassium, and blood pressure homeostasis, in Orloff J and Berliner RW (eds): *Handbook of Physiology*—Renal Physiology. Baltimore, Waverly Press, 1973, pp 831–908.
2. Streeten DHP, Anderson GH, Freiberh JM, Dalakos TG: Use of an angiotensin II antagonist (saralasin) in the recognition of "angiotensinogenic" hypertension. *N Engl J Med* 292:657–662, 1975.
3. Brunner HR, Gavras H, Laragh JH: Specific inhibition of the renin–angiotensin system: A key to understanding blood pressure regulation. *Prog Cardiovasc Dis* 17:87–98, 1974.
4. Brunner HR, Gavras H, Laragh JH, Keenan R: Hypertension in man: Exposure of the renin and sodium components using angiotensin II blockade. *Circ Res* (Suppl I) 35:35–46, 1974.
5. Case DB, Wallace JM, Keim JH, Sealey JE, Laragh JH: Limitations and usefulness of saralasin, partial competitive agonist of angiotensin II for evaluating the renin and sodium factors in hypertensive patients. *Am J Med* 60:825–836, 1976.
6. Hollenberg NK, Williams GH, Burger B, Ishikawa I, Adams DF: Blockade and stimulation of renal, adrenal, and vascular angiotensin II receptors with 1-Sar,8-Ala angiotensin II in normal man. *J Clin Invest* 57:39–46, 1976.
7. Gavras H, Brunner HR, Laragh JH, Gavras I, Vukovich RA: The use of angiotensin-converting enzyme inhibitor in the diagnosis and treatment of hypertension. *Clin Sci Mol Med* 48:57s–60s, 1975.
8. Laragh JH, Baer L, Brunner HR, Bühler FR, Sealey JE, Vaughan ED: Renin, angiotensin and aldosterone system in pathogenesis and management of hypertensive vascular disease. *Am J Med* 52:633–652, 1972.
9. Case DB, Wallace JM, Keim HJ, Weber MA, Sealey JE, Laragh JH: Possible role of renin in hypertension as suggested by renin–sodium profiling and inhibition of converting enzyme. *N Engl J Med* 296:641–646, 1977.
10. Case DB, Wallace JM, Keim JH, Weber MA, Drayer JIM, White RP, Sealey JE, Laragh JH: Estimating renin participation in hypertension: Superiority of converting enzume inhibitor over saralasin. *Am J Med* 61:790–796, 1976.
11. Sealey JE, Laragh JH: Radioimmunoassay of plasma renin activity. *Semin Nucl Med* 5:189–202, 1975.
12. Laragh JH, Soffer RL, Case DB: Converting enzyme, angiotensin II and hypertensive disease. *Am J Med* 46:147–160, 1978.
13. Colman, RW, Girey GJD, Zacest R, Talamo RC: The human plasma kallikrein-kinin system. *Prog Hematol* 7:255–298, 1971.

14. Bianchi A, Evans DB, Cobb M, Peschka MT, Schaeffer TR, Laffan RJ: Inhibition by SQ 20,881 of vasopressor response to angiotensin I in conscious animals. *Eur J Pharmacol* 23:90–96, 1973.
15. Engle SL, Schaeffer TR, Gold BI, Rubin B: Inhibition of pressor effects of angiotensin I hand augmentation of depressor effects of bradykinin by synthetic peptides. *Proc Soc Exp Biol Med* 140:240–244, 1972.
16. Bakhle YS: Inhibition of angiotensin I converting enzyme by venom peptides. *Br J Pharmacol* 43:252–254, 1971.
17. Wong PY, Talamo RC, Williams GH, Colman RW: Response of the kallikrein–kinin and renin–angiotensin systems to saline infusion and upright posture. *J Clin Invest* 55:691–698, 1975.
18. Miller ED, Samuels AI, Haber E, Barger AC: Inhibition of angiotensin conversion and prevention of renal hypertension. *Am J Physiol* 228:448–453, 1975.
19. Sancho J, Re R, Burton J, Barger AC, Haber E: The role of the renin–angiotensin–aldosterone system in cardiovascular homeostasis in normal human subjects. *Circulation* 53:400–504, 1976.
20. Ryan JQ, Roblero J, Stewart JM: Inactivation of bradykinin in the pulmonary circulation. *Biochem J* 110:795–797, 1968.
21. Bakhle YS: Converstion of angiotensin I to angiotensin II by cell-free extracts of dog lung. *Nature* 220:919–920, 1968.
22. Needleman P, Douglas JR, Jakschik BA, Blumberg AL, Isakson PC, Marshall GR: Angiotensin antagonists as pharmacological tools. *Fed Proc* 35:2488–2493, 1976.
23. Thurston H, Laragh JH: Prior receptor occupancy as a determinant of the pressor activity of infused angiotensin II in the rat. *Circ Res* 36:113–117, 1975.
24. Niarchos AP, Pickering TG, Case DB, Sullivan P, Laragh JH: Role of the renin–angiotensin system in blood pressure regulation. The cardiovascular effects of converting enzyme inhibition. in normotensive subjects. *Circ Res* 45:829–837, 1979.

Chapter 14

The Use of SQ 20,881 Converting Enzyme Inhibitor (Teprotide) for Diagnostic Purposes in Hypertension

Haralambos Gavras, Irene Gavras, Stephen Textor, Charles P. Tifft, Glenn R. Kershaw, and Hans R. Brunner

Introduction

The contribution of the renin–angiotensin system in sustaining high blood pressure is variable in different forms of hypertension and is under dispute. There is little doubt that renin profiling is helpful in detecting the few surgically curable forms of hypertension. However, since it was suggested[1] that the levels of plasma renin activity can serve as a guide to tailor specific medical treatment for a particular patient, the interest in profiling uselected hypertensive populations as well has been renewed. This prompted the search for a quick and safe screening test which might reveal whether a given hypertension is renin-dependent or not without the delay and cost necessary for measurement of plasma renin activity. One approach to this end is inhibition of angiotensin II (AII) by its competitive antagonist, saralasin.[2,3] However, the well recognized agonistic effect of this agent[4] which varies with the state of sodium balance[5] may obscure the results of angiotensin blockade. The temporary elimination of angiotensin II formation by inhibition of the enzyme converting AI to AII without any known agonistic effect or other side effect would appear theoretically to be the

HARALAMBOS GAVRAS, M.D., IRENE GAVRAS, M.D., CHARLES P. TIFFT, M.D., and GLENN R. KERSHAW, M.D. · Department of Medicine, Boston University School of Medicine, and Hypertension Section, Boston City Hospital, Boston, Massachusetts 02118. STEPHEN TEXTOR, M.D. · Research Division, Cleveland Clinic Foundation, Cleveland, Ohio 44106. HANS R. BRUNNER, M.D. · Department of Medicine, Université de Lausanne, and Department of Medicine, Hôpital Cantonal Universitaire, CH-1011 Lausanne, Switzerland.

perfect tool for this purpose. We report here our experience from 42 patients studied with the converting enzyme inhibitor teprotide.

Methods

Twenty-two of the patients were studied at the Metabolic Unit of Columbia Presbyterian Medical Center, and 20 at the Thorndike Memorial Laboratory of Boston University Medical Center. Fourteen were female and 28 male, aged 21–55 yr.

Sixteen had hypertension with a known primary cause (seven renovascular, five chronic renal failure, and four primary aldosteronism from adrenal adenoma or idiopathic adrenal hyperplasia). Eleven were hypertensive emergencies with accelerated or malignant hypertension, diastolic blood pressure of at least 125 mm Hg, and grade III or IV hypertensive retinopathy; 15 were essential hypertensives. All except six of the malignant hypertensives had been off antihypertensive medication for at least 1 week prior to admission.

Those with essential hypertension were studied according to a strict protocol described elsewhere.[6] Briefly, they were placed on a sodium-depleting regimen for 6 days, had plasma renin activity and plasma aldosterone measurements, both erect and supine, on days 5 and 6 before converting enzyme inhibition (CEI) by IV injection of teprotide and again on day 6 after CEI. Subsequently, they were repleted with sodium for 6 days, and the same procedures were carried out at the end of that period in order to study the responses of blood pressure and hormonal values to CEI and to correlate this with changes in sodium balance and posture.

The other two groups of patients, i.e., those with hypertension secondary to known organic disease and those with malignant hypertension, were given an IV injection of teprotide immediately upon admission and were not in controlled sodium balance. The doses of teprotide used were 1–4 mg/kg body weight. Full antihypertensive effect was observed with the lower doses, while higher doses prolonged the duration of the blockade but did not affect the degree of blood pressure reduction.[7] Plasma renin activity and plasma aldosterone were measured by radioimmunoassay.[8,9] In patients with essential hypertension and with hypertension secondary to organic disease, the diagnosis had been determined before admission to the present study by the usual hypertensive work-up including renal arteriography and renal or adrenal vein catheterization for differential hormonal measurements wherever appropriate.

Results

Figure 1 shows the blood pressure response to administration of the teprotide in the 16 patients with hypertension secondary to known organic

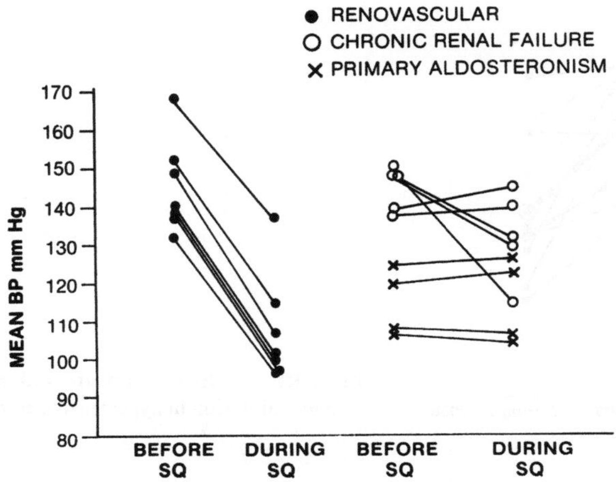

FIGURE 1. Patients with hypertension secondary to known organic disease studied with SQ 20,881 on regular sodium intake.

disease. The seven patients with renovascular hypertension had a spectacular blood pressure (BP) response from an average of 180/123 to 137/92. Out of the five with chronic renal failure, three had some BP fall. None of the four with primary aldosteronism had any BP response.

Figure 2 shows that there is a loose correlation between the levels of plasma renin activity before treatment and the fall of mean BP obtained by

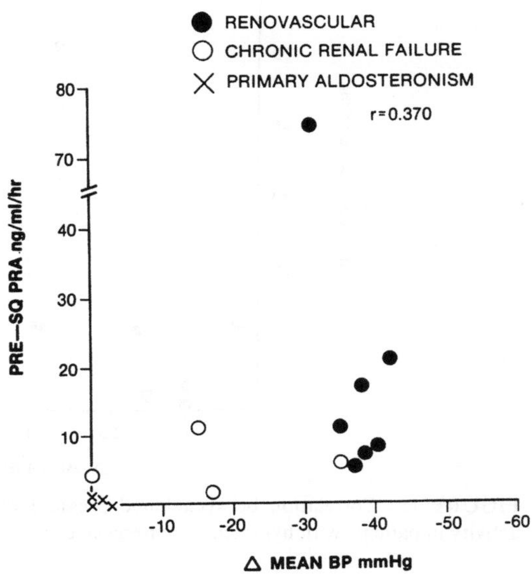

FIGURE 2. Correlation of blood pressure fall with SQ 20,881 to pretreatment plasma renin activity in patients with hypertension of known etiology.

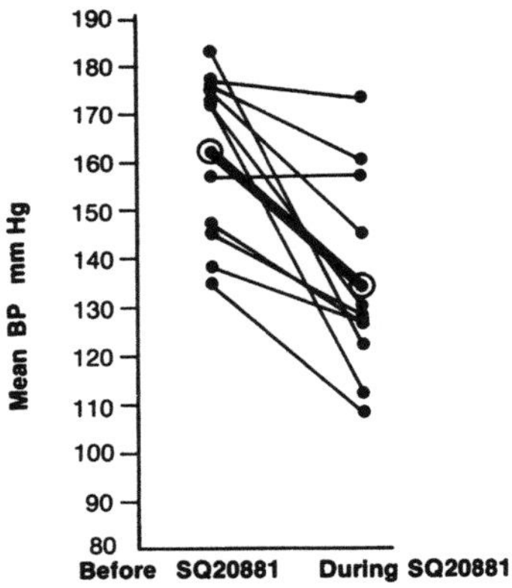

FIGURE 3. Blood pressure fall after converting enzyme inhibition in hypertensive emergencies.

teprotide. Although patients with higher plasma renin activity (PRA) tend to have greater BP falls, and most of those with low PRA have no change in BP, there is considerable individual variability, and the correlation does not attain statistical significance.

Figure 3 illustrates the blood pressure response when teprotide was administered to 11 patients with accelerated or malignant hypertension. It should be noted that several of these patients were already being treated with combination of diuretics and adrenolytic drugs at the time of

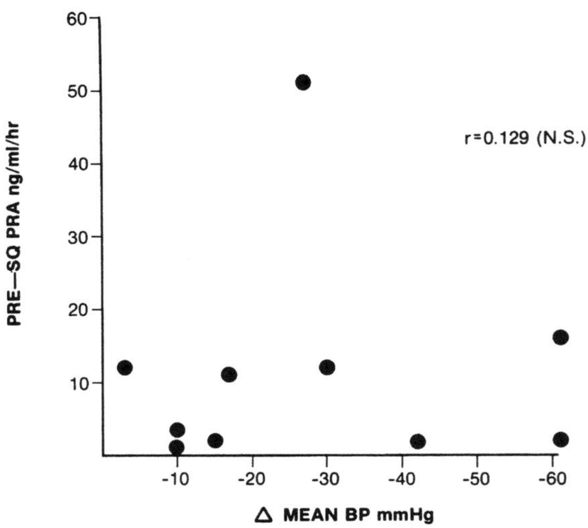

FIGURE 4. Correlation between blood pressure response and pretreatment plasma renin activity in patients with hypertensive emergencies.

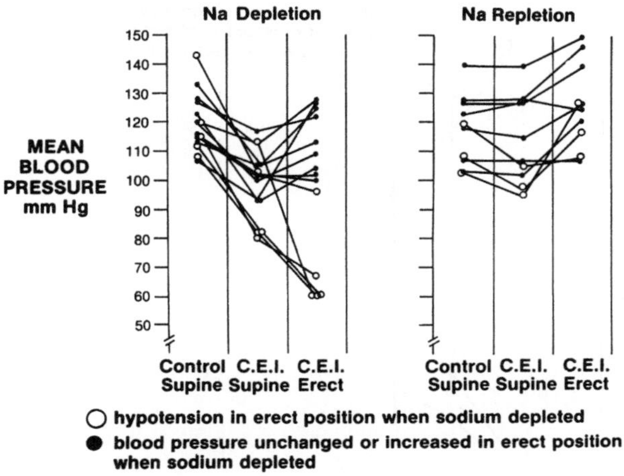

FIGURE 5. Changes of blood pressure after converting enzyme inhibition in essential hypertensives on sodium depletion and sodium repletion.

admission; therefore, their renin levels were the result of the combined stimulatory and suppressing effect of these drugs and do not represent baseline renin levels. Nine out of the 11 patients had substantial falls in BP, the overall change for the group being from 210/137 down to 180/114.

Figure 4 shows that correlation between prior levels of PRA and fall of mean BP is poor, since several patients had low PRA levels and still showed considerable fall of BP.

Figure 5 shows, in the left panel, the BP response of the essential hypertensives after sodium depletion. All patients had a fall in mean BP to a variable degree while supine. Upon standing up, five patients had a further fall in BP, most of them to the point of fainting, while the remaining 10 had an increase in BP, usually to less than preinjection levels. The right panel shows the individual BP responses to CEI after sodium repletion. Here, in the supine position, only three patients continue to have an appreciable BP fall, and these are the same ones who had become hypotensive in the previous phase when they had assumed the erect position. This time, upon standing, all patients had an increase in BP. In no case did this increase attain levels higher than the preinjection erect BP reading of each patient.

Figure 6 illustrates the changes in BP, PRA, and plasma aldosterone after CEI in the first phase of Na depletion. The upper panel shows the overall changes in mean BP for the two groups, those who became hypotensive upon standing and those whose BP increased upon standing. The middle panel shows the concomitant changes in PRA, and it is apparent that those

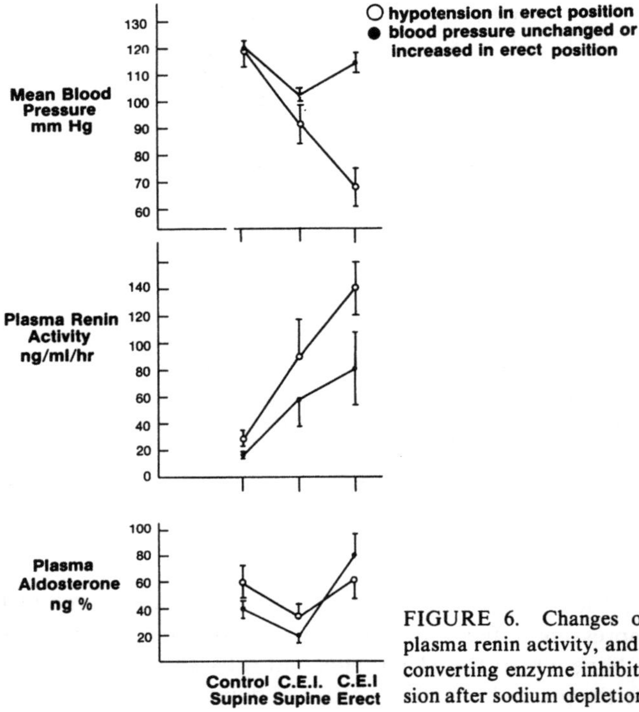

FIGURE 6. Changes of mean blood pressure, plasma renin activity, and plasma aldosterone after converting enzyme inhibition in essential hypertension after sodium depletion, lying and standing.

who develop hypotension tend to have higher PRA, although this difference is not statistically significant because of individual variability. When PRA is further stimulated, the difference becomes even more apparent, suggesting that these patients have more readiness for enhanced renin release compared with the other group. The lower panel shows that the CEI induces a decrease in plasma aldosterone, as expected, in the supine position. In the upright position, however, there is a paradoxical increase in plasma aldosterone that ranges between 50% and 400% in individual subjects.

Figure 7 shows change in the same parameters when CEI is administered after sodium repletion. The upper panel shows that there is a small decrease in BP in the supine position (which data are really attributable to three patients only). In the erect position, BP increased slightly in all patients. PRA was again stimulated in the supine position and rose further in the erect position. Plasma aldosterone also showed the same pattern: A

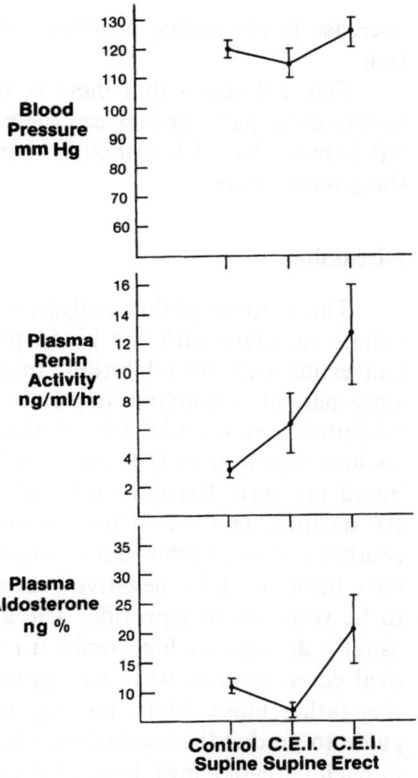

FIGURE 7. Changes of mean blood pressure, plasma renin activity, and plasms aldosterone after converting enzyme inhibition in essential hypertension after sodium repletion, lying and standing.

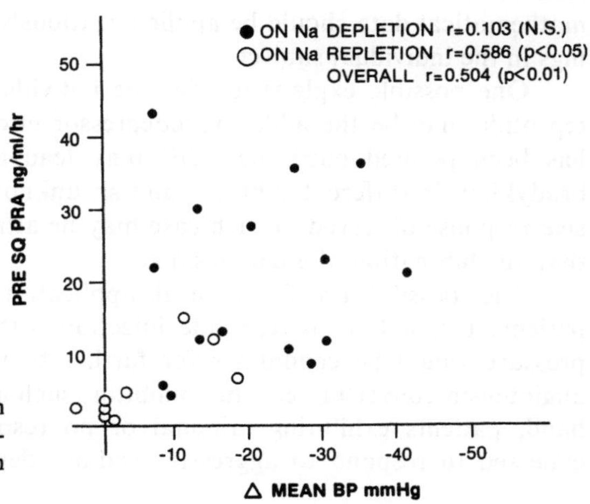

FIGURE 8. Correlation between pre-SQ 20,881 plasma renin activity and blood pressure fall in essential hypertension.

decrease in the supine position and a significant increase in the erect position.

Figure 8 shows that there is, overall, a statistically significant correlation in these patients between the pretreatment levels of PRA and the fall of BP induced by CEI, although there is a wide individual variation in both these parameters.

Discussion

The purpose of this analysis was to demonstrate how the baseline PRA values correlate with the blood pressure response elicited by angiotensin-converting enzyme inhibition. In clinical terms, the correlation was good, since patients on sodium depletion or those with high baseline PRA always exhibited a substantial fall of blood pressure after CEI, while patients on sodium repletion and/or with low PRA usually had little or no decrease in blood pressure. Exceptions to this rule consisted mostly of patients whose BP declined in spite of low preinjection PRA levels (i.e., "false positive" results) and would thus have been classified as angiotensin-dependent. There have been no "false negative" cases since no high-renin patients were found to be resistant to teprotide. The antihypertensive effect of teprotide could usually distinguish high-renin from low-renin hypertension, but the statistical correlation between nanograms of PRA and decreased BP in mm Hg was rather loose. Thus, the degree of BP lowering could not be used as a guide to predict the level of preinjection PRA. The small number of patients in each category may have affected the statistical significance of our findings, since other investigators who plotted data from larger numbers of subjects found a better correlation between these two parameters[10] However, mathematical data should be applied cautiously in interpreting clinical findings in the individual subject.

One possible explanation for the individual variability in response to teprotide may be the added vasodepressor effect of bradykinin. Indeed, it has been pointed out[11] that CEI may lead to variable accumulation of bradykinin in different subjects, and an unknown part of the antihypertensive response observed in each case may be attributable to this effect rather than to elimination of angiotensin II.

The possibilities for clinical application of this test are obvious: patients responding to teprotide injection with a substantial fall of blood pressure would be candidates for further treatment with an orally active angiotensin-converting enzyme inhibitor, such as captopril.[12,13] On the other hand, patients exhibiting minimal or no response to teprotide would be expected to respond to aggressive sodium depletion aided by intravenous and oral diuretics,[14] whereas patients with intermediate blood pressure response (i.e., over 10% reduction in diastolic pressure, but still far from normal) would be expected to require combination treatment.

In conclusion, we believe that teprotide is a potentially useful agent for the diagnosis of renin-dependency of hypertension. However, before this approach can be introduced as a reliable clinical test, more work is needed to define factors which may cause the variability of individual blood pressure responses and influence their interpretation.

ACKNOWLEDGMENTS. Haralambos Gavras is an Established Investigator of the American Heart Association. This work was partially supported by USPHS Grant No. HL-18318.

References

1. Laragh JH: Vasoconstriction–volume analysis for understanding and treating hypertension: The use of renin and aldosterone profiles. *Am J Med* 55:261, 1973.
2. Brunner HR, Gavras H, Laragh JH: Specific inhibition of the renin-angiotensin system. A key to understanding blood pressure regulation. *Prog Cardiovasc Dis* 17:87, 1974.
3. Streeten DHP, Anderson GH, Freiberg FM, Dalakos TG: Use of angiotensin II antagonist (saralasin) in the recognition of "angiotensinogenic" hypertension. *N Engl J Med* 292:657, 1975.
4. Hollenberg NK, Williams GH, Burger B, Ishikawa I, Adams DF: Blockade and stimulation of renal adrenal and vascular angiotensin II receptors with Sar-Ala[8]-Angiotensin II in normal man. *J Clin Invest* 57:39, 1976.
5. Gavras H, Ribeiro AB, Brunner HR, Gavras I: Reciprocal relation between renin-dependency and sodium-dependency in essential hypertension. *N Engl J Med* 295:1278, 1976.
6. Gavras H, Gavras I, Textor S, Volicer L, Brunner HR: Effect of angiotensin converting enzyme inhibition on blood pressure, plasma renin activity and plasma aldosterone in essential hypertension. *J Clin Endocr Metab* 46:220–226, 1978.
7. Gavras H, Brunner HR, Laragh JH, Sealey JE, Gavras I, Vukovich R: An angiotensin converting enzyme inhibitor to identify and treat vasoconstrictor and volume factors in hypertensive patients. *N Engl J Med* 291:817, 1974.
8. Sealey JE, Laragh JH, Gerten-Banes J, Aceto RM: The measurement of plasma renin activity in man. In Laragh JH (ed): *Hypertension Manual*, New York, Yorke Medical Books, 1974, p 621.
9. St Cyr MJ, Sancho JM, Melby JC: Quantitation of plasma aldosterone by radioimmunoassay. *Clin Chem* 18:1395, 1972.
10. Case DB, Wallace JM, Keim HJ, Weber MA, Sealey JE, Laragh JH: Possible role of renin in hypertension as suggested by renin–sodium profiling and inhibition of converting enzyme. *N Engl J Med* 296:641, 1977.
11. Williams GH: Angiotensin-dependent hypertension. Potential pitfalls in definition. *N Engl J Med* 296:684, 1977.
12. Gavras H, Brunner HR, Turini GA, Kershaw GR, Tifft, CP, Cuttelod S, Gavras I,

Vukovich RA, McKinstry DN: Antihypertensive effect of the oral angiotensin converting enzyme inhibitor SQ 14,225 in man. *N Engl J Med* 298:991–995, 1978.

13. Brunner HR, Gavras H, Waeber B, Kershaw G, Turini G, Vukovich R, McKinstry DN, Gavras I: Long-term treatment of hypertensive patients by the oral administration of an angiotensin converting enzyme inhibitor (SQ 14,225). *Ann Intern Med* 90:19–23, 1979.
14. Tifft C, Gavras H, Kershaw GR, Gavras I, Brunner HR, Liang C, Chobanian AV: Converting enzyme inhibition in hypertensive emergencies. *Ann Intern Med* 90:43–47, 1979.

Chapter 15

Clinical Experience with Blockade of the Renin–Angiotensin–Aldosterone System by an Oral Converting Enzyme Inhibitor (SQ 14,225, Captopril) in Hypertensive Patients

David B. Case, Steven A. Atlas, John H. Laragh, Jean E. Sealey, Patricia A. Sullivan, and Doris N. McKinstry

Introduction

Although the role of the renin–angiotensin system in the pathogenesis of hypertension remains a subject of active investigation and debate, there is increasing recognition that pharmacological inhibition of the system can be a potent mechanism by which blood pressure can be lowered. Bühler and coworkers,[1] in examining the renin-lowering effect of β-adrenergic blockade in patients with essential and malignant hypertension, found that propranolol in low to moderate doses lowers blood pressure in high an normal renin forms of hypertension but does not significantly lower blood pressure in low renin hypertensive pateints. These findings have been confirmed by many investigators using propranolol and a variety of other β-blocking agents.[2-4] It is also now apparent that propranolol can actually raise blood pressure in some patients with low levels of renin activity.[5]

Reprinted from *Progress in Cardiovascular Diseases* 21(3):195–206, 1978, by permission of the authors and the publisher, Grune & Stratton.

DAVID B. CASE, M.D., STEVEN A. ATLAS, M.D., JOHN H. LARAGH, M.D., JEAN E. SEALEY, Ph.D., and PATRICIA A. SULLIVAN, R.N. · Cardiovascular Center and Division of Cardiology, New York Hospital–Cornell Medical Center, New York, New York 10021. DORIS N. McKINSTRY, Ph.D. · The Squibb Institute for Medical Research, New Jersey 08540.

Soon afterward, the octapeptide sar^1-ala^8-angiotensin II (saralasin) was introduced as a competitive antagonist of angiotensin II. Although this agent lowers blood pressure in humans and animals with high renin activity, [6-8] further studies revealed that the magnitude of depressor responses to saralasin underestimates the degree to which angiotensin sustains elevated blood pressure because the drug has significant partial agonist properties.[8,9]

Another class of compounds has recently been developed that blocks angiotensin II formation by competitive inhibition of the dipeptidyl carboxypeptidase that converts angiotensin I to angiotensin II (angiotensin-converting enzyme). A nonapeptide inhibitor was synthesized (SQ 20,881 or teprotide) which, unlike saralasin, has no intrinsic agonist properties. Studies of large numbers of patients revealed that SQ 20,881 lowers blood pressure acutely in normal and high renin hypertension but not in low renin hypertension.[10] Moreover, the magnitude of the reduction in blood pressure is directly related to the pretreatment level of plasma renin activity (PRA). The ability of this latter compound to lower blood pressure in a large proportion of hypertensive patients has been a major stimulus to the development of other compounds of the same type that might be active orally.

Recently, Ondetti and his colleagues[11] reported the synthesis of a potent orally active inhibitor of converting enzyme (SQ 14,225 or captopril). The blockade of converting enzyme by captopril has been demonstrated in studies in man[12] and animals[13] in which the pressor effect to exogenously administered angiotensin I was inhibited. Studies in animals[13] have further confirmed the specificity of this action, since captopril does not block the pressor action of infused angiotensin II or norepinephrine. As with SQ 20,881, this drug could potentially lower blood pressure by other means, since hydrolysis by angiotensin-converting enzyme is one of the pathways by which kinins may be degraded.[14] It remains to be established, however, whether captopril can invoke sustained elevations of either blood or tissue kinins in vivo since, unlike the unique action of converting enzyme on angiotensin I, alternate pathways of kinin degradation exist.

The availability of this new agent for clinical use has provided investigators with the opportunity for the first time to study the long-term effects of direct angiotensin blockade. An early report[15] of the action of captopril in a small group of hypertensive patients indicated potent antihypertensive action which, however, could not be associated with the pretreatment PRA. In contrast, analysis of the data reported here indicates that inhibition of angiotensin II formation very likely plays a major role in the antihypertensive effect. Thus, we found that acute and long-term reductions in blood pressure induced by captopril are directly related to the pretreatment PRA and to the degree to which the renin axis is inhibited (i.e., to the relative suppression of aldosterone and its physiological effects). Moreover, these studies demonstrate that captopril blockade of the renin–angiotensin–aldosterone axis may have widespread potential as an effective, well tolerated, and safe means of treatment for both common and unusual forms of hypertension.

Design of the Study

Nineteen patients with established hypertension were entered into the study of long-term treatment with captopril; all were either refractory to or unable to tolerate conventional therapy. Diagnoses were based on complete clinical examination, serum electrolytes, urinary metanephrines, cortisol and aldosterone, renin-profiling,[16] renal vein renin sampling, and, where clinically indicated, renal arteriography. Six patients had renal artery stenosis and high renin profiles (3 unilateral, 3 bilateral), and the remaining 13 had essential hypertension (2 low renin, 9 medium renin, and 2 high renin).

After a period of 3 wk without medication, patients were admitted to the Clinical Research Center of the New York Hospital. Each patient received an 1800-calorie diet containing 60 mEq of potassium and 10 mEq of sodium. To this diet, 90 mEq of sodium was added each day using sodium chloride tablets. Daily 24-hr urinary sodium and potassium were measured throughout the study.

The study was begun 5 days following admission, at which time all patients were in sodium and potassium balance. Patients were given placebo 4 time daily for 3 days prior to administration of captopril. Blood pressure was measured 7 times daily after 5 min in the supine position and again after 2 min standing. On the last placebo day, blood pressure was also measured in the seated position at 2-min intervals using an Arteriosonde. These recordings were analyzed by averaging the values over a 30-min period after blood pressure had stabilized. On this day, blood samples were collected for measurement of plasma renin activity,[17] plasma aldosterone,[18,19] and serum potassium at 8 AM after the patient had been supine overnight, and again at 12 PM, after 4 hr ambulation. The 24-hr rate of urinary aldosterone excretion[20] was also measured.

On the first day of treatment, patients were seated in a lounge chair for 1 hr before 10 mg captopril was administered orally while blood pressure was monitored by Arteriorsonde. Blood was obtained for plasma renin activity (PRA) and plasma aldosterone just prior to and 90 min following the first dose. The dose was subsequently increased from 10 to a maximum of 250 mg 4 times daily over the next 2–3 days until a decline of at least 10 mm Hg mean arterial pressure was maintained or the maximum allowed dose was reached (1000 mg daily). In the course of the study, the maximum allowed dose was reduced to 400 mg daily. Patients were maintained on the same dose of captopril for 7 days of maintenance therapy (9–10 days of drug) before discharge from the hospital. Measurements of Arteriosonde blood pressure, urinary aldosterone excretion, supine and upright PRA, plasma aldosterone, and serum potassium were repeated on the third and seventh day of maintenance therapy as they had been on the last placebo (control) day. Additional measurements of urinary aldosterone were made daily prior to captopril and on alternate days during inpatient treatment. For calculation of cumulative sodium and potassium balance, insensible losses were determined as the average difference between intake and excretion for the 3 days prior to beginning captopril.

In the analysis of the responses to the first dose, one other patient was included who, at the time of data analysis, had just entered the same long-term treatment protocol as the 19 patients. In addition, blood pressure and pretreatment PRA data were included from 8 other patients who received only a single oral dose in the same manner. Thus, there were a total of 28 patients for analysis of blood pressure responses to the first dose, and 20 patients in whom there were measurements of both PRA and plasma aldosterone following that dose.

The data are expressed as means ± SEM. Nonparametric statistical methods were used to detect differences between groups (paired and unpaired Wilcoxon tests). Regression lines were determined by the method of least squares. The significance of correlation coefficients was always con-

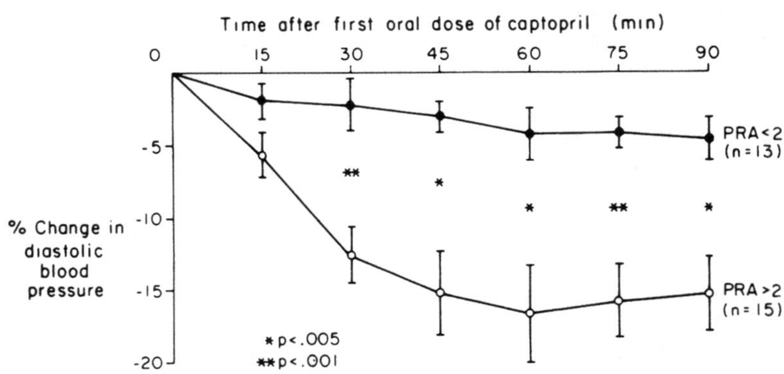

FIGURE 1. Percent change in diastolic blood pressure after the first oral dose of captopril in 28 hypertenisve patients. The solid symbols represent 13 patients whose pretreatment PRA was less than 2, and the open symbols represent the 15 patients whose PRA was greater than 2 ng Al/ml per hr. Blood pressure was measured continuously by Arteriosonde. After 15 min, the group with PRA > 2 had significantly larger depressor responses.

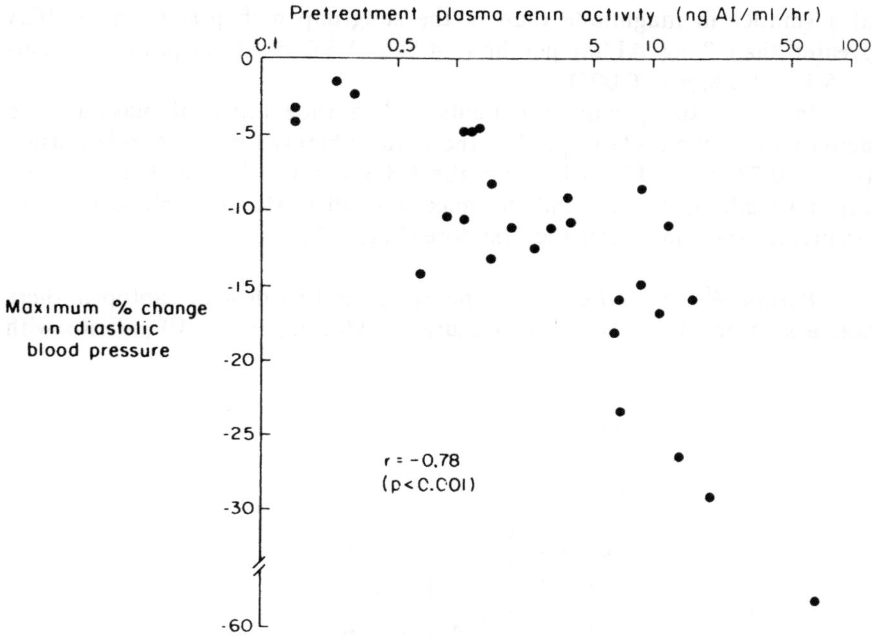

FIGURE 2. Relationship between the pretreatment (seated) PRA and the maximum percent change in diastolic blood pressure induced by the first oral dose of captopril in 28 hypertensive patients. Blood pressure was measured continuously by Arteriosonde. The average of diastolic pressure 10 min on either side of the nadir was compared with the average for 20 min prior to drug. A significant ($r = -0.78, p < 0.001$) relationship was found.

firmed using the Spearman rank correlation; these latter values are given throughout.

Results

Responses to the First Dose

Blood Pressure. Figure 1 illustrates the time course of the blood pressure response after the first dose of captopril. Because of the small number of patients profiled as low-renin, the patients were subdivided for analysis into those with PRA less than or greater than 2 ng AI/ml per hr. In the subgroup of patients who had pretreatment PRA levels greater than 2 ng AI/ml per hr, blood pressure began to fall within 15 min and reached a nadir between 60 and 90 min. Patients in the subgroup with pretreatment PRA less than 2 ng AI/ml per hr had a more gradual decline in blood pressure; after 90 min treatment, the depressor response in this group was also smaller in magnitude than in the subgroup with pretreatment PRA greater than 2 ng AI/ml per hr ($-4.5 \pm 1.5\%$ diastolic pressure versus $-15.1 \pm 2.6\%$, $p < 0.005$).

In this entire group of patients with a wide range of plasma renin activity (0.1–69 ng AI/ml per hr), there was a highly significant relationship ($r = -0.78$, $p < 0.001$) between the PRA measured immediately before captopril administration and the maximal fall in diastolic blood pressure occurring 60–90 min after the first dose (Figure 2).

Plasma Renin Activity. In response to the first dose of captopril, there was a significant rise in PRA measured at 90 min. In the 10 patients with

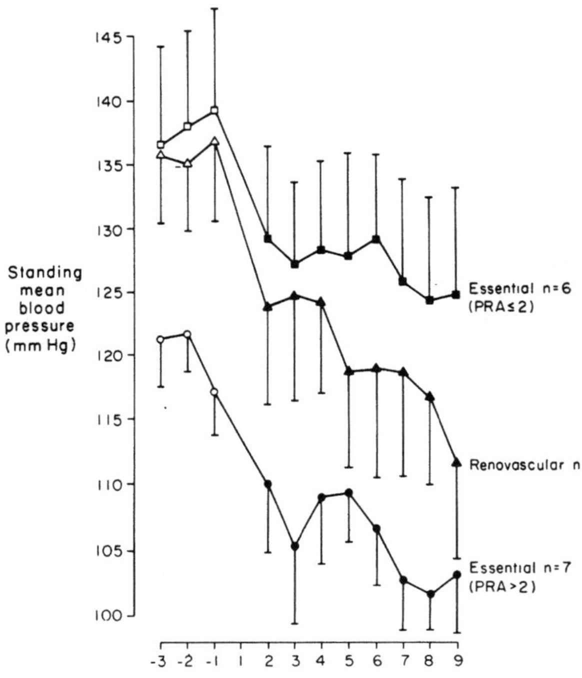

FIGURE 3. Blood pressure responses to captopril over the first 9 days of treatment. The daily average mean pressure was calculated from seven determinations for each patient. The open symbols represent the average standing mean pressures before captopril and the solid symbols those pressures while on captopril. The squares represent patients with essential hypertension with pretreatment PRA ≥ 2 (mean PRA 1.0 ± 0.9 ng Al/ml per hr); the circles are values of patients with essential hypertension with PRA ≤ 2 (mean PRA 4.4 ± 0.9 ng Al/ml per hr); and the triangles represent those with renovascular hypertension (mean PRA 10.9 ± 3.6 ng Al/ml per hr).

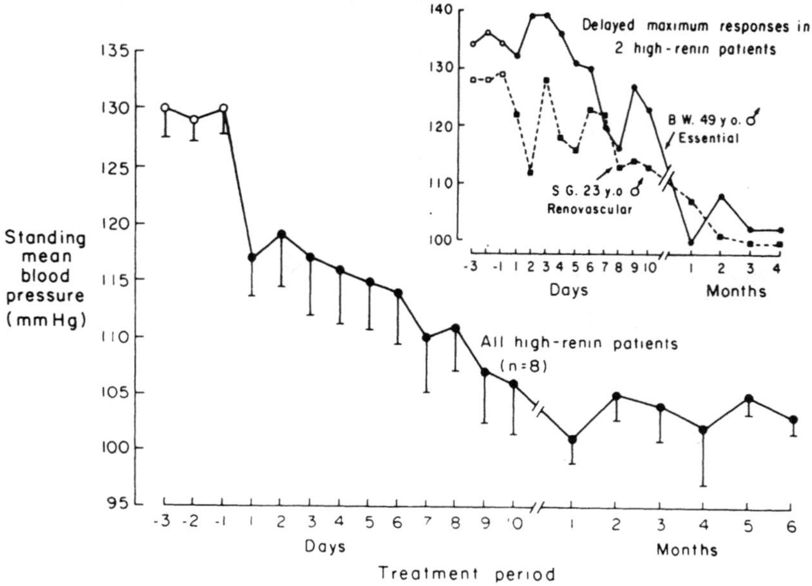

FIGURE 4. Time course of blood pressure changes in all (n = 8) high-renin patients. The open symbols represent pretreatment values, and the closed symbols represent values during captopril treatment. The inset shows the responses of two high-renin patients (see text).

control PRA less than 2, PRA rose from a mean of 1.0 ± 0.2 to 1.7 ± 0.4 ng AI/ml per hr ($p < 0.01$), or by 63%. However, in the subgroup of 10 patients with PRA greater than 2, PRA rose from 7.6 ± 1.3 to 31.6 ± 10.9 ng AI/ml per hr ($p < 0.01$), or by 253%. For all patients together, mean PRA rose from 4.3 ± 1.0 to 16.6 ± 6.3 ng AI/ml per hr ($p < 0.01$), or by 158%. The level to which PRA rose correlated both with the concurrent fall in mean arterial pressure ($r = 0.72$, $p < 0.001$) and also with the pretreatment plasma renin activity ($r = 0.98$, $p < 0.001$).

Plasma Aldosterone. Plasma aldosterone fell significantly at 90 min after the first oral dose of captopril in all patients, with an average decline in plasma aldosterone of 46.2 ± 4.4% of control ($p < 0.001$). The subgroup of 10 patients with PRA less than 2 had a mean plasma aldosterone of 9.3 ± 1.5 ng/100 ml, which fell to a mean of 5.4 ± 1.1 ($p < 0.005$; −42%). Similarly, in the subgroup of 10 patients with PRA greater than 2, plasma aldosterone declined by 50%, from a mean of 14.8 ± 2.6 ng/100 ml to 7.2 ± 1.4 ($p < 0.001$). There was no correlation between the reduction in blood pressure and either the absolute or relative induced changes in plasma aldosterone after the first oral dose of captopril.

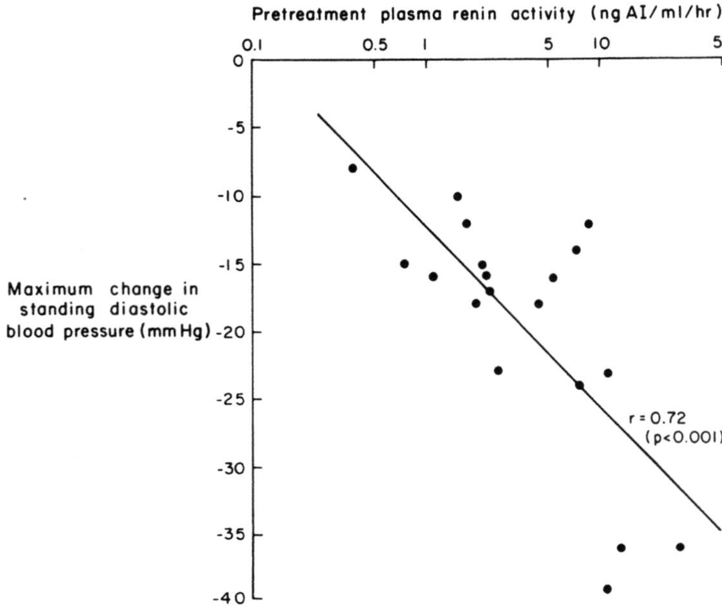

FIGURE 5. Relationship between the pretreatment (upright) PRA and the maximum change in standing diastolic blood pressure after 1 wk of treatment with captopril. The daily average standing diastolic pressure (mean of 7 readings) on the day prior to treatment was compared with the lowest daily average pressure occurring between day 8 and 10 of inpatient treatment.

Responses to Continued Administration of Captopril

Blood Pressure. Among the 19 patients in whom the drug was given continuously for 9 days or longer, standing blood pressure fell by at least 10% in all except one who had very low pretreatment PRA. The response of the subgroup of essential hypertensives with PRA < 2 was apparent by the second day and declined only slightly more during the ensuing week of inpatient treatment (Figure 3). In contrast, among patients with pretreatment PRA > 2 with either essential or renovascular hypertension, blood pressure fell to an initial level within the first 1–2 days of treatment and remained stable for 2–5 days. Subsequently, there was a secondary decline in blood pressure which, in most patients, reached its maximum in 7–10 days or afterward. While blood pressure was generally lower at this time than following the first dose, there was a good correlation ($r = 0.89$, $p < 0.001$) between the initial response and this longer term response.

The time course of the blood pressure response in the 8 high-renin patients (who exhibited very substantial depressor responses) is illustrated in Figure 4. In this subset, blood pressure, after an initial drop, continued to fall more gradually, reaching a minimum after 10 days. In general, the blood pressure levels on day 10 were representative of the long-term response (6 mo continuous treatment). Two exceptions are depicted in the inset of Figure 4, one with high-renin essential hypertension. Each of these patients exhibited an initial depressor response, but after 1–2 days, blood pressure returned toward control before pursuing a more gradual decline over the following 8–9 days. Moreover, after discharge from the hospital, while on captopril alone and an unrestricted diet, both of these patients experienced further decrements in blood pressure.

For all 19 patients, there was a significant relationship between the pretreatment levels of PRA and the magnitude of the fall in diastolic blood pressure during treatment (Figure 5). Significant relationships were also found between control plasma renin activity and the percent or absolute changes in mean arterial pressure and the percent change in diastolic pressure ($r < 0.64, 0.61, 0.68$, respectively; $p < 0.01$ for all).

Aldosterone Secretion and Potassium Metabolism. After 10 days, urinary aldosterone excretion decreased in all but 1 of the 19 patients, on average by 41.9 ± 5.0%. As seen in Figure 6, the percent decrease (from control) of urinary aldosterone excretion also correlated well with the induced change in mean arterial pressure ($r = 0.61$, $p < 0.01$). Sixteen patients developed positive potassium balance (range 10–275 mEq) during this period; the magnitude of induced potassium retention was inversely related to the percent change in urinary aldosterone excretion (Figure 7). Two patients who had a marked natriuresis during captopril treatment did not retain potassium despite maintained suppression of urinary aldosterone. These changes in potassium balance were associated with parallel changes in

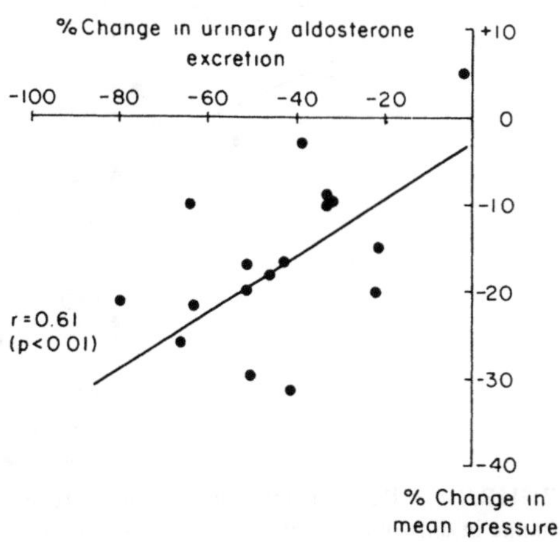

FIGURE 6. Relationship between the percent change in daily urinary aldosterone excretion and the percent changes in mean blood pressure after 7 days of maintenance treatment with captopril. Arteriosonde blood pressure readings and urinary aldosterone measurements for that day were compared with control (day −1) determinations.

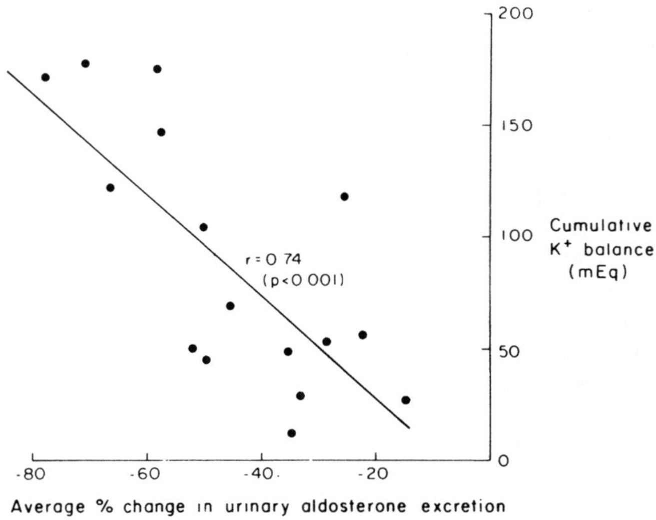

FIGURE 7. Relationship the average percent change in urinary aldosterone excretion and the cumulative potassium balance after 9 days of treatment with captopril. The average change in urinary aldosterone was determined by comparing the control value (mean of 3 consecutive days prior to receiving drug) with the average treatment value (mean of 5 determinations made on alternate days during treatment.)

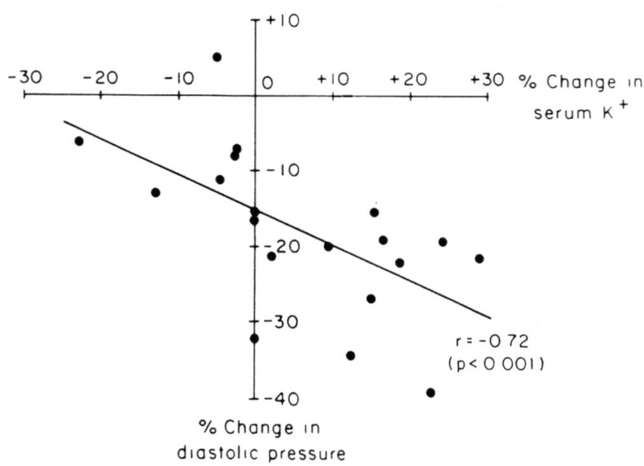

FIGURE 8. Relationship between the percent change in serum potassium and the percent change in diastolic pressure after 7 days of maintenance treatment with captopril.

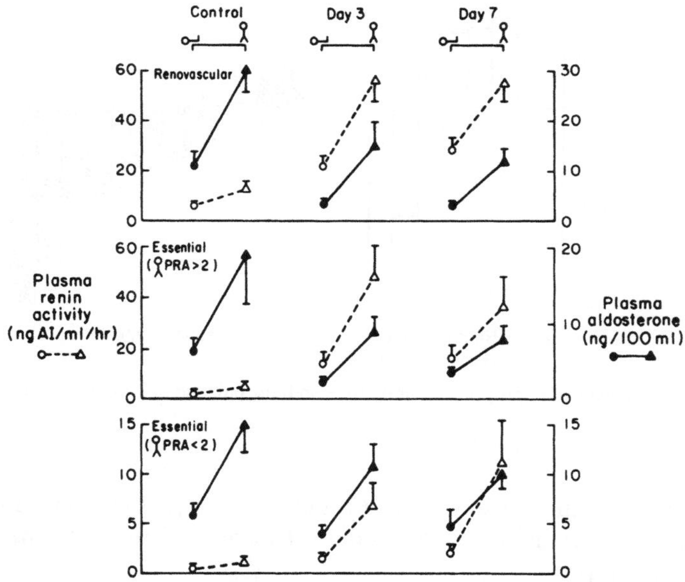

FIGURE 9. Posturally induced changes in PRA and plasma aldosterone before and during treatment with captopril. Circles represent 8 AM supine values, and triangles represent 12 PM upright values for PRA (O---Δ) and plasma aldosterone (●——▲) in patients with renovascular (upper panel), essential hypertension with PRA > 2 (middle panel), and PRA < 2 (lower panel). Paired values (mean ± SEM) are shown for the day prior to captopril treatment (control) and for the third and seventh day of maintenance treatment.

serum potassium which also correlated ($r = -0.72$, $p < 0.001$) with the observed changes in arterial pressure (Figure 8).

Both 8 AM supine and 12 PM upright plasma aldosterone levels fell after 3 and 7 days of maintenance therapy in all patients, although to a relatively smaller extent in the group with PRA < 2 (Figure 9). PRA remained elevated for as long as treatment was continued, both in supine and upright positions. In addition, assumption of the upright posture produced parallel rises ($r = 0.57$, $p < 0.05$) in both PRA and plasma aldosterone during treatment (Figure 9).

Changes in Sodium Balance. Captopril induced changes in sodium balance in all but one low-renin patient (Figure 10). Of the 6 patients with renovascular hypertension, 3 went into positive sodium balance (mean + 168 ± 9 mEq), while the other 3 went into negative sodium balance (mean −223 ± 59 mEq) despite comparable reductions in mean arterial pressure (−23.7 ± 4.1% versus −23.5 ± 8.8%). Of the patients with essential

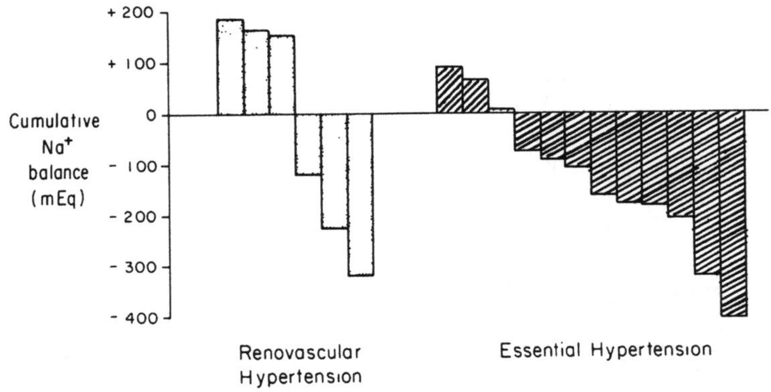

FIGURE 10. Effect of captopril on cumulative sodium balance in 19 patients after 9 days of treatment.

hypertension, 2 retained sodium (+67 and +90 mEq), 1 was unchanged (+7 mEq), and the remaining 9 lost sodium (range −76 to −410 mEq, mean −194 ± 37 mEq).

Enhanced Therapeutic Response with Addition of Diuretic. Continued treatment with captopril resulted in acceptable blood pressure control in 14 of the 19 patients (Table 1), and they were therefore continued on this regimen in long-term followup; one patient was withdrawn from treatment for nonmedical reasons. The remaining 4 patients continued to have elevated blood pressures despite the use of maximal allowed dosage. Accordingly, these 4 patients were also given chlorthalidone, 50 mg daily. The addition of the diuretic resulted in acceptable control of blood pressure (Table 1) which fell to the same level as in those patients who were controlled on captopril alone. Effective blood pressure control was maintained in all patients, varying upward only when dietary sodium intake increased greatly, as reflected by the 24-hr urinary sodium excretion.

Untoward Effects. Untoward effects from captopril treatment were uncommon. All patients reported that they felt as well as or better than before treatment was instituted. Two patients complained of mild lightheadedness during exercise, and one patient associated more frequent bowel movements (nondiarrheal in character) with drug administration. Four patients who had recurrent headaches have noted partial or complete relief while on captopril. None of the patients reported changes in mood or mental activity, impaired sexual desire or performance, symptoms of orthostatic hypotension, chest pain, or palpitations.

TABLE 1. Long-Term Effects of Captopril on 19 Hypertensive Patients

				Blood pressure (mm Hg)[c]					
				Inpatient			Outpatient		
Diagnosis	Patient no.	Age/ sex	Renin profile[b]	Admission	Day before captopril	On captopril 9 days	On captopril 1 month	On captopril and chlorthalidone	Dose (mg/day)
Essential hypertension	1	56F	Low	217/148	193/137	197/144	—	152/105	800
	2	56M	Low	190/110	157/101	135/93	146/93	—	400
	3	55M	Medium	178/129	167/121	162/120	150/108	120/80	400
	4	35M	Medium	168/122	132/98	110/84	120/90	—	400
	5	40M	Medium	182/118	185/118	160/107	164/104	104/93	400
	6	47F	Medium	131/93	139/89	112/77	135/84	—	400
	7	59F	Medium	250/116	242/114	155/95	—	—	200
	8	30M	Medium	150/105	134/88	122/82	124/93	—	400
	9	61M	Medium	159/99	139/95	124/90	138/87	—	400
	10	40M	Medium	178/129	147/98	133/93	138/96	—	100
	11	51F	Medium	154/98	154/98	127/83	135/83	—	200
	12	46M	High	176/120	144/103	119/80	114/85	—	100
	13	55M	High	200/128	156/119	157/108	119/86	—	800
Renovascular hypertension	14	26M	High	160/106	150/109	134/95	140/84	—	400
	15[a]	52F	High	225/135	227/131	197/122	—	144/88	800
	16	63F	High	210/92	188/99	172/82	181/77	—	800
	17	46M	High	142/96	149/104	116/77	119/83	—	400
	18[a]	41F	High	180/107	173/109	110/66	125/75	—	1000
	19[a]	20F	High	168/118	161/118	130/86	133/82	—	400

[a] Bilateral renal artery stenosis.
[b] Based on nomogram relating upright plasma renin activity to the 24-hr rate of urinary sodium excretion.
[c] Average supine and standing blood pressures for that day.

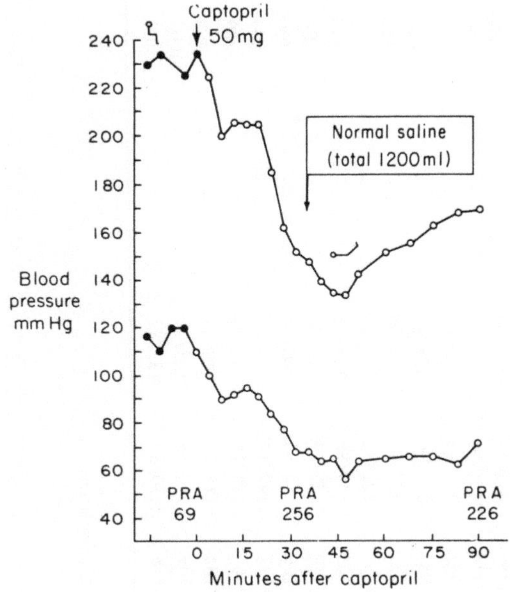

FIGURE 11. Effect of captopril in an elderly woman with high-renin hypertension who had been given furosemide 10 mg IV 30 min earlier. Symptomatic hypotension occurred that was promptly reversed by restoration of central blood volume (see text).

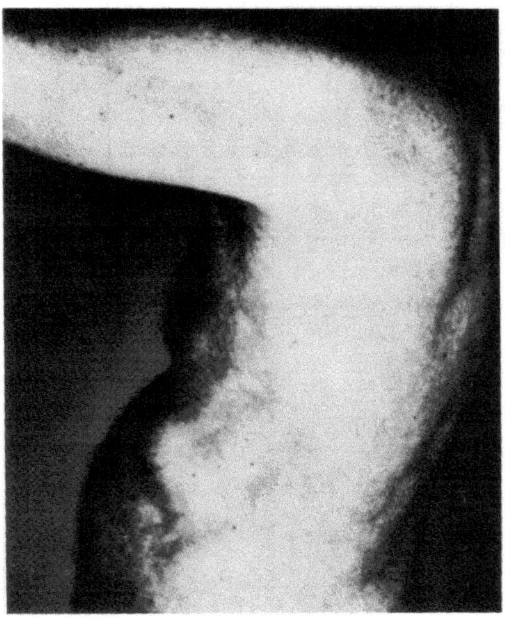

FIGURE 12. Macular rash that appeared 8 days after captopril treatment was begun (600 mg/day). The rash was nonpruritic, extended over the forearms, anterior trunk, and upper thighs, and was associated with a temperature of 38°. Three days after the dose was reduced to 150 mg/day, the fever and rash had cleared.

Three potential problems with the use of the drug were encountered: one is related to the potency of the agent in inducing abrupt falls in blood pressure in high-renin patients, the second was a mild, reversible reaction manifested by fever and rash, and the third was the appearance of proteinuria.

Figure 11 illustrates the blood pressure response of a 78-yr-old nurse who presented with complaints of dyspnea and headache. Blood pressure was 290/150, and there were signs of mild pulmonary edema. She was given 10 mg furosemide intravenously without effect on blood pressure or urine flow. Thirty minutes later, she was given 50 mg captopril orally. Within 10 min, she noted relief of dyspnea as her blood pressure fell progressively to 135/60. At this time she complained of feeling faint and nauseated. She was placed in the reverse Trendelenberg position, and 1200 cc of normal saline was infused over 1 hr. Her symptomatic hypotension was relieved as blood pressure rose without cardiac decompensation. It was subsequently learned that PRA had been 80 ng AI/ml per hr prior to furosemide.

This case illustrates that patients with extremely high levels of PRA, either native or diuretic-induced, may be extremely sensitive to angiotensin blockade, and also that the excessive reduction in arterial pressure in such circumstances may be attenuated or partially reversed by rapid isotonic fluid replacement.

The syndrome of rash and fever has occurred in two patients in this Center. After 7–10 days of drug administration, these 2 patients complained of myalgias and nonshaking chills. Within 24 hr, a diffuse macular rash erupted over the trunk (Figure 12) in association with a low-grade fever. Leukocytosis and eosinophilia were absent. In one patient who had received 1000 mg daily, the syndrome cleared within 2 days after the drug was temporarily withdrawn. In the other patient, these signs resolved in 72 hr after the dosage was reduced from 600 to 150 mg/day.

Proteinuria ($>$ 200 mg/day) appeared in 3 of these patients. The onset of the proteinuria was noted in the third month of treatment, and peak protein excretion occurred between the fifth and sixth months (range 2–7 g/day). In two of these patients, proteinuria receded and completely cleared 4 to 6 months after onset despite continued therapy in the same dosage. In the third patient, the proteinuria has persisted but in lesser amounts. Renal function was unchanged in the 3 patients developing proteinuria.

Discussion

These studies define a broad antihypertensive effectiveness for this new orally active angiotensin-converting enzyme inhibitor. While the experience to date with long-term therapy is limited, our findings in 19 patients, many of whom were refractory to traditional modes of therapy, suggest that this therapeutic agent is effective to a greater extent and in a greater proportion of hypertensive patients than any other single drug. Besides this demonstrated efficacy, these results during long-term therapy provide additional evidence for the participatory role of the renin–angiotensin–aldosterone system in maintaining elevated pressure in a majority of patients with essential hypertension. Of course captopril may not lower blood pressure exclusively by reducing angiotensin II levels, since the possibility that decreased kinin degradation might occur and play some role cannot be excluded. However, in this study, we have shown that long-term treatment with captopril causes reductions in blood pressure that are directly related in magnitude to (1) the pretreatment PRA, (2) the degree of suppression of urinary aldosterone excretion, and (3) the consequent changes in serum potassium. Moreover, in the relationships of the response to the baseline PRA, there is a similarity between the longer term action of captopril and the acute effects of the nonapeptide converting enzyme inhibitor, and a parallelism between the effects of both these agents and the effects of saralasin and β-blockade. Altogether these parallel responses reinforce the view that a major action of all four therapeutic agents is inhibition of the renin system.

Blood pressure began to fall within 15 min after administration of the first oral dose of captopril (Figure 1). This rapid response was associated with evidence of blockade of angiotensin II formation—namely, a fall in plasma aldosterone in the face of a reactive rise in PRA. The relationship between the pretreatment level of PRA and this acute fall in blood pressure (Figure 2) is similar to that described with the nonapeptide converting enzyme inhibitor SQ 20,881.[10] Reinforcing the predictive value of renin levels for the immediate responses was the finding that baseline PRA levels were also predictive of the longer term blood pressure response to the drug (Figure 5). This relationship is impressive when one considers all of the potential secondary effects of lowering angiotensin and the compensatory influences that might be invoked during the long-term response.

It should be pointed out, however, that the relationships between the baseline renin and the response may go unrecognized in a small sample size,[15] unless patients with a wide range of PRA values are studied. At both ends of the spectrum, the pretreatment PRA becomes increasingly predictive of the magnitude of the depressor response. Thus, all 4 patients with PRA less than 0.5 ng AI/ml per hr had less than 5% fall in diastolic blood pressure with the first dose (Figure 2). In contrast, 9 of the 11 patients with PRA greater than 6 ng/ml per hr had 15% or more falls in diastolic pressure. A corollary of this observation is that a striking depressor response can provide immediate information about the presence and degree of the renin factor participating in the hypertension.

Despite the prompt initial response, in most patients blood pressure either stabilized or tended to revert toward control levels during the first few days of treatment. Then, after a variable period, blood pressure gradually fell to levels equal to, and frequently exceeding, the initial response. The reason for this delayed response is unclear. It is possible that the uniformly observed reactive rises in PRA may at times overcome the angiotensin-lowering effect of converting enzyme blockade. However, it seems unlikely that this would account entirely for the delayed response, since PRA remains in the same range (Figure 9) while blood pressure continues to fall. Another possibility is that initially there is a transient compensatory neurogenic tone or baroreceptor-mediated reflex, similar to that reported to antagonize the initial antihypertensive response to β-blockers such as propranolol.[5] This counterreactive α-tone appears to abate during long-term propranolol therapy,[21] thereby allowing the antirenin and other antihypertensive actions of the drug to be expressed.

Another possible factor in the delayed depressor response may involve induced changes in sodium balance. This seems possible since the longer term blood pressure responses were related to the degree of aldosterone suppression (Figure 6) and to the concurrent changes in serum potassium (Figure 8). Notwithstanding these relationships, it was not possible to relate the depressor responses either temporally or quantitatively to induced changes in sodium balance per se. This is probably because sodium excretion depends not only on aldosterone but also on renal perfusion pressure and flow. It therefore remains to be established to what degree suppression of aldosterone plays a direct role in the antihypertensive effect of captopril. Whatever the case, changes in urinary aldosterone probably are a good estimate of the degree to which angiotensin II has been reduced.

While the reasons for the delayed response to captopril are not fully clarified, this delay must be taken into account when investigating how the drug works. This is especially true since the secondary falls in blood pressure are relatively more pronounced inthe medium- and high-renin subgroups (Figures 5 and 6). Thus, quite different conclusions might be drawn if therapeutic responses are assessed early in the course of treatment after the initial response has waned.

Continued administration of captopril produced sustained reduction of blood pressure in 18 of 19 patients who had been poorly controlled on conventional therapy (Table 1). One patient with a very low pretreatment renin exhibited an insignificant response to captopril until diuretic was added. Three other patients whose pressures were lowered by captopril but still remained elevated were fully corrected by addition of a diuretic (Table 1). In all of these patients, control of hypertension was achieved without significant side effects other than proteinuria. Despite large reductions in blood pressure, patients did not complain of fatigue, weakness, or orthostatic dizziness. In fact, 4 patients observed definite reductions in or disappearance of headaches during captopril treatment.

The pathogenesis of the infrequently observed syndrome of rash and fever remains obscure. It has been completely reversible by reductions of the dose or by discontinuation of the drug. Perhaps more serious is the possibility of profound depressor responses in high-renin states (Figure 11). At this stage, it seems prudent to withhold the drug from patients who have undergone prior sodium depletion or who are currently receiving diuretics or vasodilators. However, if the depressor response to captopril is not adequate, it may be safely augmented by subsequent addition of a diuretic.

The occurrence of proteinuria is potentially a more serious problem. More detailed studies of larger numbers of patients are required to define carefully the incidence, severity, and mechanism of this finding.

Summary

Nineteen patients with treatment-resistant essential (13) or renovascular (6) hypertension were treated with an orally active inhibitor of angiotensin-converting enzyme, D-2-methyl-3-mercaptopropanoyl-L-proline (captopril), for periods up to 6 mo. The compund alone produced moderate to marked sustained reductions in blood pressure, often to normal levels. One patient who had a low renin level exhibited no significant response. In 4 patients with a partial response, addition of a diuretic produced satisfactory blood pressure control. No serious side effects were noted. A syndrome of rash and fever was observed in 2 patients but resolved following reduction of the dose or withdrawal of drug. Reversible proteinuria occurred in 3 patients.

The mechanism of action remains to be fully elucidated, but the data indicate that a major action involves suppression of the renin–angiotensin–aldosterone system. Thus, the degree of blood pressure reduction was correlated (1) with the level of pretreatment plasma renin activity, (2) with the induced suppression of urinary aldosterone excretion, and (3) with the consequent changes in potassium balance and serum potassium. Sustained converting enzyme blockade produced natriuresis in a majority of patients on a normal sodium intake, a factor that may contribute to the blood pressure response.

The evidence suggests that at the doses currently used, the induced blockade of angiotensin II formation is incomplete, since during therapy aldosterone appears to remain responsive to physiologic changes in renin activity, although at a lower level. Indeed, reactive increases in renin secretion may, in some patients, diminish the antihypertensive action of the drug.

These results with an oral agent over a longer time closely resemble the acute effects of the intravenous nonapeptide inhibitor. The effects of these two agents in turn are in many respects similar to those obtained with other agents that block the renin system, namely saralasin and β-adrenergic blockers. Accordingly, from a conceptual standpoint, these new findings provide another dimension in the growing body of evidence indicating a significant involvement of the renin–angiotensin–aldosterone system in most hypertensive patients. This in turn provides the basis for a new approach to therapy based on the identification and containment of the renin factor by specific pharmacological agents.

ACKNOWLEDGMENTS. The work reported herein was supported in part by a grant from the Squibb Institute for Medical Research.

References

1. Bühler FR, Laragh JH, Baer L, et al: Propranolol inhibition of renin secretion: A specific approach to diagnosis and treatment of renin-dependent hypertensive diseases. *N Engl J Med* 287:1209–1214, 1972.
2. Hollifield JW, Sherman K, Vander Zwag R, et al: Proposed mechanism of propranolol's antihypertensive effect in essential hypertension. *N Engl J Med* 295:68–73, 1976.
3. Menard J, Bertagna X, N'Guyen PT, et al: Rapid identification of patients with essential hypertension sensitive to acebutolol (a new cardioselective beta-blocker). *Am J Med* 60:886–890, 1976.
4. MacGregor GA, Dawes P: Antihypertensive effect of propranolol and spironolactone in relation to plasma angiotensin II. *Clin Sci Mol Med* 50:18p, 1976.
5. Drayer JIM, Keim HY, Weber MA, et al: Unexpected pressor responses to propranolol in essential hypertension. *Am J Med* 60:897–903, 1976.
6. Streeten DHP, Anderson GH, Freiberg JM, et al: Use of an angiotensin II antagonist (saralasin) in the recognition of "angiotensinogenic" hypertension. *N Engl J Med* 292:657–662, 1975.
7. Brunner HR, Gavras H, Laragh JH, et al: Hypertension in man: Exposure of the renin and sodium components using angiotensin II blockade. *Circ Res* 34(suppl 1):35–43, 1974.
8. Case DB, Wallace JM, Keim HJ, et al: Usefulness and limitations of saralasin, a partial competitive agonist of angiotensin II, for evaluating the renin and sodium factors in hypertensive patients. *Am J Med* 60:825–836, 1976.
9. Hollenberg NK, Williams GH, Burger B, et al: Blockade and stimulation of renal, adrenal, and vascular angiotensin II receptors with 1-sar-8-ala-angiotensin II in normal man. *J Clin Invest* 57:39–46, 1976.
10. Case DB, Wallace JM, Keim HJ, et al: Possible role of renin in hypertension as suggested by renin-sodium profiling and inhibition of converting enzyme. *N Engl J Med* 296:641–646, 1977.
11. Ondetti MA, Rubin B, Cushman DW: Design of specific inhibitors of angiotensin-converting enzyme: New class of orally active antihypertensive agents. *Science* 196:441–444, 1977.

12. Ferguson RK, Turini GA, Brunner HR, et al: A specific orally active inhibitor of angiotensin-converting enzyme in man. *Lancet* 1:775–778, 1977.
13. Murthy VS, Waldron TL, Goldberg ME, et al: Inhibition of angiotensin converting enzyme by SQ 14225 in conscious rabbits. *Eur J Pharmacol* 46:207–212, 1977.
14. Colman RW, Girey GJD, Zacest R, et al: The human plasma kallikrein–kinin system. *Prog Hematol* 7:255–298, 1971.
15. Gavras H, Brunner HR, Turini GA, et al: Antihypertensive effect of the oral angiotensin converting enzyme inhibitor SQ 14225 in man. *N Engl J Med* 298:991–995, 1978.
16. Laragh JH, Baer L, Brunner HR, et al: Renin, angiotensin, aldosterone system in pathogenesis and management of hypertensive vascular disease. *Am J Med* 52:633, 1972.
17. Sealey JE, Laragh JH: How to do a plasma renin assay. *Cardiovasc Med* 2:1079–1092, 1977.
18. Bühler FR, Sealey JE, Laragh JH: Radioimmunoassay of plasma aldosterone, in Laragh JH (ed): *Hypertension Manual.* New York, Dun-Donnelley, 1974, pp 655–669.
19. MacKenzie JK, Clements JA: Simplified radioimmunoassay of serum aldosterone utilizing increased antibody specificity. *J Clin Endocrinol Metab* 38:622–627, 1974.
20. Sealey JE, Bühler FR, Laragh JH, et al: Aldosterone excretion: Physiologic variations in man measured by radioimmunoassay or double isotope dilution. *Circ Res* 31:367–378, 1972.
21. Tarazi RC, Dustan HP: Beta-adrenergic blockade in hypertension: Practical and theoretic implications of long term hemodynamic variations. *Am J Cardiol* 29:633–640, 1972.

Index

Acebutolol, 17–18
Acetylcholine, 107, 116, 128
ACh, *see* Acetylcholine
ACTH, *see* Adrenocorticotropic hormone
Actomyosin, 64
Adrenal gland, 174–176
 -renal interaction, 174–176
β-Adrenergic blocking drugs, 174
Adrenocorticotropic hormone, 15, 43
Aldosterone, 41–43, 57, 58, 103, 127, 128, 152, 157, 159, 165–167, 174–178, 182, 202, 206, 207, 211–230
 -angiotensin system, 90, 211–230
 excretion, urinary, 157, 219, 220, 226
 primary, 174, 178, 186, 202
 -renin system, 175–176, 211–230
 secretion, 219
 -sodium profiling, 177–178
 and tumor, 18
Amphibian, 59
Anastomosis, ureterovenous, 26
Anephric patient, *see* Kidney
Angiotensin, 51, 69, 82, 84
 I, 60, 89–92, 97–99, 104, 107, 115, 116, 173
 II (Saralasin), 52, 60, 68, 69, 89–92, 97, 98, 103, 104, 107, 115, 116, 149, 150, 167, 173–177, 180, 182, 185–190, 195, 196, 201, 212, 226
 III, 103, 104
 -aldosterone system, 90, 211–230
 anephric patient, 194
 blockade, 194, 212
 and blood pressure, 197
 -converting enzyme, 89–170, 191–197, 212
  active site, model of, 104–106
  biochemistry, 91–93
  blockade, *see* inhibitor
Angiotensin (Continued)
 -converting enzyme (continued)
  and blood pressure, 167, 188–191, 204–205
  carbohydrate composition, 95
  is a COOH-terminal dipeptidyl exopeptidase, 98
  immunology, 93–98
  inhibitor, 67, 103–113, 173–230
   design of, 106–109
   list of, 108
   peptide as, 103–104
   see also Teprotide (SQ 20,881)
  physiology, 89–102
  of rabbit tissue extract, 94–96
  a zinc-containing metalloprotein, 105
 equine, 89
 renal
  blood flow reduced by, 62
  circulation, 69
  function, 57–75
  perfusion, 57–75
 renin release inhibited by, 51
 -salt hypertension, 31
Antibody against antirabbit enzyme, 98
Antihypertensive action, 32
Antihypertensive drugs, listed, 181
Antihypertensive effect, chronic, 127
Aorta, 6
Arterial blood pressure, *see* Blood pressure
Arteriole, efferent, 68
Artery, 6, 78
 necrosis, fibrinoid, 34
 waterlogging of, 78
Autoregulation, 78
 between vasoconstriction and vasodilatation, 8

Barium chloride, 116
Baroreceptor, 10
D-2-Benzylsuccinic acid, 106, 110, 111
Beta-blockade, 180
  agents for, 168, 183, 211
  with propranolol, 46
Blood
  circulation, systemic, 5
  flow
    equation, 3–4
    laminar, 3
    to organ system, 7
    resistance to, 4
  pressure, 127, 167, 188–191, 204–205
    arterial, 5, 10, 11, 16, 176
    change, 188–191, 216–217
    with teprotide, 204
    equation, 3–4
    fall, 156
    homeostasis, 3–13
    mean, 117–120, 206–207, 211
    normotensive, 119
    profile, 162–163
    and resistance, 81
  see also Hypertension, Captopril
Bothrops jararaca, venom of, 90
Bradykininase, 91, 115
Bradykinin, 91, 92, 96–99, 103, 107, 115, 129, 182, 195, 208
  -potentiating factor, 90

Capoten, *see* Captopril
Captopril (SQ14,225), 91, 108–111, 115–230
  and aldosterone secretion, 219
  animal tests, 116–119, 137–147
  and blood pressure, 119–128, 153–154, 215, 218–219
  clinical use, 173–230
  development of, 182
  human studies with, 149–170
  and hypertensive patients, 213–214, 223, 227
  potassium metabolism, 219
  sodium balance changes, 221
  therapy and renin, 180–199
  time-response curve, 153
Carboxyhydrolase, 115
Carboxypeptidase A, 109, 111
  inhibition of, 110
  pancreatic, 105
Cardiovascular reflex, primitive, 79
Cervical cord transection, 43–45
  tilting patient with, 45
Chemoreceptor, 10
Chloralose anesthesia for cats, 130
Chlorthalidone, 157
Chronic renal failure, 166
Circadian rhythm, 40
Circulatory system
  a closed-loop system, 3
  flow of blood through, 3
  Poiseuille's law applied to, 4
Cirrhosis of the liver, 65
Congestive heart failure, *see* Heart failure, congestive
Conn's tumor, 50
Converting enzyme, *see* Angiotensin-converting enzyme
Cord, cervical, transection, 43–45
Cortisol, 41–43
Creatinine, 138
  clearance, 138

Deoxycorticosterone acetate–saline hypertension
  in dog, 18
  in rat, 15
Dexamethasone, 42, 43
Dihydralazine, 157
Diuresis, *see* Diuretics
Diuretics, 123, 128, 152, 157, 164, 168, 181, 227
  for therapy, 180
  see also individual diuretics
Dog, 116, 120–123
  pharmacokinetics, 140, 146
  safety
    cardiovascular, 138, 141
    renal, 138, 141
  toxicity, acute oral, 137, 138, 141, 142
Dopamine, 116
Dipeptidyl peptidase, bacterial, 91

Eel, 57
Electrolyte
  -active steroid, 22
  regulation, 174
Encephalopathy, hypertensive, 34
Epinephrine, 44, 46, 139, 142, 166

Escherichia coli, dipeptidyl exopeptidase of, 93
Essential hypertension, *see* Hypertension, essential
Exopeptidase, dipeptidyl, 93, 98

Feedback gain, 11
Fever and rash syndrome, 225, 228
Filtration, 64
Fish, 57, 59
  bony, 59
Fluid retention, 176
Frank–Starling curve, 82
Furosemide, 157–161, 224, 225

Gaucher's disease, 91
Globulin, immune, 97
Glomerulus, 58, 64
  circulation, 59
  diagram of, 41
  filtration rate, 65
Glucose tolerance, 139
Glycerol, 69
Glycoprotein, 99
Goat, antienzyme antibody from, 93
Granule, juxtaglomerular, 58–59
Guanethidine, 19, 64, 123

Heart failure
  congestive, 128, 150, 163, 165
    chronic, 168
    refractory, 151
  hallmark of, 78
  treatment, 82
Hemodialysis, 150, 151, 161, 168, 186
Hepatic cirrhosis, 65
Hippuryl-L-histidyl-L-leucine as substrate, 109
Histamine, 116
Hydralazine, 82–84, 123, 127, 145
Hydrochlorothiazide, 123, 145
Hyperaldosteronism, 50
  primary, 151, 161, 166
Hypertension
  angiotensin–salt-caused, 31
  and bladder, full, 43
  and contraceptives, oral, 178
  diagnosis with teprotide, 201–210
  dialysis-resistant, 166
  drugs for therapy, listed, 181

Hypertension (Continued)
  and encephalopathy, 34
  essential, 65, 68, 104, 149–151, 166, 178, 186, 202, 205, 206, 213, 223, 226
  genetic (spontaneous), 124–127
  and heart failure, 79
  humoral, 1–86
  and hyperaldosteronism, primary, 151
  malignant, 104, 166, 175–176, 202
  pathogenesis, 150
  physiological, 1–86
  renal, 121
    medulla and, 25–38
  renin-caused, 178, 197, 209
  renovascular, 104, 149, 151, 178, 203, 223
  and salt, role of, 21, 31
  and sodium, role of, 150
  spontaneous (genetic), 124–127
  and steroids, electrolyte-active, 15–23
    hypothesis, 21
  teprotide for diagnosis, 201–210
  therapy, 78–79
    drugs, listed, 181
    see also Captopril
Hypogeusia, 166
Hypokalemia, 15
Hypotension syndrome, postural, 47
Hypothalamus, 8

Ileum of guinea pig, excised, 116
Immunoaffinity technique, 95
Immunoglobulin, 97
Indomethacin, 128
Isoproterenol, 83, 116, 128
Ischemia, 63

Juxtaglomerular apparatus, 63
Juxtaglomerular granule, 58–59

Kaliuresis, 176
Kidney, 25–27, 175
  adaptation to salinity of ocean, 57
  anephric patient, 193–194
  antihypertensive nonexcretory function, 36
  blood flow to, 62
  cells, 59
  evolution, 57
  hypertensive action of, 25
  hypertensive state and, 25
  medulla, 27

Kidney (Continued)
  nonexcretory antihypertensive function, 36
  role for, 183
  salinity of ocean, adaptation to, 57
Kininase II (converting enzyme), 35, 115, 149, 195

Lipid and antihypertensive action, 32, 33, 36
Liver
  cirrhosis, 65
  function, 139
Lungfish, 59

Macula densa, 41, 58, 59
Malignant hypertension, *see* Hypertension, malignant
Melanin-producing cell, 48
2-Mercaptoacetyl amino acid, 109
Mercaptoalkanoyl amino acid, 109
D-3-Mercapto-2-methylpropanoyl-L-proline, *see* Captopril (SQ 14,225)
3-Mercaptopropanoyl-L-proline is SQ 13,863, 111
Methyldopa, 145
D-2-Methylglutaryl-L-proline is SQ 14,102, 111
D-2-Methylsuccinyl-L-proline is SQ 13,297, 111
Metyrapone, 16, 18
  acebutolol pretreatment, 17–18
  administration, 20
  and hypertension in dog, 15
Minoxidil, 83
Monkey and oral toxicity studies, 137, 138, 141, 142
Mouse and acute toxicity studies, 137, 140, 145
Muscle, arteriolar smooth, contraction of, 52

Nadolol, 145
Natriuresis, 128
Necrosis, fibrinoid, arterial, 34
Nephrectomy, 18
  partial, 30
Nephron, 64
  in relation to habitat, 58
Nervous system, peripheral, 19
Nicotine, 116
Nitrate, 82
Nitroglycerin, 82–84
Nitroprusside, 84
Norepinephrine, 19, 21, 44–46, 78, 98, 116, 117, 128, 165, 166

Peptidase, bacterial, 91
Peptide
  vasoactive, 97
  venomous, 93
Phentolamine, 82–83
Plasma renin, *see* Renin
Poiseuille's law of hydraulics, 4
Postural change and its effects, 43
Potassium, 78, 220, 226
PRA, *see* Renin, plasma activity
Pressoreceptor, 10
L-Proline, 107
  derivatives, 111
Propranolol, 46, 50, 66, 157, 179, 180, 211, 227
Prostaglandins, 116, 128, 129
Proteinuria, 225

Rabbit with hypertension, 33
Radioimmunoassay, competition, 94
Rash and fever syndrome, 225, 228
Rat, 116, 119, 121, 124
  absorption, 140, 145
  clip of one-kidney, 25
    unclipping effect, 26
  excretion, 140, 145
  hypertension, 126
    spontaneous, 125, 127, 130
    two-kidney renal, 126, 129
  normotensive, 116
  toxicity, acute, 137, 140
    one-month study, 138, 142
Reflex mechanism, cardiovascular, 9
Renal–adrenal axis is a hormonal cascade, 176
Renal arteriolar necrosis and rupture, 176
Renal blood flow, 61–65
  autoregulation, 61
Renal circulation, control of, 69
Renal failure, 202
  chronic, 166
Renal hypertension, 121
  in rat, 121–122
Renal insufficiency (uremia), 34
Renal medulla, 27
Renal plasma flow, 152

Renin, 130, 152, 159, 162, 164, 165, 175–177, 180
  activity, 167
  -adrenal interaction, 174–176
  -aldosterone system, 175–176, 211–230
  and angiotensin, 33–36, 51, 57, 58, 63, 65, 77, 92, 211–230
    phylogeny, 57
  axis, 176
  baseline value, 180, 226
  blockade in hypertension, 185–199
    with drugs, 185–199
  and blood pressure changes, induced, 173–184, 191, 196
  changes in plasma activity, chronic, 50–52
    and propranolol, 46
    in tetraplegic patient, 44
  and contraceptive, oral, 63
  drugs, 68, 69
  and hypertension, 173–184
  and neural defect, 39–56
  plasma activity (PRA), 50–52, 89, 127–128, 145, 155, 156, 166, 185, 186, 190, 212
    suppressed, 15
  and potassium restriction, 63
  profiling, 196–197, 201
  release, 39, 40, 52, 60–61
    inhibitors of, 51
    mechanisms, listed, 40
  renal circulation, 69
  and sodium
    cooperation, 150
    deprivation, 50, 63
    profiling, 177–179, 186, 188
  volume, 50, 180
  therapy, *see* Captopril
Renomedullary interstitial cell (RIC), 25, 28–30, 32
Reserpine, 64
Retention of fluid, 76
Rhythm, circadian, 40
RIC, *see* Renomedullary interstitial cell

Saralasin, *see* Angiotensin II
Sarcoidosis, 91
Serotonin, 116, 128
Shy–Drager syndrome, 47–49
  resembles characteristics of tetraplegic patients, 48
Sodium, 68, 78, 127, 128, 159, 167
  balance, 185, 196, 221
    cumulative, 222
  depletion, 50, 176, 189, 197, 205
  dietary, 20
  excretion, 156, 178, 186, 191, 227
  hypertension, 21, 31, 150
  homeostasis, 57
  intake, 189
  profiling, 177–178
Sodium nitroprusside, 82, 83
Spearman's coefficient of correlation, 188, 215
Spironolactone, 50, 51, 145, 157, 161
SQ compounds
  12297, 108
  13297, 107, 110, 111
  13493, 107, 108
  13745, 106, 108, 111
  13863, 108, 109, 110, 111
  14102, 107, 108, 110, 111
  14116, 107, 108
  14225, *see* Captopril
  14534, 108, 109
  20881, *see* Teprotide
Steroid, electrolyte-active, 15–23; *see also* Metyrapone
Succinyl-L-proline is SQ 13,745, 106, 109

Teprotide (SQ 20,881), 66, 68, 90, 103, 108, 111, 115, 116, 129, 130, 149, 185–210
  and diagnosis of hypertension, 201–210
Tetraplegic patient, 49
  with full bladder, 46–47
  effect of tilting, 49
Thiazide, a diuretic, 50, 129
Tonin, 93
Toxicity studies, 137–145
Tumor-producing aldosterone, 18
Tyramine, 128

Uremia, 34
Urine flow, 65

Vascular resistance, systemic, 77–86
  and heart failure, 78–79
  and left ventricular function, 77–86
  and vasodilator drugs, 80–85
Vasculitis, 176
Vasoconstriction, 179–180

Vasoconstriction (Continued)
  balance with vasodilation, 8, 78
  volume hypothesis, 179
Vasodilatation, 52
  afferent in kidney, 49
  balance with vasoconstriction, 8, 78
Vasodilators, listed, 80–83
Vasopressin, 128
Venom peptide, 93
Ventricle, left, and vasodilators, 80–83
Vessel, 7
Viscera, arterioles of, 34

Wilcoxon's two-sample test, 188, 214

Zinc ion, 107, 111
  metalloprotein, 105
Zona glomerulosa, adenoma of, 159

MIX
Papier aus verantwortungsvollen Quellen
Paper from responsible sources
FSC® C105338

If you have any concerns about our products,
you can contact us on
ProductSafety@springernature.com

In case Publisher is established outside the EU,
the EU authorized representative is:
Springer Nature Customer Service Center GmbH
Europaplatz 3, 69115 Heidelberg, Germany

Printed by Libri Plureos GmbH
in Hamburg, Germany